Nerve Repair and Transfers from Hand to Shoulder

Editors

AMY M. MOORE
SUSAN E. MACKINNON

HAND CLINICS

www.hand.theclinics.com

Consulting Editor
KEVIN C. CHUNG

May 2016 • Volume 32 • Number 2

ELSEVIER

1600 John F. Kennedy Boulevard • Suite 1800 • Philadelphia, Pennsylvania, 19103-2899

http://www.theclinics.com

HAND CLINICS Volume 32, Number 2
May 2016 ISSN 0749-0712, ISBN-13: 978-0-323-44519-1

Editor: Jennifer Flynn-Briggs
Developmental Editor: Kristen Helm

Hand Clinics (ISSN 0749-0712) is published quarterly by Elsevier Inc., 360 Park Avenue South, New York, NY 10010-1710. Months of publication are February, May, August, and November. Business and Editorial Offices: 1600 John F. Kennedy Blvd., Ste. 1800, Philadelphia, PA 19103-2899. Customer Service Office: 3251 Riverport Lane, Maryland Heights, MO 63043. Periodicals postage paid at New York, NY and at additional mailing offices. Subscription price is $390.00 per year (domestic individuals), $687.00 per year (domestic institutions), $100.00 per year (domestic students/residents), $445.00 per year (Canadian individuals), $799.00 per year (Canadian institutions), $530.00 per year (international individuals), $799.00 per year (international institutions), and $256.00 per year (international and Canadian students/residents). Foreign air speed delivery is included in all *Clinics* subscription prices. All prices are subject to change without notice. **POSTMASTER:** Send address changes to *Hand Clinics*, Elsevier Health Sciences Division, Subscription Customer Service, 3251 Riverport Lane, Maryland Heights, MO 63043. Customer Service (orders, claims, online, change of address): Elsevier Health Sciences Division, Subscription **Customer Service, 3251 Riverport Lane, Maryland Heights, MO 63043. Tel: 1-800-654-2452 (U.S. and Canada); 314-447-8871 (outside U.S. and Canada). Fax: 314-447-8029. E-mail: journalscustomerservice-usa@elsevier.com (for print support); journalsonlinesupport-usa@elsevier.com (for online support).**

Reprints. For copies of 100 or more of articles in this publication, please contact the Commercial Reprints Department, Elsevier Inc., 360 Park Avenue South, New York, New York 10010-1710. Tel.: 212-633-3874; Fax: 212-633-3820; E-mail: reprints@elsevier.com.

Hand Clinics is covered in *MEDLINE/PubMed (Index Medicus), Current Contents/Clinical Medicine, EMBASE/Excerpta Medica,* and *ISI/BIOMED.*

Contributors

CONSULTING EDITOR

KEVIN C. CHUNG, MD, MS
Charles B. G. de Nancrede Professor of
Surgery, Professor of Plastic Surgery and
Orthopaedic Surgery, Chief of Hand Surgery,
University of Michigan Health System,
Assistant Dean for Faculty Affairs, Associate
Director of Global REACH, University of
Michigan Medical School, Ann Arbor, Michigan

EDITORS

AMY M. MOORE, MD
Assistant Professor of Surgery; Program
Director-Hand Fellowship, Division of Plastic
and Reconstructive Surgery, Department of
Surgery, Washington University School of
Medicine, St Louis, Missouri

SUSAN E. MACKINNON, MD
Shoenberg Professor and Chief, Division of
Plastic & Reconstructive Surgery, Department
of Surgery, Washington University School of
Medicine, St Louis, Missouri

AUTHORS

JAYME A. BERTELLI, MD, PhD
Department of Orthopedic Surgery,
Governador Celso Ramos Hospital,
Florianópolis, Santa Catarina, Brazil;
Department of Neurosurgery, Center of
Biological and Health Sciences, University
of the South of Santa Catarina (Unisul),
Tubarão, Brazil

GREGORY H. BORSCHEL, MD
Division of Plastic & Reconstructive Surgery,
The Hospital for Sick Children; Associate
Professor, Department of Surgery,
University of Toronto, Toronto, Ontario,
Canada

LISELOTTE F. BULSTRA, BS
Department of Orthopedic Surgery, Mayo
Clinic, Rochester, Minnesota; Department of
Plastic, Reconstructive and Hand Surgery,
Erasmus Medical Center, Rotterdam, The
Netherlands

GREGORY BUNCKE, MD
The Buncke Clinic, San Francisco, California

HOWARD M. CLARKE, MD, PhD
Division of Plastic & Reconstructive Surgery,
The Hospital for Sick Children; Professor,
Department of Surgery, University of Toronto,
Toronto, Ontario, Canada

CATHERINE M. CURTIN, MD
Associate Professor, Department of Surgery,
Palo Alto VA; Division of Plastic Surgery,
Stanford University, Palo Alto, California

KRISTEN M. DAVIDGE, MD, MSc
Division of Plastic & Reconstructive Surgery,
The Hospital for Sick Children; Assistant
Professor, Department of Surgery, University
of Toronto, Toronto, Ontario, Canada

GABRIELLE DAVIS, MD
Division of Plastic Surgery, Stanford University,
Palo Alto, California

IDA K. FOX, MD
Assistant Professor of Surgery, Division of
Plastic Surgery, Washington University School
of Medicine, St Louis, Missouri

MARCOS F. GHIZONI, MD, PhD
Department of Neurosurgery, Center of
Biological and Health Sciences, University of
the South of Santa Catarina (Unisul), Tubarão,
Brazil

TESSA GORDON, PhD
Senior Scientist, Department of Surgery,
Division of Plastic Reconstructive Surgery,
06.9706 Peter Gilgan Centre for Research and
Learning, The Hospital for Sick Children,
Toronto, Ontario, Canada

LORNA CANAVAN KAHN, BSPT, CHT
Milliken Hand Rehabilitation Center, The
Rehabilitation Institute of St Louis, St Louis,
Missouri

JASON H. KO, MD
Assistant Professor, Division of Plastic
Surgery, Northwestern University Feinberg
School of Medicine, Chicago, Illinois

EMILY M. KRAUSS, MSc, MD
Hand and Microsurgery Fellow, Division of
Plastic and Reconstructive Surgery,
Washington University School of Medicine,
St Louis, Missouri

STEVE K. LEE, MD
Attending Surgeon, Department of Hand &
Upper Extremity Surgery, Hospital for Special
Surgery, New York, New York

SOMSAK LEECHAVENGVONGS, MD
Department of Medical Services, Institute of
Orthopaedics, Lerdsin General Hospital,
Bangkok, Thailand

ANGELO B. LIPIRA, MD
Resident, Division of Plastic Surgery,
Harborview Medical Center, University of
Washington School of Medicine, Seattle,
Washington

SUSAN E. MACKINNON, MD
Shoenberg Professor and Chief, Division of
Plastic & Reconstructive Surgery, Department
of Surgery, Washington University School of
Medicine, St Louis, Missouri

KANCHAI MALUNGPAISHORPE, MD
Department of Medical Services, Institute of
Orthopaedics, Lerdsin General Hospital,
Bangkok, Thailand

ZINA MODEL, BA
Research Assistant, Department of Hand &
Upper Extremity Surgery, Hospital for Special
Surgery, New York, New York

AMY M. MOORE, MD, FACS
Assistant Professor of Surgery; Program
Director-Hand Fellowship, Division of Plastic
and Reconstructive Surgery, Department of
Surgery, Washington University School of
Medicine, St Louis, Missouri

**CHYE YEW NG, MBChB(Hons),
FRCS(Tr&Orth), BDHS, EBHSD**
Consultant Hand & Peripheral Nerve Surgeon;
Upper Limb Unit, Wrightington Hospital,
Wigan, United Kingdom

JENNIFER MEGAN M. PATTERSON, MD
Assistant Professor, Department of
Orthopaedic Surgery, University of North
Carolina, Chapel Hill, Chapel Hill, North
Carolina

MITCHELL A. PET, MD
Resident, Division of Plastic Surgery,
Harborview Medical Center, University of
Washington School of Medicine, Seattle,
Washington

BAUBACK SAFA, MD, MBA, FACS
The Buncke Clinic, San Francisco, California

ALEXANDER Y. SHIN, MD
Department of Orthopedic Surgery, Mayo
Clinic, Rochester, Minnesota

FRANCISCO SOLDADO, MD, PhD
Pediatric Hand Surgery and Microsurgery Unit,
Hospital Sant Joan de Déu, Universitat de
Barcelona, Barcelona, Spain

SAMIR K. TREHAN, MD
Orthopaedic Surgery Resident, Department of
Hand & Upper Extremity Surgery, Hospital for
Special Surgery, New York, New York

THOMAS H. TUNG, MD
Professor of Surgery, Division of Plastic and
Reconstructive Surgery, Washington
University School of Medicine, St Louis,
Missouri

CHAIROJ UERPAIROJKIT, MD
Department of Medical Services, Institute of
Orthopaedics, Lerdsin General Hospital,
Bangkok, Thailand

KIAT WITOONCHART, MD
Department of Medical Services, Institute of
Orthopaedics, Lerdsin General Hospital,
Bangkok, Thailand

Contents

Poor functional outcomes are frequent after peripheral nerve injuries despite the regenerative support of Schwann cells. Motoneurons and, to a lesser extent, sensory neurons survive the injuries but outgrowth of axons across the injury site is slow. The neuronal regenerative capacity and the support of regenerating axons by the chronically denervated Schwann cells progressively declines with time and distance of the injury from the denervated targets. Strategies, including brief low-frequency electrical stimulation that accelerates target reinnervation and functional recovery, and the insertion of cross-bridges between a donor nerve and a recipient denervated nerve stump, are effective in promoting functional outcomes after complete and incomplete injuries.

Direct repair and nerve autografting are primary options in the treatment of upper extremity peripheral nerve injuries. Deciding between these surgical options depends on the mechanism of injury, time since injury, and length of repair defect. Principles of direct repair and nerve autografting are reviewed. Finally, a literature-based review of the outcomes of upper extremity peripheral nerve repair and autografting is provided. Taken together, this article provides relevant and recent data for surgeons regarding patient selection, technique selection, surgical technique, surgical outcomes, and prognostic factors that will aid surgeons treating patients with upper extremity peripheral nerve injuries.

Manufactured conduits and allografts are viable alternatives to direct suture repair and nerve autograft. Manufactured tubes should have gaps less than 10 mm, and ideally should be considered as an aid to the coaptation. Processed nerve allograft has utility as a substitute for either conduit or autograft in sensory nerve repairs. There is also a growing body of evidence supporting their utility in major peripheral nerve repairs, gap repairs up to 70 mm in length, as an alternative source of tissue to bolster the diameter of a cable graft, and for the management of neuromas in non-reconstructable injuries.

This article presents a personal overview of nerve transfers and emphasizes the various factors that contribute to outcome following these surgeries. There is no "one result" for all nerve transfers. The results will vary depending on factors relating to the donor nerve and the recipient nerve, the degree of the surgical difficulty of the specific procedure, and issues relating to preoperative and postoperative rehabilitation. The general issues that influence all nerve injury and recovery, such as age of the patient, comorbidities, and time since injury, pertain to nerve transfers as well.

develop persistent pain; once incurred, pain can be even challenging to manage. This review seeks to define the types of pain following peripheral nerve injuries, investigate the pathophysiology and causative factors, and evaluate potential treatment options.

 Video content accompanies this article at http://www.hand.theclinics.com

As nerve transfers become the mainstay in treatment of brachial plexus and isolated nerve injuries, the preoperative and postoperative therapy performed to restore motor function requires continued dedication and appreciation. Through the understanding of the general principles of muscle activation and patient education, the therapist has a unique impact on the return of function in patients with nerve injuries. As surgeons continue to develop novel nerve transfers, the perioperative training, education, and implementation of the donor activation focused rehabilitation approach model is critical to ensure successful outcomes.

HAND CLINICS

THE CLINICS ARE AVAILABLE ONLINE!
Access your subscription at:
www.theclinics.com

HAND CLINICS

Preface
Inspiration for Innovation

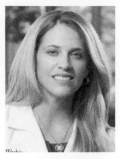   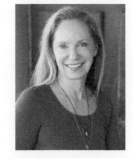

Amy M. Moore, MD   Susan E. Mackinnon, MD

Editors

Our current understanding of nerve biology, anatomy, and topography has been fueled by the fervor of both scientists and surgeons striving to improve outcomes in patients with devastating nerve injuries. These efforts have led to innovation in surgical techniques and the development of solutions to complex clinical problems.

Most recently, the advent of nerve transfers has dramatically changed the way we treat patients with nerve injuries. Nerve transfers have also changed our expectations for recovery, as we have seen function restored at unprecedented levels. Although nerve transfer surgery is now mainstream, the basics of nerve repair and graft techniques cannot be forgotten, but instead incorporated into the hand or peripheral nerve surgeon's toolbox to ensure reliable and reproducible outcomes.

When presented with the opportunity to build this issue of *Hand Clinics* on "Nerve Repair and Transfers from Hand to Shoulder," I immediately turned to my mentor, Susan Mackinnon, for help. In 2003, Susan stated that if I came to Washington University for residency she would teach me to love nerves. Fast-forward 13 years, and I can easily say she has done that and more. I love nerve surgery and am grateful for Susan's influence, support, and inspiration.

Like many of you who will read this text, I find peripheral nerve surgery to be a fascinating field: full of challenging and evolving concepts. I am excited about the opportunity to review many of these concepts with you in this issue.

Together, Susan and I have designed a comprehensive nerve surgery text encompassing the fundamentals of neurobiology, operative management of conditions affecting the nerves of the upper extremity, as well as postoperative therapy techniques to maximize patient results after nerve injury. This issue has contributions from the authorities in nerve surgery, including international nerve surgeons and specialists from multiple disciplines (plastic surgery, orthopedic surgery, neurosurgery, and physical therapy).

Our hope is that the combined efforts of the authors and editors provide you, the student, the nerve surgeon, the hand surgeon or fellow lover of nerves, with an excellent resource on which to expand your knowledge, increase your excitement, and inspire your innovation in the treatment of our patients with nerve injuries.

Amy M. Moore, MD
Division of Plastic and Reconstructive Surgery
Department of Surgery
Washington University School of Medicine
660 South Euclid Avenue
Campus Box 8238
St Louis, MO 63110, USA

Susan E. Mackinnon, MD
Department of Surgery
Washington University School of Medicine
660 South Euclid Avenue
Campus Box 8238
St Louis, MO 63110, USA

E-mail addresses:
mooream@wustl.edu (A.M. Moore)
mackinnons@wudosis.wustl.edu (S.E. Mackinnon)

Hand Clin 32 (2016) xiii
http://dx.doi.org/10.1016/j.hcl.2016.02.001
0749-0712/16/$ – see front matter © 2016 Published by Elsevier Inc.

hand.theclinics.com

Nerve Regeneration
Understanding Biology and Its Influence on Return of Function After Nerve Transfers

Tessa Gordon, PhD

KEYWORDS

- Peripheral nerve injury • Peripheral nerve regeneration • Skeletal muscle reinnervation
- Motor nerve sprouting • Perisynaptic Schwann cells • Chronic Schwann cell denervation • Axotomy

KEY POINTS

- Schwann cells support regeneration in the peripheral nervous system after nerve injuries, but functional outcomes are frequently disappointing.
- Strategies, including brief electrical stimulation at the time of surgical repair, are effective in significantly improving outcomes of peripheral nerve injury.
- Autologous nerve cross-bridges placed between a donor intact nerve and a recipient denervated nerve stump improve nerve regeneration through chronically denervated Schwann cells.
- Axonal sprouting in partially denervated muscles and skin is effective, but to a limit, in compensating for loss of innervation.
- Motor control may be compromised by a few nerves to partially denervate and partially reinnervate muscles after sprouting and/or nerve transfers.

INTRODUCTION

Poor functional outcomes are frequent after peripheral nerve injuries despite the well-recognized capacity for the Schwann cells (SCs) of the peripheral nervous system to support axon regeneration. The poor outcomes are particularly frequent for injuries that are sustained at short distances from motoneuron cell bodies in the spinal cord and lower brainstem as well as from the sensory nerves whose cell bodies lie in the dorsal root ganglia alongside the spinal cord. This review considers the biology of peripheral nerve injury, nerve regeneration, and axonal sprouting. Nerve regeneration is the growth of lost axons from the stump of the remaining crushed or transected nerve: regenerating axons grow into the denervated nerve stumps where the axons undergo Wallerian degeneration and the remaining SCs in the empty endoneurial sheaths support axon regeneration. Sprouting describes axonal outgrowth under a variety of pathologic conditions. These conditions include: first, the axonal outgrowth from the proximal stump of an injured nerve, and second, the motor and sensory axon sprouts from intact intramuscular nerve sheaths to reinnervate partially denervated muscles and skin, respectively. The review concludes with the consideration of surgical procedures that include nerve transfers to promote functional return in the context of the limits of sprouting and the reduced capacity for smooth gradation of contractile forces by fewer motoneurons.

Disclosure: The author has nothing to declare.
Division of Plastic Reconstructive Surgery, Department of Surgery, 06.9706 Peter Gilgan Centre for Research and Learning, The Hospital for Sick Children, 686 Bay Street, Toronto, Ontario M5G 0A4, Canada
E-mail address: tessat.gordon@gmail.com

Hand Clin 32 (2016) 103–117
http://dx.doi.org/10.1016/j.hcl.2015.12.001

PERIPHERAL NERVE INJURY
Neuronal Response to Axotomy

Nerves in the peripheral nervous system are subjected to injuries that damage the nerves to varying degrees.[1-3] Under circumstances where the injury results in disruption of the axonal continuity, as may be the case for crush and transection injuries, the injuries are referred to as axonotmesis and neurotmesis, respectively, using the Seddon classification scheme,[4] and second-degree and fifth-degree injuries, using the Sunderland criteria.[3]

In adults, no motoneurons are lost unless the nerve injuries are sustained close to the cell body,[5-7] but morphologic criteria of cell death indicate a loss of up to 35% of the sensory neurons.[8-10] The injured neurons undergo morphologic changes known as chromatolysis[11,12] (Fig. 1A). These changes include the movement of the nucleus from a central to an asymmetric position in the neuronal soma and the disruption of Nissl bodies that comprise the rough endoplasmic reticulum; the morphologic changes reflect the molecular response of the neuron of changed expression of hundreds of genes, including a large number of immediate early genes, transcription factors, and many novel genes.[13-15] These genes are frequently referred to as growth or regeneration associated genes (RAGs), and they include those that transcribe neurotrophic factors and their receptors, such as brain-derived neurotrophic factor (BDNF) and its neurotrophin trkB receptor and glial derived neurotrophic factor (GDNF) and its receptors GFRα1 and ret. They also include the cytoskeletal proteins, tubulin and actin,[16-21] that are transported down the axons and are essential for the extension of the growth cones from the proximal nerve stump.[22] The transcriptional upregulation of the growth-associated proteins of GAP-43, CAP-23, and SCG10 is directly correlated with the regenerative capacity of the injured neurons[23] (see Fig. 1A).

RAG expression after nerve injury is transient, the expression declining in neurons without target contact (axotomy), but the genes are upregulated a second time by the refreshment cut axotomy that is frequently performed before nerve repair in humans and in animal models.[24,25] The significance of the second upregulation is that the injured neurons respond to positive signals emanating from the injury site rather than to negative signals resulting from the isolation of the axotomized neurons from target derived neurotrophic

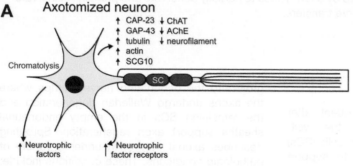

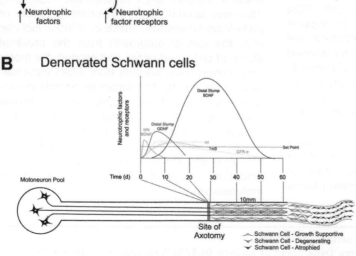

Fig. 1. Schematic illustrations of an axotomized motoneuron and denervated Schwann cells (SCs) after peripheral nerve injury. (A) The neuronal cell body that is isolated from its target (axotomy) undergoes morphologic changes known as chromatolysis. These changes reflect altered gene expression in which several RAGs are upregulated, and others, including choline-acetyltransferase (ChAT) and acetylcholine esterase (AChE), are downregulated. (B) Denervated SCs in the nerve stump distal to the site of injury (axotomy) lose their myelin, proliferate, and convert to a growth-supportive state. They express several growth factors, including glial and brain-derived neurotrophic factors (GDNF and BDNF, respectively). BDNF is also expressed in motoneurons as are the receptors for both factors, TrkB for BDNF, and GFR-α and ret for GDNF. The transient expression of the growth factors and receptors in both the axotomized neurons and denervated SCs is responsible, at least in part, for the progressive failure of neurons to regenerate after delayed nerve surgery or when injured nerves regenerate over long distances to reach denervated targets. ([B] Adapted from Furey MJ, Midha R, Xu Q-G, et al. Prolonged target deprivation reduces the capacity of injured motoneurons to regenerate. Neurosurgery 2007;60(4):730; with permission.)

factors.[24,25] The target-derived factors include BDNF and neurotrophin-4/5 (NT-4/5) expressed in denervated nerve stumps and muscles.[26,27]

Injured motoneurons are said to revert from a transmitting to a growth state as RAG upregulation occurs concomitant with downregulation of genes that transcribe transmitter-related enzymes, such as choline acetyltransferase and acetylcholine esterase.[14,15,28] Although exogenous BDNF and NT-4/5 can upregulate these genes in axotomized motoneurons,[29] it is unlikely that these factors downregulate the cytoskeletal proteins, given that a second axotomy alone is sufficient to upregulate their expression.[24,25] The downregulation and, in turn, the reduced slow transport of the cytoskeletal protein, neurofilament, accounts for the decline in the axon dimensions proximal to the injury site, the size varying with the reduced neurofilament content of the nerves.[30–32]

Wallerian Degeneration and Schwann Cell Response to Denervation

Axons separated from the cell body of their neurons continue to transmit action potentials for several hours and even days during which the slow transport of cytoskeletal and other proteins continues temporarily.[33–35] Thereafter, the axons and myelin undergo Wallerian degeneration. The SCs that formed the myelin sheaths of the large axons and surrounded groups of the small axons before injury withdraw their myelin, divide, and phagocytose myelin and axonal debris during the first days of Wallerian degeneration. The axonal and myelin debris are mitogenic for the SCs and play an essential role in their proliferation (Fig. 1B).[36,37]

Myelinating and nonmyelinating (Remak) SCs revert to a growth-supportive state in which RAGs, including neurotrophic factors and surface proteins, are upregulated,[21,38] and cytokines, such as the interleukins -1α, -1-β, and -6, and leukemia inhibitory factor are also upregulated as an innate immune response.[39,40] Macrophages that are attracted by the cytokines enter through the permeabilized nerve blood barrier[41] to become the prime cells responsible for the phagocytosis of the debris over a protracted period of 3 weeks in rodents.[42,43] The axons and their myelin also degenerate proximal to the injury, to the first node of Ranvier.[44,45]

The denervated SCs form long processes in the bands of Bungner on the basal lamina that the SCs elaborated within the endoneurial sheaths of the innervated nerves[46,47] (see Fig. 1B). The SC processes play an important role in guiding and supporting the regenerating axons across the injury site as well as into and through the denervated endoneurial sheaths.[15] The basal lamina is a 3-dimensional network of proteins and carbohydrates that is considered to be a layer of extracellular matrix within the endoneurium. It contains growth-promoting molecules that include the glycoproteins, laminin and fibronectin, as well as inhibitory molecules, the best known of which is chondroitin sulfate proteoglycan.[48–50]

NERVE REGENERATION
Axon Outgrowth from the Proximal into the Distal Denervated Nerve Stump

SCs migrate into the site of nerve injury and are misaligned within a tangle of laminin and fibronectin matrix for at least 10 days in a rat.[51] During this time, axons are growing out from the proximal nerve stump, crossing the suture line in a staggered fashion, and frequently being misdirected even backward into the proximal stump (Fig. 2A). As the glycoproteins become more organized and SCs align in parallel in the site and in the denervated distal nerve stumps, the axons progressively enter into the endoneurial tubes of the nerve stumps[51] (Fig. 2B). The femoral motoneurons that regenerate their axons over a 25-mm distance from the site of transection and microsurgical repair into the nerve branches, progressively increase in number over a period of 8 to 10 weeks (Fig. 2C). This time period of axon regeneration is surprisingly long considering an established rate of regeneration of 3 mm/d in rodents.[52] The motoneurons that regenerated their axons into the appropriate motor branch to the quadriceps muscle and/or the inappropriate saphenous sensory branch were discerned and enumerated after applying retrograde fluorescent dyes to each of the branches (see insert in Fig. 2C).[52]

Motoneurons regenerating their axons into the inappropriate sensory branch were initially the same in number as those regenerating their axons into the appropriate motor branch; the numbers that regenerated into the sensory nerve branch remained constant from 2 weeks onwards, whereas motoneurons regenerating their axons into the appropriate motor branch progressively increased in number (see Fig. 2C), a phenomenon referred to as preferential motor reinnervation by Brushart.[53] When motoneurons that regenerated their axons just across the surgical repair site were counted, it was evident that the reason for the long period of time for all femoral nerves to regenerate into their branches was because motor axons "stagger" across the suture site, the number of neurons regenerating their axons across the site increasing

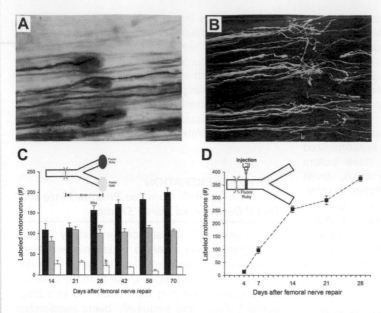

Fig. 2. Staggered axon regeneration across the site of nerve transection and surgical repair and through the distal nerve stump. (A) Asynchronous growth of silver-stained axons within the distal nerve stump. (B) The asynchronous outgrowth of axons containing green fluorescent protein on laminin (red) proceeds forward and backward at the suture site and into the denervated distal nerve stump. (C) Axotomized motoneurons regenerate axons into the branches of the femoral nerve; those regenerating their axons preferentially into the appropriate quadriceps muscle (mu) branch of the nerve increase progressively over 70 days, whereas those that grow their axons into the inappropriate saphenous cutaneous (cu) branch remain constant. The few femoral motoneurons sending axons into both branches, which were double labeled with fluororuby and fluorogold retrograde dyes, remain constant in numbers throughout the time period of regeneration. (D) The slow progressive increase in numbers of motoneurons regenerating axons 25 mm into the distal nerve stump in the graph in (C) is accounted for by the progressive increase in numbers of motoneurons that send axons across the suture site as determined after back-labeling the neurons with fluororuby dye that was injected 1.5 mm from the suture site. ([C] Adapted from Al-Majed AA, Neumann CM, Brushart TM, et al. Brief electrical stimulation promotes the speed and accuracy of motor axonal regeneration. J Neurosci 2000;20:2605; and [D] Brushart TM, Hoffman PN, Royall RM, et al. Electrical stimulation promotes motoneuron regeneration without increasing its speed or conditioning the neuron. J Neurosci 2002;22:6634; with permission.)

progressively over a 3 to 4 week period (Fig. 2D).[52,54]

The presence of inhibitory molecules plays a role in slowing the axon outgrowth and regeneration across and into the distal nerve stumps. The glycosaminoglycan side chains of the chondroitin sulfate glycoproteins are large and negatively charged.[55] Evidence that they hinder the access of neurites in vitro[56] and regenerating axons into acellular grafts and distal nerve stumps in vivo[57–60] is that their digestion by the bacterial enzyme, chondroitinase ABC, promotes neurite outgrowth and axon regeneration. Later evidence that a) proteoglycan degradation by heparinase III treatment amplifies the regenerative response with more axons entering into a nerve graft and, b) treatment with chondroitinase ABC or heparinase I promotes axonal elongation, indicates that there may be several glycoproteins involved in the inhibition.[57]

Accelerated Axon Outgrowth in Rats and Humans by Brief Electrical Stimulation

A period of 2 weeks of continuous low-frequency (20 Hz) electrical stimulation (ES) of an injured nerve proximal to the site of injury promotes axon regeneration: all the axotomized femoral motoneurons regenerated their axons over a 25-mm distance within 3 rather than 8 weeks.[52] A brief period of ES of 1 hour was shown to be as effective for promoting both motor and sensory nerve regeneration,[52,61] the efficacy of the ES being confirmed in several later studies on other rodent nerves as reviewed recently.[62] ES promotes axon outgrowth across the injury site and does not affect the rate of axonal regeneration within the distal nerve stumps.[54] The accelerated axon outgrowth in turn leads to earlier reinnervation of denervated targets and functional recovery.[63–65]

ES mediates its effect at the level of the axotomized neurons because the enhanced nerve regeneration in response to the ES was blocked by preventing the propagation of action potentials to the cell body with tetrodotoxin blockade.[52] The upregulation of BDNF and its trkB receptors followed by upregulation of cytoskeletal proteins and GAP-43 in motoneurons was accelerated by ES.[19,20] ES also elevates cyclic adenosine monophosphate (cAMP) in axotomized neurons before the accelerated upregulation of RAGs, and, its efficacy in accelerating axon outgrowth of motor and sensory nerves is mimicked by rolipram application to the site of surgical repair of a transected common peroneal nerve (**Fig. 3**).[58] The finding that the rolipram effect was not additive with the positive effect of locally placed

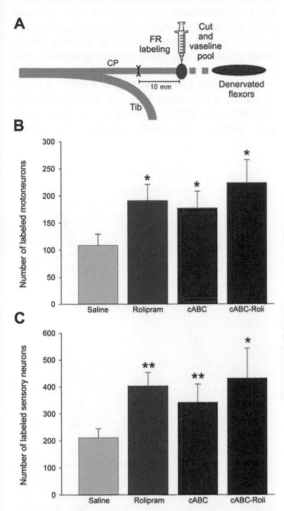

Fig. 3. After (*A*) transection and surgical repair of the common peroneal (CP) nerve, (*B*) the pharmacologic increase of cAMP by blocking phosphodiesterase mediated breakdown of cAMP with rolipram, or the breakdown of chondroitin phosphate glycoprotein with chondroitinase ABC (cABC), or the combination of rolipram and cABC increased the number of (*B*) motor and (*C*) sensory neurons that regenerated their axons a distance of 10 mm from the CP nerve transection and repair. FG, fluorogold; Roli, rolipram; Tib, tibial nerve. (Statistical significance vs saline at *$P<0.05$ and **$P<0.01$. ([*B*, *C*] *Adapted from* Udina E, Ladak A, Furey M, et al. Rolipram-Induced elevation of cAMP or chondroitinase ABC breakdown of inhibitory proteoglycans in the extracellular matrix promotes peripheral nerve regeneration. Exp Neurol 2010;223:148; with permission.)

chondroitinase ABC on numbers of neurons that regenerated their axons indicated that the efficacy of the rolipram in elevating cAMP and, in turn, promoting axon outgrowth overcomes the inhibitory effects of the molecules at the injury site (see **Fig. 3**B, C).[58]

The efficacy of the brief 1-hour period of ES in accelerating axon outgrowth is also sufficient to accelerate muscle reinnervation in humans after nerve injury.[66] Importantly, the ES was effective despite the long periods that the affected neurons remained without target contact (chronic axotomy) and the chronic denervation of the distal nerve stumps in this human study. The author has recently used an experimental rat model of delayed nerve repair to demonstrate the efficacy of the 1-hour period of 20-Hz ES in promoting axon regeneration after chronic axotomy of motor and sensory neurons and/or chronic denervation of the distal nerve stumps, the chronic axotomy, and denervation having depressed regenerative capacity before ES.[67] It remains to be determined whether this protocol of ES is effective in promoting axon regeneration over very long periods required for axons to regenerate over long distances, as, for example, after brachial nerve injuries requiring years to grow to reinnervate muscles and sense organs. As injured nerves do reinnervate chronically denervated muscles,[68–71] contrary to accepted views that the muscles undergo irreversible atrophy,[2,3] ES may very well be applicable for more proximal injuries that require nerve regeneration over long distances to reinnervate distant denervated targets.

NERVE SPROUTING
Partial Nerve Injuries and Axon Sprouting

Nerve injuries are frequently partial, involving a portion rather than entire peripheral nerves.[1] The most dramatic examples include the brachial nerve injuries, especially those in which spinal roots are avulsed as they are frequently in motorcycle accidents.[72,73] Somatic and sympathetic axons that remain without target contact may sprout to reinnervate denervated targets in muscles and skin.[74–77]

Sensory axons innervate as few as 4 and as many as 100 receptors in the skin: in salamander skin, each sensory nerve supplies many Merkel cells and the fields of innervation are organized as a mosaic with little overlap between fields.[78] Neurotrophic factors likely regulate sprouting of sensory axons in partially denervated skin because the sprouting was abolished when neurotrophic factors, including nerve growth factor (NGF), BDNF, NT-3, and/or NT-4/5, were blocked by a polyclonal antibody raised against NGF but which could not distinguish between the factors.[79] The location of the factors that stimulate sprouting was attributed to the denervated Schwann tubes of the horizontal subepidermal network that secrete the factors.[79]

Motor nerves each innervate as few as 10 muscle fibers in eye muscles and as many as thousands as in the proximal muscles of the limbs.[80] The intact motor nerves within partially denervated skeletal muscles reinnervate denervated muscle fibers by sprouting new axons from the last node of Ranvier (**Fig. 4A**). These nodal sprouts are the most common with preterminal sprouts emanating distal to the node (**Fig. 4B**), and ultraterminal sprouts from the nerve terminals

at the neuromuscular junctions being less frequent (**Fig. 4C**).[76]

The specialized perisynaptic Schwann cells (PSCs) at the neuromuscular junction are critical for motor axonal sprouting.[81,82] PSCs normally respond to transmitters released from the presynaptic terminals that prevent the cells from extending long processes, but they extend processes when transmitter release is blocked pharmacologically or the nerve is cut.[83] In partially denervated muscles, the PSCs extend processes that bridge between innervated and denervated neuromuscular junctions (**Fig. 4D**) within a week of partial denervation in a rat hindlimb muscle (**Fig. 4E**). The PSCs at the innervated junctions also extend processes despite the intact

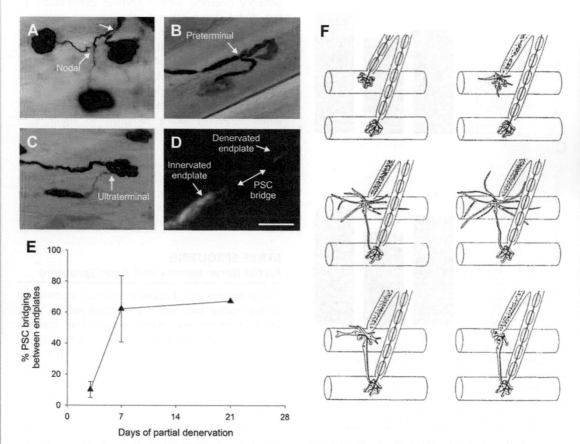

Fig. 4. Motor nerve sprouting within the intramuscular branches of partially denervated rat muscle. (*A*) Nodal sprout from the last node of Ranvier before the neuromuscular junction is the most frequently encountered, followed by (*B*) preterminal sprouts before the junction, and (*C*) ultraterminal sprouts from the nerve terminal at the junction as demonstrated with silver staining of the nerves and cholinesterase staining of the neuromuscular junction. (*D*) Perisynaptic Schwann cells (PSCs) immunostained with S-100 bridge between innervated and denervated endplates, their numbers increasing to a maximum within 7 days. (*E*) The number of PSCs that bridge between endplates as a percentage of the number of endplates counted. (*F*) The PSC bridging lead axon sprouts from the intact motor nerve to neuromuscular junctions of denervated muscle fibers. (*Adapted from* Tam SL, Gordon T. Axonal sprouting in health and disease. Encyclopedia Neurosci 2011;1–8; with permission.)

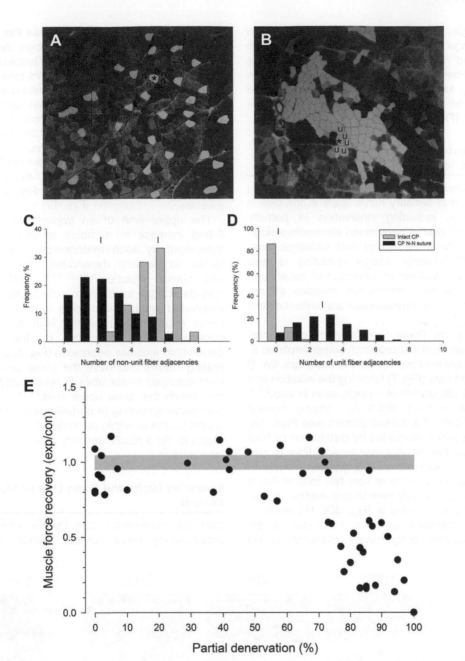

Fig. 5. (A) Axonal sprouting compensates for moderate but not extreme partial denervation because the muscle fibers innervated by a single motor axon progressively clump as the numbers of motor nerves to the muscles decrease. (A–D) Rat tibialis anterior muscle fiber innervation after transection and surgical repair of the common peroneal (CP) nerve. In muscle cross-sections in (A), the glycogen-depleted muscle fibers innervated by one axon, the unit muscle fibers (u), lie in a mosaic pattern within a defined territory in contrast to (B), the clumped distribution of glycogen depleted unit fibers in muscles reinnervated by reduced numbers of nerves. (C) The frequency distribution of non-unit (n) fiber adjacencies for the reinnervated muscles was shifted to the left of the distribution in normally innervated muscles. (D) The motor unit (u) muscle fiber adjacencies increase in the reinnervated muscles from the very low numbers in normally innervated muscles. (E) Nerve sprouting in partially denervated muscles results in full recovery of muscle force (relative to the uninjured muscles on the contralateral side of the rat) until more than approximately 75 to 80% of the nerves are cut. Mean numbers in C and D are shown are short vertical lines above the distributions. CP, common peroneal; N-N, nerve-nerve; n, non-unit; u, unit. ([E] *Adapted from* Gordon T, Tyreman N. Sprouting capacity of lumbar motoneurons in normal and hemisected spinal cords of the rat. J Physiol 2010;588:2754; with permission.)

cholinergic transmission, likely in response to short-range diffusible, sprout-inducing stimuli generated from the denervated (or inactive) muscle fibers.[84–87] The PSC processes lead the sprouting axons from the intact motor nerves to reinnervate denervated neuromuscular junctions[81,82] (**Fig. 4F**).

Reinnervation of Partially Denervated Skin and Muscle

Axon sprouting from nociceptive, touch, and heat-sensitive sensory nerve fibers in the skin is effective in providing innervation in partially denervated skin as determined electrophysiologically and from behavioral and histologic analyses.[79,88] Similarly, axonal sprouting is also effective in providing reinnervation of denervated fibers in partially denervated muscles as assessed by electrophysiological and histochemical analyses.[76]

The muscle fibers innervated by one motoneuron can be visualized as glycogen-depleted fibers in muscle cross-sections in rats (**Figs. 5A, B** and **6**) and cats (**Fig. 7**) following the isolation and repeated stimulation of a single axon in vivo.[89,90] They are normally distributed among nonunit muscle fibers in a mosaic pattern (see **Figs. 5A, 6**, and **7**) that is paralleled by distribution of fiber types (see **Fig. 6**). Any one muscle fiber is surrounded by approximately 6 non-unit muscle fibers (**Fig. 5C**) with no or very few muscle fibers of the motor unit adjacent to one another in normally innervated muscle (**Fig. 5D**). However, in partially denervated muscles, motor unit muscle fibers become progressively clumped as do muscle fibers of the same type (see **Fig. 6**). The adjacencies of non-unit muscle fibers decline as the unit fiber adjacencies increase because nodal and terminal sprouts emerging from intact motor nerves reinnervate nearby or adjacent denervated muscle fibers within a circumscribed territory (see **Fig. 6**).[91–93] The same phenomenon of progressive clumping of muscle unit fibers and fiber types occurs when reduced numbers of nerves regenerate and reinnervate muscles after nerve transection injuries, as illustrated in **Fig. 5B** for rat muscles and in **Fig. 7** for cat muscles.

The upper limit of an approximately 4- to 6-fold increase in numbers of muscle fibers innervated by each motoneuron that is quite similar in partially denervated rodents, cats, and human muscles[74,91,92,94,95] likely corresponds with the available muscle fibers to be reinnervated within the muscle territory that the nerve supplies.[93] Once the limit is reached, contractile force generated by the partially denervated muscles decreases (**Fig. 5E**). Regenerating nerves that have the same capacity to form enlarged motor units in reinnervated muscles reach the same upper limit.[68,69,90,96] Sensory nerve sprouting in partially denervated skin is also limited to within territories that each nerve supplies. As a result, sensory areas may be left insensate.[78]

Sprouting Limits and Some Loss of Motor Control

Normally movement occurs by the activation of progressively more forceful motor units in

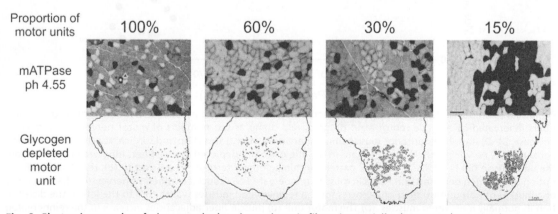

Fig. 6. Photomicrographs of glycogen-depleted muscle unit fibers in partially denervated rat muscles in cross-section that show progressive clumping accompanied by parallel progressive clumping of muscle fiber types as the number of motor units is progressively reduced from 100% to 15%. The fiber types were recognized by staining histochemically for acidic myosin ATPase. The scale bars for the mATPase staining of the muscle fibers in cross-section is 50 microns and for the glycogen depleted motor units in camera lucida drawing is 1 mm. (*Adapted from* Gordon T, Tyreman N. Sprouting capacity of lumbar motoneurons in normal and hemisected spinal cords of the rat. J Physiol 2010;588:2762; with permission.)

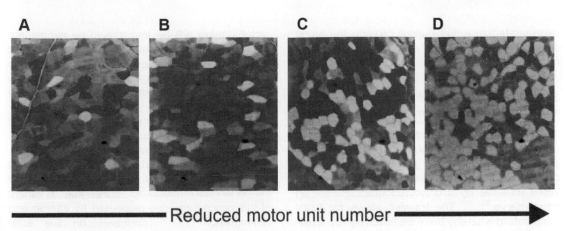

Reduced motor unit number ⟶

Fig. 7. Photomicrographs of periodic Schiff-stained cross-sections of reinnervated cat medial gastrocnemius showing the progressive clumping of the glycogen-depleted muscle fibers of single motor units when the numbers of reinnervating nerves were reduced by cutting 1 of 2 contributing ventral roots. Numbers of motor units and the numbers of muscle fibers reinnervated by a single axon, respectively, were (A) 260 and 194; (B) 229 and 293; (C) 156 and 403, and (D) 65 and 933.

appropriate muscles to exert the movement as well as by increasing the frequency at which action potentials are generated in the nerves to the muscles.[97] This control is progressively compromised when fewer nerves supply the muscles. In contrast to normally innervated muscles, the activation of reduced numbers of motoneurons that supply partially denervated and

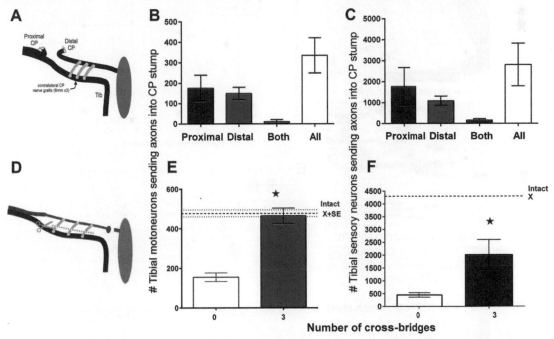

Fig. 8. (A) Placement of autologous common peroneal (CP) nerve cross-bridges between a donor intact tibial (TIB) nerve and a denervated distal CP nerve stump in a rat hindlimb results in regeneration of axons from TIB motoneurons (B) and sensory neurons (C) that grow proximal and distal to the cross-bridges in the denervated CP nerve stump with very few growing in both directions. (D) Axotomized CP neurons that regenerated their axons through nerve stumps that were either "protected" or not by cross-bridges, were backlabeled with a fluorescent dye and counted 3 months after delayed repair of the chronically injured CP nerve. TIB neurons were not labeled and counted because the bridges containing the donor TIB axons were cut at the time of the dye application. The numbers of (E) CP motor and (F) sensory neurons that regenerated their axons into the distal nerve stumps were significantly higher when cross-bridges were placed than when they were not. (Statistical significance of 3 vs 0 cross-bridges at *P<0.05). (*Adapted from* Gordon T, Hendry HM, Lafontaine CA, et al. Nerve cross-bridging to enhance nerve regeneration in a rat model of delayed nerve repair. PLoS One 2015;10(5):e0127397; with permission.)

reinnervated muscles cannot provide the same smooth gradation of muscle force during movement.

Surgical Methods Including Nerve Transfers and End-to-Side Neurorrhaphies

The surgical technique of nerve transfer, introduced by Tuttle in 1913 and brought into surgical practice by Mackinnon's group,[98] has become a popular means to reinnervate one or more denervated muscles by a dissected fascicle from an intact nerve.[98–100] The transfer allows for functional return whereby there are relatively few available nerves; this is frequently the case after spinal root avulsions, for example, in which poor functional recovery is generally anticipated as a result of the long distances of the injuries from denervated targets.[101–104] The probability that some

motor control will be lost should be anticipated as a result of the reduced availability of motor nerves from the donor nerve fascicle to reinnervate the muscle or muscles of choice. The donor nerve supply, on the other hand, may not be unduly compromised.

An end-to-side neurorrhaphy is another surgical technique with the same objective of "borrowing" from intact nerve to reinnervate denervated muscle: a denervated distal nerve stump is inserted into an intact nerve to "borrow" innervation for the denervated muscle.[105–109] However, a variant of this procedure, also pioneered by Viterbo and colleagues,[105,110–112] improves on the end-to-side neurorrhaphy because insertion of nerve autografts (nerve cross-bridges) between an innervated nerve and a denervated nerve stump "borrows" relatively few axons from the intact nerve to supply innervation to chronically

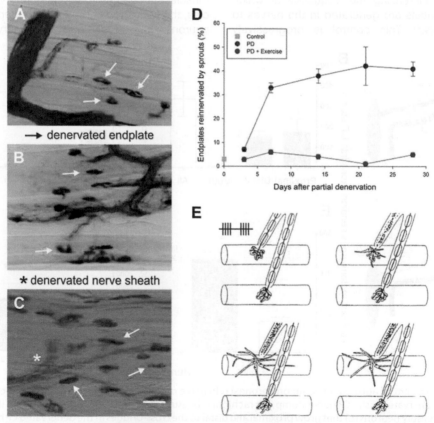

Fig. 9. Intensive exercise (of 8 hours daily) during a 4-week period inhibits sprouting in partially denervated rat muscles as shown at (A) 3 days, (B) 7 days, and (C) 28 days after partial denervation with cholinesterase staining of neuromuscular junctions and silver staining of motor axons. (D) The graph of the percentage of endplates reinnervated by axon sprouts from intact motor nerves with time after partial denervation with and without intensive daily exercise, and (E) the diagrammatic illustration shows that the failure of the PSCs to bridge between denervated and innervated endplates accounts for the failure of sprouting after excessive exercise. ([D] *Adapted from* Tam SL, Gordon T. Neuromuscular activity impairs axonal sprouting in partially denervated muscles by inhibiting bridge formation of perisynaptic Schwann cells. J Neurobiol 2003;57:226; with permission.)

denervated SCs in the denervated distal nerve stump in the time frame in which transected axons regenerate from the surgical repair site to the location of the cross-bridges (**Fig. 8A–C**).[67,113] The donor axons that regenerate through the cross-bridges, and both proximal and distal to the bridges, protect the distal nerve stumps because the insertion of the cross-bridges significantly increased the number of axotomized motor and sensory neurons that regenerated their axons after delayed surgical repair as compared with the neurons regenerating through chronically denervated nerve stumps that were not "protected" by any cross-bridges distal nerve stumps[113,114] (see **Fig. 8D–F**). This technique has been adopted in human surgery to promote the regeneration of branches of the facial nerve from one side of the face to the other to restore movement of paralyzed facial muscles, having carried out experiments in rats.[115,116]

Cautionary Notes Concerning Physiotherapy

Findings from animal studies should be noted for consideration of physiotherapy following surgical repair. Continuous ES at low frequencies does not deter muscle reinnervation after crush injuries or complete nerve transection and surgical repair in cats,[117] rabbits,[64] or mice.[118] Indeed, it accelerates target reinnervation in rabbits, mice, and humans.[64,66,118] However, ES for longer than 1 hour is ineffective in promoting sensory nerve regeneration.[61] In experiments in which the effects of neuromuscular activity generated by excessive physical exercise or daily ES of the nerves to partially denervated muscles were investigated, it was found that an 8-hour period of running wheel exercise or continuous 20-Hz ES of the nerves reduced the capacity of the intact nerves to sprout.[91] These very high levels of neuromuscular activity actually prevented the outgrowth of sprouts from the intact motor nerves. They reduced the formation of processes in the PSCs at the innervated junctions (**Fig. 9**),[119] consistent with findings that transmitters released from intact neuromuscular junctions prevent PSCs from sending out processes.[83] Moderate exercise, on the other hand, is either not harmful or might even promote sprouting, as shown by Diamond and colleagues[88] for sensory nerves.

SUMMARY

Poor functional outcomes are frequent after peripheral nerve injuries despite the regenerative support of SCs. Although motoneurons, and to a lesser extent, sensory neurons survive the injuries, outgrowth of axons across the injury site is slow and the neuronal regenerative capacity is progressively reduced when neurons remain without targets and chronically denervated SCs fail to support axon growth. Strategies, including brief low-frequency ES that accelerates target reinnervation and functional recovery and insertion of cross-bridges between a donor nerve and a recipient denervated nerve stump, are effective in promoting functional outcomes after complete and incomplete injuries. Axon sprouting from intact nerves to reinnervate partially denervated muscles and skin is effective after incomplete injuries but limited in extent. However, reduced numbers of nerves supplying partially denervated muscles and of nerves regenerating to reinnervate denervated muscles, as in the case of nerve transfers, may compromise motor control.

REFERENCES

1. Sulaiman OAR, Midha R, Gordon T. Pathophysiology of surgical nerve disorders. In: Winn HR, editor. Yeomans Neurological Surgery. 6th edition. Philadelphia: Saunders; 2011. p. 1–12.
2. Lundborg G. Nerve injury and repair. New York: Churchill Livingstone; 2004.
3. Sunderland S. Nerve and nerve injuries. Edinburgh: Livingstone; 1978.
4. Seddon HJ. Three types of nerve injury. Brain 1943; 66:238–88.
5. Gordon T, Gillespie J, Orozco R, et al. Axotomy-induced changes in rabbit hindlimb nerves and the effects of chronic electrical stimulation. J Neurosci 1991;11:2157–69.
6. Vanden Noven S, Wallace N, Muccio D, et al. Adult spinal motoneurons remain viable despite prolonged absence of functional synaptic contact with muscle. Exp Neurol 1993;123:147–56.
7. Xu QG, Forden J, Walsh SK, et al. Motoneuron survival after chronic and sequential peripheral nerve injuries in the rat. J Neurosurg 2010;112:890–9.
8. Otto D, Unsicker K, Grothe C. Pharmacological effects of nerve growth factor and fibroblast growth factor applied to the transectioned sciatic nerve on neuron death in adult rat dorsal root ganglia. Neurosci Lett 1987;83:156–60.
9. McKay Hart A, Brannstrom T, Wiberg M, et al. Primary sensory neurons and satellite cells after peripheral axotomy in the adult rat: timecourse of cell death and elimination. Exp Brain Res 2002;142:308–18.
10. Kingham PJ, Terenghi G. Bioengineered nerve regeneration and muscle reinnervation. J Anat 2006;209:511–26.
11. Lieberman AR. The axon reaction: a review of the principal features of perikaryal responses to axon injury. Int Rev Neurobiol 1971;14:49–124.

12. Gordon T, Sulaiman OA, Ladak A. Chapter 24: electrical stimulation for improving nerve regeneration: where do we stand? Int Rev Neurobiol 2009; 87:433–44.

13. Stam FJ, Macgillavry HD, Armstrong NJ, et al. Identification of candidate transcriptional modulators involved in successful regeneration after nerve injury. Eur J Neurosci 2007;25:3629–37.

14. Verhaagen J, van Kesteren RE, Bossers KA, et al. Molecular target discovery for neural repair in the functional genomics era. Handb Clin Neurol 2012; 109:595–616.

15. Fu SY, Gordon T. The cellular and molecular basis of peripheral nerve regeneration. Mol Neurobiol 1997;14:67–116.

16. Tetzlaff W, Bisby MA, Kreutzberg GW. Changes in cytoskeletal proteins in the rat facial nucleus following axotomy. J Neurosci 1988;8:3181–9.

17. Tetzlaff W, Bisby MA. Cytoskeletal protein synthesis and regulation of nerve regeneration in PNS and CNS neurons of the rat. Restor Neurol Neurosci 1990;1:189–96.

18. Tetzlaff W, Alexander SW, Miller FD, et al. Response of facial and rubrospinal neurons to axotomy: changes in mRNA expression for cytoskeletal proteins and GAP-43. J Neurosci 1991; 11:2528–44.

19. Al-Majed AA, Tam SL, Gordon T. Electrical stimulation accelerates and enhances expression of regeneration-associated genes in regenerating rat femoral motoneurons. Cell Mol Neurobiol 2004;24: 379–402.

20. Al-Majed AA, Brushart TM, Gordon T. Electrical stimulation accelerates and increases expression of BDNF and trkB mRNA in regenerating rat femoral motoneurons. Eur J Neurosci 2000;12: 4381–90.

21. Boyd JG, Gordon T. Neurotrophic factors and their receptors in axonal regeneration and functional recovery after peripheral nerve injury. Mol Neurobiol 2003;27:277–324.

22. Dent EW, Gupton SL, Gertler FB. The growth cone cytoskeleton in axon outgrowth and guidance. Cold Spring Harb Perspect Biol 2011;3.

23. Mason MR, Lieberman AR, Grenningloh G, et al. Transcriptional upregulation of SCG10 and CAP-23 is correlated with regeneration of the axons of peripheral and central neurons in vivo. Mol Cell Neurosci 2002;20:595–615.

24. Gordon T, Tetzlaff W. Regeneration associated genes decline in chronically injured rat sciatic motoneurons. Eur J Neurosci 2015. [Epub ahead of print].

25. Gordon T, You S, Cassar SL, et al. Reduced expression of regeneration associated genes in chronically axotomized facial motoneurons. Exp Neurol 2015;264:26–32.

26. Funakoshi H, Belluardo N, Arenas E, et al. Muscle-derived neurotrophin-4 as an activity-dependent trophic signal for adult motor neurons. Science 1995;268:1495–9.

27. Funakoshi H, Frisen J, Barbany G, et al. Differential expression of mRNAs for neurotrophins and their receptors after axotomy of the sciatic nerve. J Cell Biol 1993;123:455–65.

28. Gordon T. The biology, limits, and promotion of peripheral nerve regeneration in rats and human. Nerves and nerve injuries. New York: Elsevier; 2015. p. 903–1019.

29. Fernandes KJ, Kobayashi NR, Jasmin BJ, et al. Acetylcholinesterase gene expression in axotomized rat facial motoneurons is differentially regulated by neurotrophins: correlation with trkB and trkC mRNA levels and isoforms. J Neurosci 1998; 18:9936–47.

30. Davis LA, Gordon T, Hoffer JA, et al. Compound action potentials recorded from mammalian peripheral nerves following ligation or resuturing. J Physiol 1978;285:543–59.

31. Gordon T, Stein RB. Time course and extent of recovery in reinnervated motor units of cat triceps surae muscles. J Physiol 1982;323:307–23.

32. Hoffman PN, Thompson GW, Griffin JW, et al. Changes in neurofilament transport coincide temporally with alterations in the caliber of axons in regenerating motor fibers. J Cell Biol 1985;101: 1332–40.

33. Lubinska L. Early course of Wallerian degeneration in myelinated fibres of the rat phrenic nerve. Brain Res 1977;130:47–63.

34. Miledi R, Slater CR. On the degeneration of rat neuromuscular junctions after nerve section. J Physiol 1970;207:507–28.

35. Mackenzie SJ, Smirnov I, Calancie B. Cauda equina repair in the rat: part 2. Time course of ventral root conduction failure. J Neurotrauma 2012;29:1683–90.

36. Beuche W, Friede RL. The role of non-resident cells in Wallerian degeneration. J Neurocytol 1984;13: 767–96.

37. Scheidt P, Friede RL. Myelin phagocytosis in Wallerian degeneration. Properties of millipore diffusion chambers and immunohistochemical identification of cell populations. Acta Neuropathol 1987;75:77–84.

38. Jessen KR, Mirsky R, Salzer J. Introduction Schwann cell biology. Glia 2008;56:1479–80.

39. Rotshenker S. Wallerian degeneration: the innate-immune response to traumatic nerve injury. J Neuroinflammation 2011;8:109.

40. Bauer S, Kerr BJ, Patterson PH. The neuropoietic cytokine family in development, plasticity, disease and injury. Nat Rev Neurosci 2007;8: 221–32.

41. Avellino AM, Hart D, Dailey AT, et al. Differential macrophage responses in the peripheral and central nervous system during Wallerian degeneration of axons. Exp Neurol 1995;136:183–98.

42. Rotshenker S. Microglia and macrophage activation and the regulation of complement-receptor-3 (CR3/MAC-1)-mediated myelin phagocytosis in injury and disease. J Mol Neurosci 2003;21:65–72.

43. You S, Petrov T, Chung PH, et al. The expression of the low affinity nerve growth factor receptor in long-term denervated Schwann cells. Glia 1997;20:87–100.

44. Kury P, Stoll G, Muller HW. Molecular mechanisms of cellular interactions in peripheral nerve regeneration. Curr Opin Neurol 2001;14:635–9.

45. Stoll G, Jander S, Myers RR. Degeneration and regeneration of the peripheral nervous system: from Augustus Waller's observations to neuroinflammation. J Peripher Nerv Syst 2002;7:13–27.

46. Jessen KR, Mirsky R. Negative regulation of myelination: relevance for development, injury, and demyelinating disease. Glia 2008;56:1552–65.

47. Gonzalez-Perez F, Udina E, Navarro X. Extracellular matrix components in peripheral nerve regeneration. Int Rev Neurobiol 2013;108:257–75.

48. Dou CL, Levine JM. Identification of a neuronal cell surface receptor for a growth inhibitory chondroitin sulfate proteoglycan (NG2). J Neurochem 1997;68:1021–30.

49. McKeon RJ, Schreiber RC, Rudge JS, et al. Reduction of neurite outgrowth in a model of glial scarring following CNS injury is correlated with the expression of inhibitory molecules on reactive astrocytes. J Neurosci 1991;11:3398–411.

50. Zuo J, Hernandez YJ, Muir D. Chondroitin sulfate proteoglycan with neurite-inhibiting activity is up-regulated following peripheral nerve injury. J Neurobiol 1998;34:41–54.

51. Witzel C, Rohde C, Brushart TM. Pathway sampling by regenerating peripheral axons. J Comp Neurol 2005;485:183–90.

52. Al-Majed AA, Neumann CM, Brushart TM, et al. Brief electrical stimulation promotes the speed and accuracy of motor axonal regeneration. J Neurosci 2000;20:2602–8.

53. Brushart TM. Motor axons preferentially reinnervate motor pathways. J Neurosci 1993;13:2730–8.

54. Brushart TM, Hoffman PN, Royall RM, et al. Electrical stimulation promotes motoneuron regeneration without increasing its speed or conditioning the neuron. J Neurosci 2002;22:6631–8.

55. Carulli D, Laabs T, Geller HM, et al. Chondroitin sulfate proteoglycans in neural development and regeneration. Curr Opin Neurobiol 2005;15:116–20.

56. Zuo J, Neubauer D, Dyess K, et al. Degradation of chondroitin sulfate proteoglycan enhances the neurite-promoting potential of spinal cord tissue. Exp Neurol 1998;154:654–62.

57. Groves ML, McKeon R, Werner E, et al. Axon regeneration in peripheral nerves is enhanced by proteoglycan degradation. Exp Neurol 2005;195:278–92.

58. Udina E, Ladak A, Furey M, et al. Rolipram-induced elevation of cAMP or chondroitinase ABC breakdown of inhibitory proteoglycans in the extracellular matrix promotes peripheral nerve regeneration. Exp Neurol 2010;223:143–52.

59. Zuo J, Neubauer D, Graham J, et al. Regeneration of axons after nerve transection repair is enhanced by degradation of chondroitin sulfate proteoglycan. Exp Neurol 2002;176:221–8.

60. Krekoski CA, Neubauer D, Zuo J, et al. Axonal regeneration into acellular nerve grafts is enhanced by degradation of chondroitin sulfate proteoglycan. J Neurosci 2001;21:6206–13.

61. Geremia NM, Gordon T, Brushart TM, et al. Electrical stimulation promotes sensory neuron regeneration and growth-associated gene expression. Exp Neurol 2007;205:347–59.

62. Gordon T, English AW. Strategies to promote peripheral nerve regeneration: electrical stimulation and/or exercise. Eur J Neurosci 2015 [Epub ahead of print].

63. Eberhardt KA, Irintchev A, Al-Majed AA, et al. BDNF/TrkB signaling regulates HNK-1 carbohydrate expression in regenerating motor nerves and promotes functional recovery after peripheral nerve repair. Exp Neurol 2006;198:500–10.

64. Nix WA, Hopf HC. Electrical stimulation of regenerating nerve and its effect on motor recovery. Brain Res 1983;272:21–5.

65. Pockett S, Gavin RM. Acceleration of peripheral nerve regeneration after crush injury in rat. Neurosci Lett 1985;59:221–4.

66. Gordon T, Amirjani N, Edwards DC, et al. Brief post-surgical electrical stimulation accelerates axon regeneration and muscle reinnervation without affecting the functional measures in carpal tunnel syndrome patients. Exp Neurol 2010;223:192–202.

67. Elzinga K, Tyreman N, Ladak A, et al. Brief electrical stimulation improves nerve regeneration after delayed repair in Sprague Dawley rats. Exp Neurol 2015;269:142–53.

68. Fu SY, Gordon T. Contributing factors to poor functional recovery after delayed nerve repair: prolonged axotomy. J Neurosci 1995;15:3876–85.

69. Fu SY, Gordon T. Contributing factors to poor functional recovery after delayed nerve repair: prolonged denervation. J Neurosci 1995;15:3886–95.

70. Gordon T, Tyreman N, Raji MA. The basis for diminished functional recovery after delayed peripheral nerve repair. J Neurosci 2011;31:5325–34.

71. Sulaiman OAR, Gordon T. Effects of short- and long-term Schwann cell denervation on peripheral nerve regeneration, myelination, and size. Glia 2000;32:234–46.

72. Malessy MJ, Pondaag W. Obstetric brachial plexus injuries. Neurosurg Clin N Am 2009;20:1–14, v.

73. Narakas AO. The treatment of brachial plexus injuries. Int Orthop 1985;9:29–36.

74. Tam SL, Gordon T. Axonal sprouting in health and disease. Encylclopedia Neurosci 2011;1–8.

75. Gordon T, Hegedus J, Tam SL. Adaptive and maladaptive motor axonal sprouting in aging and motoneuron disease. Neurol Res 2004;26:174–85.

76. Tam SL, Gordon T. Mechanisms controlling axonal sprouting at neuromuscular junction. J Neurocytol 2003;32:961–74.

77. Diamond J, Cooper E, Turner C, et al. Trophic regulation of nerve sprouting. Science 1976;193: 371–7.

78. Diamond J. The regulation of nerve sprouting by extrinsic influences. In: Schmitt TO, Worden FG, editors. The neurosciences: fourth study program. Cambridge (MA): MIT Press; 1979. p. 937–55.

79. Diamond J, Holmes M, Coughlin M. Endogenous NGF and nerve impulses regulate the collateral sprouting of sensory axons in the skin of the adult rat. J Neurosci 1992;12:1454–66.

80. Burke RE. Motor units: anatomy, physiology and functional organization. Handbook of physiology. The nervous system. Motor control. Bethesda (MD): American Physiological Society; 1981. p. 345–421.

81. Son YJ, Thompson WJ. Nerve sprouting in muscle is induced and guided by processes extended by Schwann cells. Neuron 1995;14:133–41.

82. Son YJ, Trachtenberg JT, Thompson WJ. Schwann cells induce and guide sprouting and reinnervation of neuromuscular junctions. Trends Neurosci 1996; 19:280–5.

83. Georgiou J, Robitaille R, Charlton MP. Muscarinic control of cytoskeleton in perisynaptic glia. J Neurosci 1999;19:3836–46.

84. Slack JR, Williams MN. The absence of nodal sprouts from partially denervated nerve trunks. Brain Res 1981;226:291–7.

85. Pockett S, Slack JR. Source of the stimulus for nerve terminal sprouting in partially denervated muscle. Neurosci 1982;7:3173–6.

86. Brown MC, Holland RL, Ironton R. Is the stimulus for motoneurons terminal sprouting localized? [Proceedings]. J Physiol 1978;282:7P–8P.

87. Brown MC, Holland RL, Ironton R. Degenerating nerve products affect innervated muscle fibres. Nature 1978;275:652–4.

88. Nixon BJ, Doucette R, Jackson PC, et al. Impulse activity evokes precocious sprouting of nociceptive nerves into denervated skin. Somatosens Res 1984;2:97–126.

89. Tötösy de Zepetnek JE, Zung HV, Erdebil S, et al. Innervation ratio is an important determinant of force in normal and reinnervated rat tibialis anterior muscles. J Neurophysiol 1992;67:1385–403.

90. Rafuse VF, Gordon T. Self-reinnervated cat medial gastrocnemius muscles. II. Analysis of the mechanisms and significance of fiber type grouping in reinnervated muscles. J Neurophysiol 1996;75: 282–97.

91. Tam SL, Archibald V, Tyreman N, et al. Increased neuromuscular activity reduces sprouting in partially denervated muscles. J Neurosci 2001;21: 654–67.

92. Rafuse VF, Gordon T, Orozco R. Proportional enlargement of motor units after partial denervation of cat triceps surae muscles. J Neurophysiol 1992; 68:1261–75.

93. Gordon T, Tyreman N. Sprouting capacity of lumbar motoneurons in normal and hemisected spinal cords of the rat. J Physiol 2010;588:2745–68.

94. Yang JF, Stein RB, Jhamandas J, et al. Motor unit numbers and contractile properties after spinal cord injury. Ann Neurol 1990;28:496–502.

95. Gordon T, Yang JF, Ayer K, et al. Recovery potential of muscle after partial denervation: a comparison between rats and humans. Brain Res Bull 1993; 30:477–82.

96. Rafuse VF, Gordon T. Incomplete rematching of nerve and muscle properties in motor units after extensive nerve injuries in cat hindlimb muscle. J Physiol 1998;509:909–26.

97. Milner-Brown HS, Stein RB, Yemm R. The orderly recruitment of human motor units during voluntary isometric contractions. J Physiol 1973;230:359–70.

98. Fox IK, Davidge KM, Novak CB, et al. Nerve transfers to restore upper extremity function in cervical spinal cord injury: update and preliminary outcomes. Plast Reconstr Surg 2015;136:780–92.

99. Midha R. Nerve transfers for severe brachial plexus injuries: a review. Neurosurg Focus 2004;16:E5.

100. Nath RK, Mackinnon SE. Nerve transfers in the upper extremity. Hand Clin 2000;16:131–9, ix.

101. Tung TH, Novak CB, Mackinnon SE. Nerve transfers to the biceps and brachialis branches to improve elbow flexion strength after brachial plexus injuries. J Neurosurg 2003;98:313–8.

102. Malessy MJ, de Ruiter GC, de Boer KS, et al. Evaluation of suprascapular nerve neurotization after nerve graft or transfer in the treatment of brachial plexus traction lesions. J Neurosurg 2004;101: 377–89.

103. Malessy MJ, Thomeer RT. Evaluation of intercostal to musculocutaneous nerve transfer in reconstructive brachial plexus surgery. J Neurosurg 1998;88: 266–71.

104. Tung TH, Mackinnon SE. Brachial plexus injuries. Clin Plast Surg 2003;30:269–87.

105. Viterbo F, Amr AH, Stipp EJ, et al. End-to-side neurorrhaphy: past, present, and future. Plast Reconstr Surg 2009;124:e351–8.

106. Yuksel F, Karacaoglu E, Guler MM. Nerve regeneration through side-to-side neurorrhaphy sites in a rat model: a new concept in peripheral nerve surgery. Plast Reconstr Surg 1999;104:2092–9.

107. Zhang Z, Soucacos PN, Bo J, et al. Evaluation of collateral sprouting after end-to-side nerve coaptation using a fluorescent double-labeling technique. Microsurgery 1999;19:281–6.

108. Zhang F, Fischer KA. End-to-side neurorrhaphy. Microsurgery 2002;22:122–7.

109. Sawamura Y, Abe H. Hypoglossal-facial nerve side-to-end anastomosis for preservation of hypoglossal function: results of delayed treatment with a new technique. J Neurosurg 1997;86:203–6.

110. Viterbo F, Teixeira E, Hoshino K, et al. End-to-side neurorrhaphy with and without perineurium. Sao Paulo Med J 1998;116:1808–14.

111. Viterbo F, Trindade JC, Hoshino K, et al. End-to-side neurorrhaphy with removal of the epineurial sheath: an experimental study in rats. Plast Reconstr Surg 1994;94:1038–47.

112. Viterbo F, Trindade JC, Hoshino K, et al. Latero-terminal neurorrhaphy without removal of the epineural sheath. Experimental study in rats. Rev Paul Med 1992;110:267–75.

113. Ladak A, Schembri P, Olson J, et al. Side-to-side nerve grafts sustain chronically denervated peripheral nerve pathways during axon regeneration and result in improved functional reinnervation. Neurosurgery 2011;68:1654–65.

114. Gordon T, Hendry M, Lafontaine CA, et al. Nerve cross-bridging to enhance nerve regeneration in a rat model of delayed nerve repair. PLoS One 2015;10:e0127397.

115. Placheta E, Wood MD, Lafontaine C, et al. Enhancement of facial nerve motoneuron regeneration through cross-face nerve grafts by adding end-to-side sensory axons. Plast Reconstr Surg 2015;135:460–71.

116. Placheta E, Wood MD, Lafontaine C, et al. Macroscopic in vivo imaging of facial nerve regeneration in Thy1-GFP rats. JAMA Facial Plast Surg 2015;17:8–15.

117. Gordon T, Thomas CK, Munson JB, et al. The resilience of the size principle in the organization of motor unit properties in normal and reinnervated adult skeletal muscles. Can J Physiol Pharmacol 2004;82:645–61.

118. Ahlborn P, Schachner M, Irintchev A. One hour electrical stimulation accelerates functional recovery after femoral nerve repair. Exp Neurol 2007;208:137–44.

119. Tam SL, Gordon T. Neuromuscular activity impairs axonal sprouting in partially denervated muscles by inhibiting bridge formation of perisynaptic Schwann cells. J Neurobiol 2003;57:221–34.

Nerve Repair and Nerve Grafting

Samir K. Trehan, MD, Zina Model, BA, Steve K. Lee, MD*

KEYWORDS

• Nerve injury • Nerve repair • Nerve autograft • Nerve grafting • Nerve repair outcomes

KEY POINTS

• Depending on the mechanism of injury, time since injury, and defect length, direct repair or nerve autografting are primary options for upper extremity peripheral nerve injuries.
• Principles of direct repair and nerve autografting, including donor selection, are reviewed.
• The outcomes, and factors associated with outcomes, of upper extremity peripheral nerve repair and autografting are reviewed.

DIRECT REPAIR

Introduction

The mechanism of injury (eg, closed crush injury vs sharp laceration), location of injury, zone of injury, time since injury, and degree of neurologic impairment are important decision-making factors in the treatment of upper extremity peripheral nerve injuries. An epidemiologic study in the United Kingdom reported that upper extremity peripheral nerve injuries more commonly occurred in males (3:1), in the distal extremity, and secondary to sharp laceration in a domestic or industrial setting.[1] The most commonly injured upper extremity peripheral nerves were the index radial digital nerve and small finger ulnar digital nerve.[1]

Timing

Direct end-to-end repair of a lacerated nerve is ideally performed in the acute setting (ie, within 3 days). The advantages of acute repair include the ability to perform intraoperative nerve stimulation, to optimize motor nerve recovery, and to adequately gain exposure and mobilize nerve

ends without scar tissue hindrance.[2] From a biomechanical standpoint, nerve ends have been reported to still contain neurotransmitters within 72 hours of injury.[2] From a histopathologic standpoint, nerve ends have symmetrically apposed fascicles immediately after transection but then become increasingly difficult to match, as Schwann cell proliferation, fibrosis, and angiogenesis occur at each end.[3]

The primary disadvantage of early nerve repair is the inability to accurately assess the zone and extent of injury (eg, in the setting of crush injuries). Direct nerve repair after longer time intervals has been described as delayed primary suture (up to 3 weeks) and secondary suture (greater than 3 weeks; requiring resection of neuroma proximally and glioma distally).[4] However, numerous studies have reported that a well-performed primary nerve repair has a significantly better outcome than either delayed end-to-end repair or delayed nerve grafting.[5–7] The importance of early repair has been reported in multiple upper extremity peripheral nerves, including the median, radial, ulnar, and musculocutaneous nerves.[5,8–10]

Disclosure Statement: No disclosures (S.K. Trehan and Z. Model); Arthrex (royalties; consulting), BioMedical Enterprises (consulting), AxoGen (consulting; research support), Checkpoint (consulting; research support), Integra (research support) (S.K. Lee).
Department of Hand & Upper Extremity Surgery, Hospital for Special Surgery, 535 East 70th Street, New York, NY 10021, USA
* Corresponding author.
E-mail address: lees@hss.edu

0749-0712/16/$ – see front matter © 2016 Elsevier Inc. All rights reserved.

hand.theclinics.com

Technique

Several technical principles of direct nerve repair must be highlighted. First, adequate visualization of relevant neural, vascular, and musculoskeletal structures is required for precise end-to-end nerve repair. Although large nerves can be repaired under high-powered loupe magnification (ie, at least 3.5×), smaller branches usually benefit from use of the microscope (12× to 15× magnification).[11] Adequate exposure also entails injured nerve end resection in order to visualize healthy nerve tissue and facilitate fascicle apposition. Given the healing process initiated at the nerve ends after traumatic injury, more end resection is required as the time from injury increases. How much nerve to resect because of neuroma and/or damage is controversial and ultimately based on the surgeon's experience and preference. Common methods used are external and internal visualization (eg, fascicular structure and bleeding), palpation, pliability, intraoperative histology, and intraoperative nerve studies (eg, nerve action potentials and somatosensory evoked potentials). At the authors' institution, they use all of the aforementioned methods; but in cases whereby there is uncertainty, they used intraoperative histology. The authors' threshold for adequate nerve health is at least 75% preservation of fascicular architecture.[12,13]

Secondly, the nerve ends must be neurolysed from the surrounding scar tissue bed. During this step, it is critical to avoid physical damage (ie, crushing or tearing) to the nerve ends.[3] In addition, nerve repairs should be performed in a well-vascularized tissue bed.[14] Third, repair must be achieved with minimal tension.[15] Minimal tension is emphasized because even in the setting of a fresh nerve laceration, some tension exists because of the elastic nature of nerves. Nerve repairs under tension have been shown to result in nerve ischemia and repair mechanical failure in a rat model.[16] Assessing repair tension intraoperatively is an important component of repair, and multiple technical recommendations have been described. Unfortunately these technical recommendations have yet to be comparatively tested in a rigorous scientific fashion. de Medinaceli and colleagues[17] reported that failure to hold an end-to-end repair with a single 9-0 suture was a sign of undue tension. For nerves of the wrist and forearm, one can place a single 7-0 nylon epineural suture with wrist flexed less than 30° and determine whether the suture holds the ends together without epineural tearing and/or blanching of the epineural vessels.[4] The importance of minimizing tension on the nerve repair must be considered

postoperatively as well because certain repairs will require splint immobilization to prevent joint range of motion. In addition, Bertelli and colleagues[18] and Kechele and colleagues[19] have advocated the use of polypropylene mesh to augment direct epineural repairs ("epineural splinting") in order to minimize tension at the repair site.[18,19]

Finally, nerve repair can be performed by suture placement in either the epineurium or the perineurium. The theoretic advantage of perineural sutures is that these repairs repair individual fascicles, thus allowing identification of sensory versus motor fascicles and allowing appropriate alignment and potential improvement in outcomes.[20] The theoretic disadvantage is that placement of these sutures requires greater dissection and trauma to the nerve, increased operative time, increased suture material, and is technically demanding.[11] Epineural repair, on the other hand, aligns the nerve ends only. Several investigators have demonstrated no difference between fascicular and epineural repairs for peripheral nerve injuries.[21–23]

Author's Preferred Method

The senior author's preferred indication for direct nerve repair is an acute nerve laceration with minimal gap, easily mobilized nerve ends after resection, and minimal repair tension without restricted adjacent joint range of motion. An operative microscope is usually used for all nerve repair cases as it aids in accurate placement of epineural sutures and minimizes damage to nerve tissue. A few epineural sutures are placed (**Fig. 1**), the preferred suture material being nylon with caliber typically 8-0 or 9-0. The repair is performed on a blue

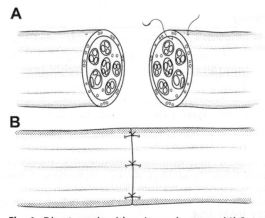

Fig. 1. Direct repair with epineural sutures. (*A*) Suture passed through epineural tissue only (ie, not fascicles). (*B*) Direct repair with epineural sutures resulting in nerve end approximation.

background made from a small piece cut from a Mayo stand cover. For any nerve larger than a digital nerve, the repair is augmented with fibrin glue. Fibrin glue is dripped on the repair, and then the blue background is wrapped around the nerve in a burrito fashion in order to create a layer of glue around the repair site. The repair should be on the looser rather than tighter side. The most destructive error is a repair that is too tight, whereby opposing fascicles actually pass each other (**Fig. 2**). Repairing the back wall first in a slightly loose fashion is helpful to initially align the nerve ends and to keep the back wall fascicles contained. Repairing the remainder of the nerve so that the fascicles *barely* touch is the goal. At the end of the repair, there should be no deformity to the nerve. At the repair site, the edges of the nerve should be flush without any kinks. No fascicles should be escaping the repair site; this is a sign that the repair is too tight and the fascicles are past pointing (see **Fig. 2**). If minimal, this situation can be salvaged by a minimal trimming of escaping fascicles. Otherwise, the repair should be repeated but looser. This description may seem to go into excessive detail, but the senior author feels strongly that poor technique is at least partly responsible for poor results that sully the outcomes of nerve repair and, thus, the overall perception of the value of nerve surgery.

At the completion of repair, it is imperative that there is minimal tension on the repair sites when the involved body part is put through passive range of motion on the operating room table. Postoperatively the body part should be immobilized so that the repair sites do not have traction on them for 4 weeks.

AUTOGRAFT
Donor Options

If direct nerve repair is not feasible (eg, unable to achieve tension-free repair, delayed presentation, and/or presence of a segmental defect), nerve grafting should be considered. The gold standard graft material is autograft. The advantages of autograft, as a graft material, include preserved nervous architecture and biology (ie, Schwann cells and vasculature). In addition, autograft is the preferred graft option (as opposed to allograft or conduits) for motor and mixed nerves.[2] The disadvantages of autograft include potential donor site morbidity (from surgical harvest itself and/or resulting nerve deficit or painful stump neuroma formation) and limited availability.

Donor nerve selection is based on minimizing postoperative deficit, size match to the injured nerve, and ease of harvest. Peripheral nerves frequently used for autograft include the sural nerve, medial brachial and antebrachial cutaneous nerves, and lateral antebrachial cutaneous nerve.[4,11,24] Higgins and colleagues[25] examined the suitability of several donor site options for digital nerve segments based on fascicle number and cross-sectional area. Distal to the common digital nerve bifurcation, the lateral antebrachial cutaneous nerve was most similar. From the wrist to the common digital nerve bifurcation, the sural nerve was most appropriate based on these two criteria (ie, fascicle number and cross-sectional area).[25,26]

Finally, nerve grafting should be done with caution in an altered soft tissue environment with impaired vascularity (eg, burns, radiation). In cases whereby nerve injury is accompanied by significant soft tissue injury, soft tissue coverage in the form of rotational or free flaps may be required, either before or concomitantly with nerve reconstruction. In these cases, unique donor options may be available. For example, Bresnick and colleagues[27] described using a rectus abdominis free flap for soft tissue coverage of upper extremity injuries and using associated intercostal nerves as the autograft.

In the major nerves of the upper extremity (ie, axillary, radial, ulnar, median, and musculocutaneous nerves, nerve roots), the sural nerve is the senior author's preferred donor nerve choice.[11] For smaller nerves, ipsilateral cutaneous nerves of the upper extremity can be used.[4]

Technique

After the appropriate amount of nerve is resected back to healthy proximal and distal ends, the gap is measured. Donor nerve is then harvested at a length 20% longer than was measured. This length allows for the elasticity of the nerve and also for trimming of the nerve ends. The donor nerve can be exposed but is not sacrificed until ready for transfer into the nerve gap and suturing. Schwann

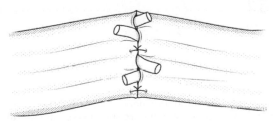

Fig. 2. Poor repair with past pointing. Fascicles escaping the repair site indicate that the nerve repair is too tight.

cells have limited survival time ex vivo. When the recipient site is completely ready, the donor nerve is explanted and prepared on the back table. The nerve graft is cut into segments and cabled once reversing the polarity to reduce the amount of axonal loss that would leave branch points if the nerve graft was placed in an antegrade fashion (**Fig. 3**).

Fibrin glue is applied to the nerve ends only so that repair is facilitated, but glue is not placed along the entire length of nerve graft in order to allow diffusion of blood, cells, and growth factors into the central portion of the graft. The cable graft is then laid into place. If the length is correct, the graft ends will touch the nerve ends and the blood in the field will stick the ends together. Different from direct repair, a no-tension repair should be achieved. At the completion of repair, it is imperative that there is minimal tension on the repair sites when the involved body part is put through passive range of motion on the operating room table. Postoperatively the body part should be immobilized

so that the repair sites do not have traction on them for 4 weeks.

OUTCOMES

Studies on the outcomes of upper extremity peripheral nerve repair and/or autograft are heterogeneous in terms of patient age, injury mechanism, time since injury, nerves injured, level of nerve injury, repair technique, and length of follow-up. However, valuable information can be drawn from these studies to inform surgical decision making and predict prognosis.

In reporting the outcomes of primary nerve repair in 2000, Allan[14] reported that the most important determinants of outcome were patient age for median and/or ulnar nerve injuries at the wrist/forearm and age and mechanism for digital nerve injuries. Young patients with simple lacerations had the best prognosis; few patients had complete return of normal sensation, even after digital nerve repair.[14] Improved clinical outcomes

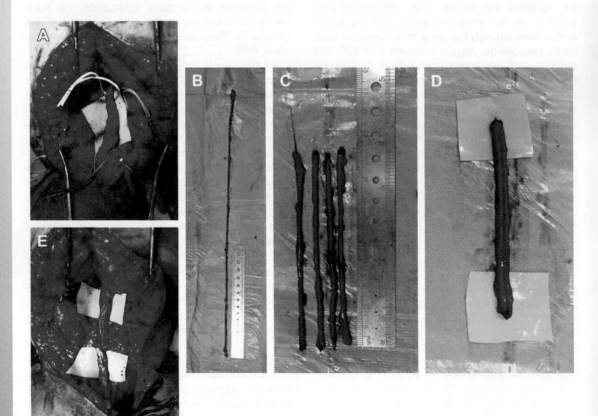

Fig. 3. Intraoperative pictures of patients with peroneal nerve lesion requiring sural nerve autograft repair given defect length. (*A*) Peroneal nerve exposed proximal and distal to zone of injury before sural nerve harvest. (*B*) Maximal length of sural nerve was harvested. (*C*) Sural nerve was cut into segments (measuring 20% longer than defect length) to allow cable graft. (*D*) Cable graft assembled. (*E*) Tension-free reconstruction of peroneal nerve defect with sural nerve cable graft.

have been previously reported in younger patients (compared with adults and even adolescents) following primary repair or grafting of median and/or ulnar nerve injuries.[28–31] Chemnitz and colleagues[28] reported in a series of 45 patients (38 primary repair and 8 sural nerve autograft) with median and/or ulnar nerve injury in the forearm with a 21- to 41-year follow-up that children experienced almost full sensory and motor recovery. In a meta-analysis of nerve repair outcomes, Rujis and colleagues[9] reported the results of 23 studies (623 median and/or ulnar nerve injuries) and found that negative prognosticators included age (ie, >40 years old), site of injury (ie, proximal vs distal), injured nerve (ie, ulnar nerve motor recovery probability was 71% less than the median nerve), and delay in surgery (incremental effect per month).

Other factors that have been implicated as negative prognosticators for upper extremity peripheral nerve repair include hypertrophic scar/keloid formation, surgeon inexperience, and concomitant bone and/or soft tissue injury.[32,33]

In settings where a segmental defect prevents primary repair, nerve grafting with autograft is one of the best options along with nerve transfer, depending on the clinical scenario. In a study of 220 upper extremity peripheral nerve lesions, Kalomiri and colleagues[31] concluded that superior axonal growth and nerve recovery could be achieved via nerve grafting without tension versus primary repair under undue tension. In this study, the investigators also found that younger age and earlier surgical treatment were positive prognosticators.[31] Another series, including 132 median nerve injuries at the level of the wrist (34 treated with primary repair and 98 with nerve grafting) and 10.4 years of mean follow-up, demonstrated good/excellent outcomes in 49%.[29] Factors that significantly affected prognosis included age, width of nerve contusion, length of grafting (greater than 7 cm correlated with poor outcome), preoperative delay, and level of injury (>56 cm proximal to fingertip correlated with poor results).[29] Other investigators have reported the importance of earlier surgical intervention (eg, less than 4 weeks) in achieving improved outcomes with nerve grafting.[34,35] Another important consideration in the setting of nerve autograft is donor site morbidity, which has been reported in up to 10% of patients.[36] In this study by Meek and colleagues,[36] it should be noted that 17% of patients also developed neuromas at the acceptor site (ie, site of the graft).

The significant functional and societal implications of upper extremity peripheral nerve injuries have been previously reported. In a study of 220 patients who underwent primary repair of ulnar and/or median nerve injuries at the wrist and forearm, 24% were unable to return to preinjury level of employment at a mean of 17.7 months follow-up. Negative prognosticators for return to work included poor sensory recovery, poor motor recovery, more proximal nerve lesion, type of work (ie, manual laborers), presence of nerve-related complications (eg, thenar atrophy, clawing, cold intolerance, paresthesia), and lack of hand therapy.[37] In another study, Bruyns and colleagues[38] reported the outcomes of 96 patients who underwent primary repair of ulnar and/or median nerve injuries. Forty-one percent of patients were unable to return to work at the 1-year follow-up. Negative prognosticators for return to work included combined nerve injury, poor compliance with hand therapy, lower level of education, and manual labor–type occupation. In addition, physical examination signs representing return of nerve function (ie, grip strength, pinch strength, sensation) differed between groups.[38]

In a meta-analysis of 33 studies comparing median and/or ulnar nerve defect repair with conduit versus autograft, Yang and colleagues[39] concluded that sensory nerves recovered better than motor nerves and the median nerve recovered better than ulnar nerve. Likewise, Rosen and Lundborg[40] concluded that motor recovery was inferior after ulnar nerve injury as compared with median nerve injury. Finally, in a comparison of nerve graft repairs after missile-induced peripheral nerve injuries, Roganovic and Pavlicevic[41] concluded that sensory recovery potential was the same across all nerves studied, although there was significant variability in motor recovery. Specifically, the proximal radial nerve recovered better than the ulnar nerve; the mid-musculocutaneous and radial nerves recovered better than the median and ulnar nerves; and distally, motor recovery potential was similar for all nerves.

Isolated, closed radial nerve injury may occur in the setting of humeral shaft fracture.[42] The indications and timing of operative exploration for these injuries are beyond the scope of this article, but excellent results have been reported in 78% to 90% of patients.[42,43] Similarly encouraging outcomes have been reported for radial nerve lesions requiring operative intervention, besides just those in the setting of humeral shaft fracture.[44] The outcome of delayed primary repair or grafting for radial nerve injuries has been correlated with the time since injury.[30] In addition, several studies have correlated clinical outcomes with the level of radial nerve injury.[8,45,46] Pan and colleagues[45] divided radial nerve injuries into 4 regions (infraclavicular, humeral shaft, from lateral arm to antebrachial fossa, and posterior interosseous nerve) and found improved outcomes at a mean of 21.5 months follow-up in the most distal subgroup (ie, posterior interosseous nerve injuries) as well as injuries treated within 5 months of injury. Similarly, Roganovic and Petkovic[46] reported the results of 131 missile-induced radial nerve injuries and concluded that the outcomes of proximal radial nerve injuries were worse than intermediate/distal injuries.[46] In addition, consistent with previous studies, they found that the length of repair defect, time interval between injury and surgery, and age significantly correlated with outcome.[46] Similar series of median and ulnar nerve injury repairs determined that level of repair, time until surgery, and length of repair defect were significant predictors of outcome.[47,48] In Roganovic's[47] series of ulnar nerve injury repairs, age and associated median nerve injury were also significant predictors of outcome. Finally, Shergill and colleagues[8] reported a series of 260 radial nerve injury repairs and determined that "violence of injury" (ie, comorbid arterial injury) was the most important prognosticator. Other negative prognosticators included repair defect greater than 10 cm and greater than a 14-day delay until surgery. Consistent with previous studies, good outcomes were reported in the subset of patients with posterior interosseous nerve (ie, distal) injuries.[8]

With regard to the musculocutaneous nerve, Osborne and colleagues[10] reported the outcomes 85 patients with traumatic lesions requiring repair: 13 underwent primary repair and 72 were grafted. The investigators reported that improved outcomes were associated with early repair (ie, <14 days) and graft length less than 10 cm, whereas worse outcomes were associated with arterial or bony injury.

SUMMARY

In conclusion, the outcomes of upper extremity peripheral nerve surgery depend on multiple factors, including patient age, mechanism of injury (ranging from a sharp laceration to a closed crush injury), injured nerve, level of nerve injury (ie, proximal to distal), time interval between injury and surgery, repair method (ie, primary repair vs grafting), surgeon expertise, and participation in hand therapy. Furthermore, upper extremity peripheral nerve surgery outcomes can be measured in terms of sensory, motor, and/or functional outcomes. Thus, maximizing success requires appropriate patient selection, setting of patient expectations, technique selection, surgical technical expertise, and postoperative recovery.

REFERENCES

1. McAllister RM, Gilbert SE, Calder JS, et al. The epidemiology and management of upper limb peripheral nerve injuries in modern practice. J Hand Surg Br 1996;21(1):4–13.
2. Moore AM, Wagner IJ, Fox IK. Principles of nerve repair in complex wounds of the upper extremity. Semin Plast Surg 2015;29(1):40–7.
3. Merle M, de Medinaceli L. Primary nerve repair in the upper limb. Our preferred methods: theory and practical applications. Hand Clin 1992;8(3):575–86.
4. Birch R. Chapter 32: nerve repair. In: Wolfe S, Pederson W, Hotchkiss R, et al, editors. Green's operative hand surgery. 6th edition. Philadelphia: Churchill Livingstone; 2011. p. 1035–74.
5. Birch R, Raji AR. Repair of median and ulnar nerves. Primary suture is best. J Bone Joint Surg Br 1991; 73(1):154–7.
6. Leclercq DC, Carlier AJ, Khuc T, et al. Improvement in the results in sixty-four ulnar nerve sections associated with arterial repair. J Hand Surg Am 1985; 10(6 Pt 2):997–9.
7. Merle M, Amend P, Foucher G, et al. Plea for the primary microsurgical repair of peripheral nerve lesions. A comparative study of 150 injuries of the median or the ulnar nerve with a follow-up of more than 2 years. Chirurgie 1984;110(8–9):761–71.
8. Shergill G, Bonney G, Munshi P, et al. The radial and posterior interosseous nerves. Results of 260 repairs. J Bone Joint Surg Br 2001;83(5):646–9.
9. Ruijs AC, Jaquet JB, Kalmijn S, et al. Median and ulnar nerve injuries: a meta-analysis of predictors of motor and sensory recovery after modern microsurgical nerve repair. Plast Reconstr Surg 2005;116(2): 484–94 [discussion: 495–6].
10. Osborne AW, Birch RM, Munshi P, et al. The musculocutaneous nerve. J Bone Joint Surg Br 2000;82(8): 1140–2.
11. Pederson WC. Median nerve injury and repair. J Hand Surg Am 2014;39(6):1216–22.
12. Wolfe SW, Johnsen PH, Lee SK, et al. Long-nerve grafts and nerve transfers demonstrate comparable outcomes for axillary nerve injuries. J Hand Surg Am 2014;39(7):1351–7.
13. Murji A, Redett RJ, Hawkins CE, et al. The role of intraoperative frozen section histology in obstetrical brachial plexus reconstruction. J Reconstr Microsurg 2008;24(3):203–9.
14. Allan CH. Functional results of primary nerve repair. Hand Clin 2000;16(1):67–72.
15. Millesi H. Interfascicular nerve grafting. Orthop Clin North Am 1981;12(2):287–301.
16. Clark WL, Trumble TE, Swiontkowski MF, et al. Nerve tension and blood flow in a rat model of immediate and delayed repairs. J Hand Surg Am 1992;17(4): 677–87.

17. de Medinaceli L, Prayon M, Merle M. Percentage of nerve injuries in which primary repair can be achieved by end-to-end approximation: review of 2,181 nerve lesions. Microsurgery 1993;14(4):244–6.

18. Bertelli JA, Kechele PR, Ghizoni MF, et al. Mesh epineural splinting for late median nerve repair in older patients: a preliminary report. Microsurgery 2011;31(6):441–7.

19. Kechele PR, Bertelli JA, Dalmarco EM, et al. The mesh repair: tension free alternative on dealing with nerve gaps-experimental results. Microsurgery 2011;31(7):551–8.

20. Kato H, Minami A, Kobayashi M, et al. Functional results of low median and ulnar nerve repair with intraneural fascicular dissection and electrical fascicular orientation. J Hand Surg Am 1998;23(3):471–82.

21. Bora FW Jr, Pleasure DE, Didizian NA. A study of nerve regeneration and neuroma formation after nerve suture by various techniques. J Hand Surg Am 1976;1(2):138–43.

22. Cabaud HE, Rodkey WG, McCarroll HR Jr, et al. Epineurial and perineurial fascicular nerve repairs: a critical comparison. J Hand Surg Am 1976;1(2):131–7.

23. Young L, Wray RC, Weeks PM. A randomized prospective comparison of fascicular and epineural digital nerve repairs. Plast Reconstr Surg 1981;68(1):89–93.

24. Pilanci O, Ozel A, Basaran K, et al. Is there a profit to use the lateral antebrachial cutaneous nerve as a graft source in digital nerve reconstruction? Microsurgery 2014;34(5):367–71.

25. Higgins JP, Fisher S, Serletti JM, et al. Assessment of nerve graft donor sites used for reconstruction of traumatic digital nerve defects. J Hand Surg Am 2002;27(2):286–92.

26. Slutsky DJ. The management of digital nerve injuries. J Hand Surg Am 2014;39(6):1208–15.

27. Bresnick S, Lineaweaver W, Hui K. Acute reconstruction of traumatic injuries of median and ulnar nerves by grafting with intercostal nerves from the rectus muscle: case reports. J Reconstr Microsurg 1997;13(7):503–6.

28. Chemnitz A, Bjorkman A, Dahlin LB, et al. Functional outcome thirty years after median and ulnar nerve repair in childhood and adolescence. J Bone Joint Surg Am 2013;95(4):329–37.

29. Kallio PK, Vastamaki M. An analysis of the results of late reconstruction of 132 median nerves. J Hand Surg Br 1993;18(1):97–105.

30. Kallio PK, Vastamaki M, Solonen KA. The results of secondary microsurgical repair of radial nerve in 33 patients. J Hand Surg Br 1993;18(3):320–2.

31. Kalomiri DE, Soucacos PN, Beris AE. Nerve grafting in peripheral nerve microsurgery of the upper extremity. Microsurgery 1994;15(7):506–11.

32. Gurbuz H, Aktas S, Calpur OU. Clinical evaluation of ulnar nerve repair at wrist level. Arch Orthop Trauma Surg 2004;124(1):49–51.

33. Mailander P, Berger A, Schaller E, et al. Results of primary nerve repair in the upper extremity. Microsurgery 1989;10(2):147–50.

34. Kalomiri DE, Soucacos PN, Beris AE. Management of ulnar nerve injuries. Acta Orthop Scand Suppl 1995;264:41–4.

35. Kokkalis ZT, Efstathopoulos DG, Papanastassiou ID, et al. Ulnar nerve injuries in Guyon canal: a report of 32 cases. Microsurgery 2012;32(4):296–302.

36. Meek MF, Coert JH, Robinson PH. Poor results after nerve grafting in the upper extremity: quo vadis? Microsurgery 2005;25(5):396–402.

37. Jaquet JB, Luijsterburg AJ, Kalmijn S, et al. Median, ulnar, and combined median-ulnar nerve injuries: functional outcome and return to productivity. J Trauma 2001;51(4):687–92.

38. Bruyns CN, Jaquet JB, Schreuders TA, et al. Predictors for return to work in patients with median and ulnar nerve injuries. J Hand Surg Am 2003;28(1):28–34.

39. Yang M, Rawson JL, Zhang EW, et al. Comparisons of outcomes from repair of median nerve and ulnar nerve defect with nerve graft and tubulization: a meta-analysis. J Reconstr Microsurg 2011;27(8):451–60.

40. Rosen B, Lundborg G. The long term recovery curve in adults after median or ulnar nerve repair: a reference interval. J Hand Surg Br 2001;26(3):196–200.

41. Roganovic Z, Pavlicevic G. Difference in recovery potential of peripheral nerves after graft repairs. Neurosurgery 2006;59(3):621–33 [discussion: 621–33].

42. DeFranco MJ, Lawton JN. Radial nerve injuries associated with humeral fractures. J Hand Surg Am 2006;31(4):655–63.

43. Lowe JB 3rd, Sen SK, Mackinnon SE. Current approach to radial nerve paralysis. Plast Reconstr Surg 2002;110(4):1099–113.

44. Kim DH, Kam AC, Chandika P, et al. Surgical management and outcome in patients with radial nerve lesions. J Neurosurg 2001;95(4):573–83.

45. Pan CH, Chuang DC, Rodriguez-Lorenzo A. Outcomes of nerve reconstruction for radial nerve injuries based on the level of injury in 244 operative cases. J Hand Surg Eur Vol 2010;35(5):385–91.

46. Roganovic Z, Petkovic S. Missile severances of the radial nerve. results of 131 repairs. Acta Neurochir (Wien) 2004;146(11):1185–92.

47. Roganovic Z. Missile-caused ulnar nerve injuries: outcomes of 128 repairs. Neurosurgery 2004;55(5):1120–9.

48. Roganovic Z. Missile-caused median nerve injuries: results of 81 repairs. Surg Neurol 2005;63(5):410–8 [discussion: 418–9].

Autograft Substitutes
Conduits and Processed Nerve Allografts

Bauback Safa, MD, MBA*, Gregory Buncke, MD

KEYWORDS

- Conduit • Allograft • Peripheral nerve injury • Peripheral nerve repair • Autograft alternative
- Autograft substitute

KEY POINTS

- Regardless of the repair methodology (direct suture, autograft, conduit or allograft), the same principles of good nerve repair should be rigorously adhered to in order to achieve the best possible outcome.
- Manufactured tube conduits are seeing a decreasing role in gap repair and an increasing role as an aid to coaptation.
- Use of processed nerve allografts seems to be increasing based on published clinical data showing high success rates and favorable comparisons with alternative techniques.
- Current studies and ongoing research help to clarify the role of processed nerve allografts and their limitations as a substitute for nerve autograft and direct suture.

INTRODUCTION

Why do clinicians care about substitutes for nerve autograft? Berger and Millesi[1] popularized grafting techniques by demonstrating their superiority to a tensioned direct repair. This popularity is for good reason, because nerve autografts provide a readily available source of patient-specific tissue, with a peripheral nerve-specific microenvironment, basal lamina scaffolding, guidance cues, and supportive Schwann cells. For these reasons, autograft has been the workhorse of peripheral nerve gap repair for decades. Surgeons therefore must ask themselves why, with all of these benefits, there is a need for a substitute? The apparent answer is that, for all of its benefits, there are some clear shortcomings and limitations associated with nerve autograft that can be detrimental to patients' quality of life and therefore have to be considered. Clinical outcomes are often less than are considered desirable, with roughly a 50/50 chance of returning M4 function or sensory discrimination.[2] Furthermore, there is a limited supply, and that supply can be of variable caliber, at times supplying subpar tissue with regard to the cross section of the nerve tissue that provides scaffolding for regeneration.[3] Also, there may be diminished Schwann cell viability after harvest.[4] In addition, in certain situations the supply of expendable donor tissue is not adequate or even available.[5] In addition, the autograft harvest site creates a new nerve injury that leaves the patient with a permanent deficit, often requires a second incision to access the donor tissue, can lead to the formation of a potentially symptomatic neuroma at the proximal donor site,[6] and can add considerable time and cost to the procedure.[7,8]

Because of these compromises, alternatives to the classic nerve autograft have been sought and have recently been increasing in popularity.

Disclosure: Dr B. Safa and Dr G. Buncke are research advisors for AxoGen, Inc.
The Buncke Clinic, 45 Castro Street #121, San Francisco, CA 94114, USA
* Corresponding author.
E-mail address: bauback@drsafa.com

Hand Clin 32 (2016) 127–140
http://dx.doi.org/10.1016/j.hcl.2015.12.012

Millesi[9] proposed that the ideal nerve graft should contain the following characteristics: be available in large quantity, have structural and mechanical properties consistent with the nerve's natural extracellular matrix, contain capillaries and a few fibroblasts, and contain a large number of Schwann cells originating from the nerve to be repaired. To help address these criteria, tissue and biomedical engineering has focused on development of biomaterials and advancements in tissue processing technologies to create a variety of devices and substrates to support peripheral nerve regeneration. Over the past few decades, the development of biocompatible materials and tissue processing that mimic or preserve the microenvironment of nerve tissue has produced advances. With these advances, processed nerve allograft (PNA) and manufactured conduits have become increasingly accepted alternatives in clinical practice.

MANUFACTURED CONDUITS

The manufacture of conduits can be traced back to Gluck and colleagues[10] in the 1880s when they fashioned a tube of decalcified bone to aid the approximation of transected nerve ends. This coupling of the nerve ends within the tubular device compensated for the lack of proper instrumentation in an era before the advent of microsurgery. This practice continued with modest enthusiasm until Dahlin and Lundborg's[11] landmark work with silicone tubes. Their work explored the application of tubes in peripheral nerve repair and, perhaps most importantly, characterized the mechanism of action of regeneration within the lumen of the tube.

A conduit works by encasing the distal and proximal nerve ends within the tube and providing gross macroalignment for the nerve and containment of the fluid leaking from the transected nerve ends, gathering it within the inner chamber. This fluid forms a rudimentary fibrin matrix between the nerve ends. If robust enough, the matrix forms a cable to support cellular migration between the nerve ends. As cells invade the cable, linear bands of Büngner form within the disorganized fibrin matrix. The neurite growth cone follows these bands and, with maturation, microfasciculation within the newly formed pseudo–nerve sheath occurs.[11] This mechanism depends on the volumetric output from the nerve stumps.[11–13] If the gap is too long or the inner lumen too large, the cable that forms is often thin, and, because of the mechanical contraction of the fibrin matrix, takes on a classic hourglass appearance. This alteration limits the area for axonal regeneration, with the maximum area for axonal regeneration being directly proportional to the cross-sectional area of the thinnest aspect of the fibrin cable. This characteristic is a limitation inherent to conduits that do not provide a laminin-rich endoneural scaffold, and has been observed in both the early silicone tube research and in subsequent advances with collagen-based biomaterials and synthetic polymers.[11–14] Even with this limitation, the theoretic benefits and ease of use are readily apparent. The tube creates a microchamber to contain the axoplasm and milieu; provides a barrier to invasion from wound bed inflammation[11]; limits the potential escape of neurites from the repair site, which may result in neuroma formation; and splints the nerve coaptation by loading the force during active range of motion onto the juncture between the suture and the tube versus the end-to-end coaptation.[15] Based on these benefits and promising research in animal models, Lundborg and colleagues[16] transitioned to clinical research with silicone tubes. They researched a series of mixed nerve repairs in the forearm, and with 5 years of follow-up data showed that the conduit repairs were comparable with direct suture and trended toward greater sensory recovery in gaps less than 5 mm in length. Although they were able to show the applicability of a conduit in short gaps, the silicone material resulted in patient complications caused by the nonpermeable, permanent nature of the silicone. In documented cases, superficial soft tissue irritation, fibrotic encapsulation, and mild compression necessitated the exploration and planned removal of several of the silicone tubes. Although practical application of their research was limited by the technology of the time, it spawned a renewed interest in tubular repair with a multitude of assorted biomaterials.

Modern biomaterials now play a role in manufactured conduits replacing the rigid sheath with semipermeable, biodegradable materials such as denatured collagen and polyesters. The purpose of these materials is to provide an outer sheath that allows diffusion of oxygen and micronutrients across their outer walls and into the fibrin matrix. Weber and colleagues[17] published on the first commercially available conduit, a woven polyglycolic acid tube for digital nerve repair. The study evaluated sensory outcomes compared with a control group of mainly direct suture repair and, secondarily, a small cohort of 8 autograft repairs. The study found that, in defects less than 4 mm, the conduit provided significantly better return of sensory function compared with the direct suture repair, with 91% providing excellent return of 2-point discrimination versus 49% in the suture-only group. This benefit was not seen in gaps larger than 4 mm, for which overall outcomes reported a 34% failure rate in the conduit group versus 24% in the standard group. The study concluded that conduits have utility for nerve gaps up to 30 mm in length. However, the longest gap treated with a conduit was less than 25 mm, and the mean nerve gap was only 7 mm. This finding brings into question the utility of conduits in larger gap repairs, but does highlight their potential benefits as an adjunct to the coaptation for gaps less than 4 mm. Following the polyglycolic acid conduit, denatured collagen, polycaprolactone, and decellularized porcine submucosa tubes have also been commercialized. Denatured collagen conduits are available from multiple manufacturers. NeuraGen (Integra Lifesciences, Princeton, NJ) was commercialized in 2001, and has been examined by numerous investigators for digital nerve gap repair and as a coaptation aid in major peripheral nerve repair (**Table 1**). Outcomes in digital nerve repair were first described by Lohmeyer and colleagues[18] in 2009, followed closely by Taras and colleagues[19] in 2011. Lohmeyer and colleagues[18] found that, in short digital nerve gaps less than 15 mm, collagen conduits provided consistent functional recovery. However, in gaps more than 15 mm, no return of function was observed. In 2010, Wangensteen and Kalliainen[20] reported on a large, single-center, multisurgeon registry of nerve injuries repaired with collagen conduits, and concluded that although the material can be used in multiple regions of the body, clinically meaningful outcomes were only observed in 43% of the cases and 31% of the subjects needed revisions. Haug and colleagues[21] reported 40% return of static 2-point discrimination in digital nerve gap repairs up to 20 mm, and Lohmeyer and colleagues[18] reported on 40 patients, finding that recovery was more reliable when the gaps were less than 12 mm. Most recently, Lohmeyer and colleagues[22] reported on the outcomes of 2 prospective randomized controlled studies in digital nerve gap repair. In their updated series, 65% of subjects reported useful return of sensory function, with a change in their recommendation to now state that gaps less than 10 mm performed significantly better than gaps more than 10 mm.[22,23]

Data on collagen conduits in major peripheral nerve repair are limited to a single industry-sponsored clinical study in median and ulnar nerve repairs at the wrist. The published data set examined the use of conduits as an alternative to the classic epineurial suture repair. The study found that 2-year outcomes were not different between the direct-suture group and the conduit-assisted group. However, overall success ranges for either group were not published, and the investigators cautioned that the gap must be restricted to no more than 6 mm.

In addition to the length limitation, other considerations include the degradation of the material and the body's response to it. Both Moore and colleagues[12] and Liodaki and colleagues[14] published case series of failed collagen conduits in mixed nerve repair and digital nerve repair respectively.[12,14] Moore and colleagues[12] observed remnants of the conduit remaining in the repair site that adhered to the nerve. Both found inadequate regenerate, with the classic hourglassing of the internal fibrin cable, as well as fibrosis and scarring between the material, the nerve, and the surrounding tissue bed. Histologic assessment found neuromatous formations and a foreign body reaction. No clinical data are available for the other collagen conduits (NeuroMatrix, NeuroFlex, Stryker Orthopedics, Mahwah, NJ) in the upper extremity.

The polycaprolactone (PCL) conduits (NeuroLac, NeuroLac TW, Polyganics, Netherlands) are polymer-based tubes and have the benefit of being transparent in nature, allowing visualization of the nerve stumps within the chamber of the tube. The material goes through a hydrolysis degradation and fractures into small particles over a period of 3 to 24 months until fully resorbed. In addition, the conduit may experience circumferential swelling after implantation and selection of an appropriate size to compensate for this swelling is recommended. Mechanically, the conduit is stiff and requires a long hydration period in warm saline to improve the suppleness of the material. Piercing with a large needle is recommended to provide a tract for the more delicate microsuture.[24] Clinically, Bertleff and colleagues[25] investigated them in a digital nerve repair model and found outcomes comparable with direct suture repair in gaps less than 20 mm. The use of autografts were foregone in longer gaps in favor of performing a direct suture repair, which potentially confounds the comparison with the control group data. Two complications related to the PCL conduit were reported, with irritation and extrusion from the wound necessitating revisions for each.[25] Chiriac and colleagues[26] published on a series of 29 PCL conduit repairs in both sensory and mixed nerves with an average gap of 11 mm and a range of 2 to 25 mm. They reported that only 31% of the sensory nerve repairs provided useful outcomes, and only 8% of the mixed nerve repairs provided useful function. The investigators reported a very high complication rate (8 out of 23 subjects), the worst being fistulization of the conduit requiring removal and wound care. Based on the limited functional

Table 1
Review of manufactured conduit clinical evidence

Reference	Nerves (N)	Age (y) Mean	Age (y) Range	Nerve Location	Nerve Type	Repair Type	Defect Length (mm) Mean	Defect Length (mm) Range	Follow-up (mo) Mean	Follow-up (mo) Range	Publication Recovery Classification	Publication Reported Outcomes	Standardized Meaningful Recovery[a]	Complication Rate (%)	Complications
Weber et al,[17] 2000	46	36	22–50	Digital	Sensory	PGA	7	0–25	9	3–12	S4 ≤6 mm; S3+ ≤15 mm	Gaps<4 mm, 100% Gaps 5–25 mm, 66%	Gaps<4 mm, 100% Gaps 5–25 mm, 66%	—	3 tube extrusions requiring revision
Lohmeyer et al,[18] 2009	12	38	13–66	Digital	Sensory	Collagen	13	6–18	12	—	S4 ≤6 mm; S3+ ≤15 mm	75%	75%	0	None
Wangensteen and Kalliainen,[20] 2010	86	33	7–79	Global	Sensory/mixed	Collagen	12.8	2.5–20	8.5	—	Sensory and motor improvement and qualitative evaluation	43% Postoperative improvement	—	13	11 complications reported; 1 desmoplastic melanoma with focal perineural extension; 10 neuromas
Moore et al,[12] 2009	7	16	3–43	Upper	Mixed (motor)	Collagen and PGA	27	20–30	24	9–48	Various: nerve conduction studies, 2PD, muscle testing, pain assessment	0%	0%	100	In all cases failure of reinnervation was reported. Two patients underwent revision surgery with excision of neuroma and reconstruction with nerve autograft
Taras et al,[19] 2011	22	44	22–72	Digital	Sensory	Collagen	12	5–17	20	12–59	Taras classification	59% Excellent 14% Good	91%	0	None
Rinker and Liau,[7] 2011	36	33	SD 10.4	Digital	Sensory	PGA	9	4–25	6	—	Static and moving 2PD	Static 2PD, 8 mm; Moving 2PD, 7 mm	94%	8	3 complications were reported: 1 postoperative wound infection; 2 implant extrusions

Chiriac et al,[26] 2012	16	33	26–61	Digital	Sensory	PCL	11	3–25	22	3–45	Weber 2PD <30 Weber SWM <75	44%	31%	11	8 complications reported; of the 8, 2 fistulizations of guide and 1 incidence of ulnar nerve irritation
Chiriac et al,[26] 2012	12	32	17–62	Upper extremity	Mixed (motor)	PCL	11	2–25	22	3–45	Weber 2PD <30 Weber SWM <75	25%	8%	—	8 complications reported; of the 8, 2 fistulizations of guide and 1 incidence of ulnar nerve irritation
Liodaki et al,[14] 2013	4	34.5	13–50	Digital/ upper extremity	Sensory/ mixed	Collagen	17	10–30	12	6–17	Sensory or motor improvement	0%	0%	100	4 complications reported; 1 perineural fibrosis/ scar neuroma; 1 fibrosis/scar formation, foreign body reaction, and chronic inflammation; 2 scar neuroma
Haug et al,[21] 2013	42	47	11–83	Digital	Sensory	Collagen	12	5–26	12	—	Sensory composite score	10% Very good 50% Good	40%	13	6 patients experienced paresthesias, with 2 patients experiencing wound healing problems; both patients had conduit removed
Lohmeyer et al,[23] 2014	40	38	17–75	Digital	Sensory	Collagen	12	5–25	12	—	ASSH modified guidelines	8% Excellent 43% Good 13% Fair	64%	Not discussed	Not discussed
Buncke et al,[27] ASSH 2015	23	42	19–76	Digital	Sensory	Collagen and PGA	15	4–20	13	6–40	2PD <15 mm and/ or SWM <4.31 (2g)	48%	48%	—	1 patient with 4 repairs with neuromas and dense scaring around collagen conduits

Abbreviation: PCL, polycaprolactone.
a MRCC Scale ≥ S3+/M3.
Data from Refs.[7,12,*4,17–21,23,26,27]

outcomes and the safety concerns, Chiriac and colleagues[26] did not recommend the use of the PCL conduit for nerve reconstruction in the hand.

Recently the authors presented the outcomes of a multicenter peripheral nerve registry designed to track outcomes of multiple nerve gap repair modalities. The cohort of conduit repairs included 23 sensory nerve repairs with an average gap of 15 mm. At an average of 14 months' follow-up, 48% of the subjects reported useful return of sensation. When stratified by gap length, 75% of the repairs less than 10 mm reported meaningful outcomes, whereas only 33% reported meaningful outcomes in gaps between 11 and 20 mm.[27]

In summary, conduits provide a convenient off-the-shelf alternative in peripheral nerve repair. Modern conduits are biocompatible, mechanically splint the nerve repair, and provide a protective environment for nerve regeneration. Although early studies proposed their benefits as a substitute for the classic nerve autograft,[17,28] the available clinical data now currently find their role more in line with Gluck,[10] Lundborg[11] and Boeckstyn's[29] original premise, as an alternative or augmentation to the classic epineurial suture repair.[10,16,29] This view is reinforced by the preclinical models[15,30–32] and the growing body of clinical evidence on their use as a coaptation aid.[16,17,33–35]

Given these results, the authors recommend the use of conduits in noncritical short-gap digital nerve repairs of less than 1 cm in length. Caution should be exercised when considering the use of polycaprolactone conduits.

NERVE ALLOGRAFTS

The concept of nerve allograft is an attractive option, offering many of the benefits of conduits (biocompatible, off-the-shelf convenience, wealth of supply, and avoidance of a donor defect). By their nature, allograft contains the microenvironment (microarchitecture, neurotrophic factors, and guidance cues) inherent in peripheral nerve tissue. In addition to those attributes, the ability to choose donor nerve tissue with a higher ratio of endoneural surface area to connective tissue offers the potential of a greater amount of active scaffolding for supporting axonal regeneration. As an example, the lateral antebrachial cutaneous (LABC) nerve is 1 to 2 mm in diameter and has roughly 20% of its cross section composed of fascicular surface area, the remainder being connective tissue. The radial nerve in the proximal forearm is at least 4 to 5 mm in diameter and has roughly 50% of its cross section composed of fascicular surface area. This differential leaves a similar-diameter cable graft of LABC having 40%

less fascicular scaffolding than the radial nerve in need of repair. This deficit is reduced to 25% if a sural cable graft is chosen.[3,36] Although this concept of matching architecture and nerve substructures is often difficult to visualize, it applies the reconstructive principle of matching like structures with like structures. These cumulative attributes have led to a proliferation of research assessing the role of nerve allografts in peripheral nerve repair.

Albert[37] published his initial experience with whole-nerve allograft in 1885. Over the next 100 years, numerous reports explored the merits and limitations of allograft tissue.[38] Immune response, primarily to major histocompatibility complexes (MHCs) on the surface of the Schwann cells, limited their clinical effectiveness.[38,39] Through advancements in immunosuppressive therapies, donor-recipient matching, and cold storage mediums, whole-nerve allograft found a role in the reconstructive ladder.[40] This advancement afforded patients with massive nerve defects the opportunity for return of function. Nerve gaps up to 37 cm have been successfully repaired with both cables of allograft only and in combination with autograft to augment the size of the cable graft to more appropriately match the injured nerves. Most patients tolerated the treatment well, but rejection was seen in noncompliant patients. However, whole allograft is marred by the need for short-term or long-term treatment with potentially life-threating immunosuppressive medications, precluding its widespread utility.

Given these drawbacks, tissue engineering has focused on methodologies to mitigate the potential risks and accentuate the potential benefits of nerve allograft. Extraction techniques to remove the MHCs, myelin, and cellular debris while preserving the neurotropic architecture of the endoneurium have shown promise in providing an immune-tolerant allograft.[41–44] However, current methods that render the tissue nonimmunogenic remove the supportive Schwann cells, potentially limiting the material's regenerative capacity. These decellularized nerve allograft (DCA) scaffolds serve as the basis for researching methodologies that can augment regeneration through either the addition of regenerative stimulants[45,46] or the removal of endogenous inhibitory components.[47] Subsequent research has focused on surface modification of the basal laminal tubes, mostly through enzyme-mediated degradation of inhibitory proteoglycans.[48,49] Chondroitin sulfate proteoglycans, a family of glycosaminoglycans (GAGs), are known inhibitors of axonal regeneration because they block or diminish neurite extension and increase risk of aberrant regeneration.[48–50] By selectively removing these inhibitory components from the inner surface of the basal lamina, laminin activity is subsequently increased.[51,52] This process has been shown to increase the amount of axonal extension into the proximal graft,[52] decrease the risk of retrograde and aberrant regeneration,[53] and allow regeneration across longer distance than non–enzyme-treated grafts.[54] The most promising processing methods seem to mimic the body's own wallerian degeneration process by facilitating removal of myelin, neurofilament, cellular debris, and inhibitory GAGs within the scaffold.

DCAs function by providing laminin-rich endoneural tube architecture as a physical scaffold to bridge nerve defects.[55] Cellular regenerate populates onto the cleansed endoneural tube. The proliferating Schwann cells from the repaired nerve migrate along the organized tubes to form bands of Büngner.[43] Neurites extend along these tubes, using the base scaffold to physically support and organize the linear progression of the growth cone. Simultaneously, the material revascularizes through inosculation from the proximal and distal nerve stumps.[39] This mechanism is similar to that of the nerve autograft. The major differences involve the existing cells in the nerve autograft and the need for the autograft to undergo wallerian degeneration, whereas the DCA is acellular and predegenerated at time of implant. Both grafts populate with the proliferating Schwann cells, regenerating axons, and vascular ingrowth from the repaired nerve. One major limitation to DCAs is the distance the repopulating Schwann cells migrate along the scaffold. In animal studies, grafts processed with a chondroitinase treatment have been shown to support myelinated fibers across a 4-cm rat sciatic nerve defect.[54] However, 6-cm defects in non–chondroitinase-treated grafts had a higher rate of senescent Schwann cells and exhausted regeneration.[56] However, clinical correlation from the rodent model to human regeneration is not clearly established or understood and will certainly be the focus of future research.

In the United States, the Avance nerve graft (AxoGen, Alachua, FL) is the only commercially available PNA. These PNAs are processed with a combination of both detergent extraction, to cleanse the scaffold, and chondroitinase predegeneration of the inhibitory GAGs. Karabekmez and colleagues[57] first described the clinical use of PNA in a series of 10 digital nerve repairs. All repairs reported return of 2-point discrimination to at least 6 mm in gaps ranging from 10 to 30 mm. Taras and colleagues[8] reported similar results, with all patients returning 2-point discrimination to 8 mm or less, in a series of 18 nerve repairs with

gaps from 5 to 30 mm. Similarly, reports from both Vögelin and Juon[58] and Gou and colleagues[59] found that all subjects reported S3+ or better sensation; however ,Vögelin and Juon's[58] series included 32 nerve repairs at longer gap lengths, ranging from 10 to 70 mm. In 2012, Cho and colleagues[60] reported from an ongoing observational registry of peripheral nerve repair outcomes (the RANGER [Registry Study of Avance Nerve Graft Evaluating Recovery Outcomes] study). The digital nerve cohort contained 35 digital nerve gaps ranging from 5 to 40 mm, and there was meaningful recovery ($\geq$S3) in 89% of the repairs.[61] This study was followed by Rinker and colleagues,[62] in 2015, reporting on 37 short-gap sensory repairs after which 92% of subjects showed meaningful recovery. Given the wealth of available clinical data, PNA seems to be established as a consistent and reliable alternative for sensory nerve repair.

Outcomes from the use of PNA in major peripheral nerve repairs are less prevalent in the literature, but seem equally promising. Cho and colleagues[60] reported recovery of M3 or better motor function in 75% of median nerve repairs and 66% of ulnar nerve repairs in the mid to distal forearm. Overall, M4 or better recovery was observed in 54% of major mixed nerve repairs and 71% of major motor nerve repairs, which was similar to historical outcomes for nerve autograft.[2] Fleming and colleagues[5] reported return of motor and sensory function, as well as electrodiagnostic confirmation of reinnervation, through a 70-mm PNA ulnar nerve repair just proximal to the elbow. Outcomes for PNAs are summarized in **Table 2**.

Not all outcomes are as positive. Cho and colleagues[60] reported that 2 of their subjects, one with 491-day-old median nerve injury, the other a high-energy blast injury to the ulnar nerve repaired with 20-mm PNA, reported no functional recovery. Berocal and colleagues[63] reported a single case of a failed PNA repair for a 17-mm ulnar nerve repair following high-energy fracture of the distal ulna. The repair was revised 6 months later and, after more aggressive debridement, a 4-cm-long sural nerve cable graft was required to span the defect. The reasons for these failures are not clearly understood. However, positive outcomes have been reported in longer, more complex injures, therefore factors other than the just the PNA's performance may be involved. This finding is common with other repair modalities.[6,13,64] As with all nerve repairs, factors such as chronicity of the injury, adequacy of debridement of damaged nerve, controlling tension, and the overall health of patient and wound bed should be considered.

Table 2
Review of nerve allograft clinical evidence

Reference	Nerves (N)	Age (y) Mean	Age (y) Range	Nerve Location	Nerve Type	Repair Type	Defect Length (mm) Mean	Defect Length (mm) Range	Follow-up (Mo) Mean	Follow-up (Mo) Range	Publication Recovery Classification	Publication Reported Outcomes	Standardized Meaningful Recovery[a]	Complications	Complication Rate (%)
Karabekmez et al,[57] 2009	10	43	23–65	Digital	Sensory	PNA	22	5–30	9	5–12	Mackinnon Modified MRCC	50% Excellent S4 50% Good S3+	100%	None	0
Brooks et al,[61] 2012	13	38	SD 19	Not specified	Mixed	PNA	29	SD 12	7	SD 3.8	Modified Mackinnon Classification M3–M5	77%	77%	None	0
Brooks et al,[61] 2012	7	45	SD 20	Not specified	Motor	PNA	29	SD 13	11	SD 2.4	Modified Mackinnon Classification M3–M5	86%	86%	None	0
Cho et al,[60] 2012	35	46	23–68	Digital	Sensory	PNA	19	5–40	10	2–24	Mackinnon Modified MRCC	89%	76%	4 revisions deemed unrelated to the nerve graft. 2 Neuromas proximal to the original repair site, 2 with residual foreign bodies in wound	0
Guo et al,[59] 2013	5	29	18–39	Digital	Sensory	PNA	23	18–28	13.2	12–15	Mackinnon Modified MRCC	100%	100%	None	0

Study												Average score			
Ducic et al,[71] 2012	3	—	—	—	Sensory	PNA	18	10-50	6	4-18	QuickDash	19.8 ± 10	—	0	None
Taras et al,[8] 2013	18	39	18-76	Digital	Sensory	PNA	11	5-30	15	5-30	Taras Classification	39% Excellent 44% Good	100%	0	None
Vögelin and Juon,[58] 2013	24	36	18-60	Digital	Sensory	PNA	22	10-70	17	12-28	Mackinnon Modified MRCC	100%	100%	4	None
Squintani et al,[67] 2013	14	33	18-58	Brachial plexus	Motor	DCA	72	40-100	24	—	Mackinnon Modified MRCC	100% ≥ M3	100% ≥ M3	0	None
He et al,[69] 2015	95	33	18-61	Digital	Sensory	DCA	18	1-50	6	—	Mackinnon Modified MRCC	72%	72%	0	None
Zuniga,[66] 2015	23	33	9-67	Sensory	Sensory	PNA	34	8-70	14	6-20	Mackinnon Modified MRCC	87%	87%	0	None
Rinker,[62] 2015	37	43	23-81	Digital	Sensory	PNA	11	5-15	16	—	Mackinnon Modified MRCC	92% MR S3 or greater; 84% MR S3+ or S4	92% MR S3 or greater; 84% MR S3+ or S4	0	None
Buncke et al,[27] ASSH 2015	40	36	18-65	Digital	Sensory	PNA	12	4-20	11	6-21	2PD: <15 mm and/or SWM: <4.31 (2g)	90%	90%	0	None
Safa et al,[65] ASSH 2015	14	34	19-77	Upper	Mixed/ motor	PNA	30	10-65	12	9-20	MRCC ≥ M3	86%	86%	0	None

Abbreviations: 2PD, Two Point Discrimination; ASSH, American Society for Surgery of the Hand; MRCC, Medical Research Council Classification of Recovery; PGA: Polyglycolic Acid; SD, Standard Deviation; SWM, Semmes-Weinstein Monofilaments.

a MRCC Scale ≥ S3+/M3.

Data from Refs[8,27,57–62,66,67,69,71]

As with the previously discussed conduit data, the authors recently presented updated outcomes from a multicenter peripheral nerve registry that included PNAs. Outcomes were stratified by nerve function and gap length. The update included 146 PNA repairs, 124 sensory nerves, and 22 major nerves in the upper extremity for gap lengths up to 65 mm. A group of sensory nerve repairs matched to the conduit group referenced earlier reported 90% return of meaningful recovery and were noted to be a statistically significant improvement compared with the conduit group. PNA repairs in major peripheral nerves reported M3 or better recovery in 86% of repairs and M4 or better in 58% of repairs. The average reported gap was 30 mm, with a range from 15 to 65 mm. Compared with matched contemporary cases of sural nerve autograft repairs, no difference was detected between groups. However, the autograft group had an average gap of 40 mm with a range from 20 to 60 mm.[27,65]

Clinical length limitations in PNAs have been debated. The available clinical data suggest that the general trends follow those for nerve autograft. Cho and colleagues[60] reported a 10% decrease in recovery rates for gaps between 30 and 50 mm (90%), compared with those for gaps of 15 mm or less (100%); however, the result was not statistically significant. Clinical evidence for the use of PNAs in longer gap lengths is less prevalent in the literature, but not absent. RANGER and independent reports from Zuniga,[66] Vögelin and Juon,[58] and Fleming and colleagues[5] have documented functional sensory and motor recovery in gap lengths between 50 and 70 mm. Fleming and colleagues[5] also state that the military has used PNAs at distances much larger than 70 mm with promising outcomes.[5] Although there is clinical support for the role of PNAs in gaps up to 70 mm, the final determination for the upper length limit in clinical use of PNAs is not yet established, and the upper length limit will continue to be followed.

In addition to PNAs, tissue processors in both Italy and China have published outcomes from institution-specific decellularized nerve allografts. These allografts are decellularized, but do not undergo the same processing steps for safety sterilization and enzyme mediated removal of growth inhibitors that are used in commercially available PNAs. Squintani and colleagues[67] published on 10 extracted and cryoprotected DCAs. Ten brachial plexus lesions were repaired with DCAs between 40 and 100 mm in length. All subjects reported recovery of M3 to M4 motor function. A series of studies from China document clinical experience of DCAs processed with detergent

treatments.[42,68–70] These studies combine to report outcomes on 131 nerve repairs. Outcomes were reported as generally favorable and not different than the control groups.

Nerve allografts provide a readily available tissue source for peripheral nerve repair. PNAs currently offer the most prolific clinical evidence and have been evaluated in both sensory and major nerve repairs with promising outcomes. In addition to spanning traumatic nerve injuries or augmenting the caliber of cable grafts, Ducic and colleagues[71] also suggested they play a role in reconstruction of nerve donor sites, nerve biopsy sites, and in neuroma management.[71,72] PNAs have also been used as extender grafts in nerve transfers and reverse end-to-side transfers.[73] For management of recurrent stump neuromas, interest has grown in the use of PNAs as a so-called graft to nowhere placed on the freshened proximal stump. The goal of the procedure is 2-fold: first, relocating the hot end of the nerve (proximal stump) to a more suitable area away from the point of irritation and, second, to provide a controlled and organized environment for the extending axons. The endoneurium of the PNA serves as that environment, and, without the contributions from the distal nerve stump, regeneration is hampered and the growth cone has an opportunity to exhaust itself within the protected length of the graft.

Given these results, the authors recommend PNAs for a variety of nerve reconstructions. PNAs have utility to span nerve defects, augment the size of cable grafts, extend the length of nerve transfers, reposition stump neuroma, and repair biopsy or donor sites. Consideration should be given to the function of the nerve, the health and injury status of the patient, the goal of the procedure, and the patient's preference. As with conduit and autograft, length limitations play a role with nerve allografts. PNAs seem to provide sufficient regeneration at their current lengths; however, additional evaluations are necessary to consider in gaps greater than 70 mm. PNAs show utility in the reconstructive ladder for both simple and complex nerve repairs, with evidence suggesting they may be used in both short-gap digital nerve repair and major peripheral nerve repairs.

GENERAL CONSIDERATIONS WHEN SELECTING AUTOGRAFT ALTERNATIVES

Other variables to consider when implementing these tools in clinical practice include access, size selection, and cost. Although the placement of either product may be performed under loupe magnification, the authors prefer high-powered operative microscope. Standard nonabsorbable microsutures, between 8-0 and 10-0, should be used with either product. A tapered needle and smaller suture is recommended at the coaptation site, and a cutting or spatulated cutting needle is recommended with the stiffer conduit material. The use of a coaptation aid at the proximal and distal ends of a nerve graft should provide the same benefits observed at the primary repair site, and allows for less suture material in the coaptation.[68] Conduits are generally available in diameters from 1.5 mm to 7 mm, and lengths from 10 to 30 mm. PNAs are offered in diameters from 1 to 2 mm up to 4 to 5 mm and are available in 15-mm, 30-mm, 50-mm, and 70-mm lengths. Both materials can be trimmed to length to fit the defect. Care should be taken to ensure that there is sufficient length to avoid detrimental tension within the repair. The diameter of the conduit should be slightly larger than the nerve being repaired. If the conduit is too tight, it risks compressing the nerve following release of the tourniquet or swelling in the tissue bed. Choosing a conduit diameter that is too large has been correlated with impaired results. Isaacs and colleagues[13] characterized the impact of conduit diameter on nerve regeneration and found that the larger diameter tubes performed significantly worse than better fitting tubes. The investigators therefore recommended not increasing the size of the tube beyond an additional 2 mm. PNAs should be sized to the repaired nerve, erring on the side of slightly larger diameter rather than slightly smaller. They may be cabled or used as a single strand. When using a coaptation aid on a nerve graft, it is advisable to ensure that the tube is slightly larger than both the graft and the intended nerve stump. If a size mismatch occurs, the tube can be cinched with a microclip or stitch to better fit the nerve. **Table 3** provides a general list of material benefits for manufactured conduit, PNA, and autograft.

Cost is a major factor in modern health care decisions. Studies have assessed the cost difference between nerve repair methodologies.[7,8] The commercially available materials are fairly cost neutral, with comparable lengths costing roughly US$1000 to US$2200. Longer lengths of PNAs are available in the US$2500 to US$4000 range. Both of these may actually present a cost savings, given that operating room time alone costs US$100 to US$200 per minute.[74] Additional anesthesia time and treatment of donor site complications add to the overall cost.[6] Individual operative plans should take each of these factors into consideration.

As with any nerve transection, consideration should be given to several factors when choosing between reconstructive options. The first step is to ensure that the nerve stumps are adequately debrided of damaged nerve tissue. Fibrosis and intraneural scarring should be systematically removed until soft supple nerve tissue remains. Often fascicular bloom is not enough to visually confirm healthy tissue and, as with most wounds, bleeding from the debrided tissue should be confirmed. In nerves, this bleeding should not just be from the epineurial vessels but should also include punctate bleeding around the fascicular bundles within the nerve. After debridement to healthy tissue, the associated joint should be ranged to determine the maximum range of motion planned for the patient within the first 2 months following the repair. The nerve gap should be measured at the maximal planned range of motion to ensure a consistent, tension-free repair. Once the gap is assessed, the appropriate material for reconstruction should be selected. Consideration should be given to the internal nerve topography, to properly align sensory and motor fascicles. Protection or reinforcement with a coaptation aid may also be considered in order to reduce the risk of

Table 3
Review of material benefits

Feature	Manufactured Conduit	Processed Allograft	Nerve Autograft
Biocompatible	+	+	+
Peripheral nerve tissue	−	+	+
Three-dimensional endoneurium-based scaffold	−	+	+
Schwann cells/supportive cells	−	−	+/−
Laminin	−	+	+
Inherent nerve-specific growth factors	−	+	+
Vascularity/vascular scaffolding	−	+/	+
Mechanical properties similar to nerve	+/−	+	+
Sterile	+	+	+

repair rupture with early range-of-motion and rehabilitation protocols.

SUMMARY

The goal of peripheral nerve repair is to make the injured patient as whole and functional as possible. Taking a holistic approach to reconstruction, this sometimes means giving the patient a choice of the materials used for the reconstruction. Alternatives for the classic nerve autograft are readily available and have the added benefit of avoiding the creation of a permanent nerve injury to repair an existing one. However, these products must work well and have adequate evidence of their utility. In peripheral nerve repair, much of the available literature for manufactured conduits, allografts, and autografts is only observational. The heterogeneous nature of traumatic peripheral nerve injuries, concomitant injuries, and patient demographics make conducting level 1 studies arduous. To mitigate these challenges, reproducibility of results across multiple centers and multiple surgeons must be taken into consideration, and clinical evidence from such studies must be evaluated and scrutinized to provide the best available understanding of anticipated outcome and utility. The evidence shows that manufactured conduits and allografts have a place within the reconstructive ladder and are tools that can and should be included in the armamentarium. As with any tool, their benefits and limitations should be considered. This consideration allows these products to function as viable alternatives to the classic direct suture repair and nerve autograft. Manufactured conduits should be limited to gaps less than 10 mm, and most often should be considered as an aid to the coaptation. PNAs have shown great utility as a substitute for either conduit or autograft in sensory nerve repairs. There is also a growing body of evidence for their utility in major peripheral nerve repairs, gap repairs up to 70 mm in length, as an alternative source of tissue to bolster the diameter of a cable graft, and for the management of neuromas in nonreconstructable injuries.

Nerve repair can be a complex but rewarding endeavor, and requires a vigilant approach to the factors that are controllable. Regardless of the materials chosen, by applying good nerve repair principles of appropriately timed surgical intervention, adequate resection of damaged tissue, avoiding tension, choosing a suitable bridging material, and proper protection for early rehabilitation protocols, surgeons can greatly increase the odds of meaningful outcomes for their patients.

REFERENCES

1. Berger A, Millesi H. Nerve grafting. Clin Orthop Relat Res 1978;133:49–55.
2. Ruijs AC, Jaquet JB, Kalmijn S, et al. Median and ulnar nerve injuries: a meta-analysis of predictors of motor and sensory recovery after modern microsurgical nerve repair. Plast Reconstr Surg 2005;1162:484–94.
3. Sunderland S. Nerves and nerve injuries, 2nd edition. London: Churchill Livingstone; 1978.
4. Janssen I, Reimers K, Allmeling C, et al. Schwann cell metabolic activity in various short-term holding conditions: implications for improved nerve graft viability. Int J Otolaryngol 2012;2012:742183.
5. Fleming ME, Bharmal H, Valerio I. Regenerative medicine applications in combat casualty care. Regen Med 2014;9:179–90.
6. Ijpma FF, Nicolai JP, Meek MF. Sural nerve donor-site morbidity: thirty-four years of follow-up. Ann Plast Surg 2006;57:391–5.
7. Rinker B, Liau JY. A prospective randomized study comparing woven polyglycolic acid and autogenous vein conduits for reconstruction of digital nerve gaps. J Hand Surg Am 2011;36:775–81.
8. Taras JS, Amin N, Patel N, et al. Allograft reconstruction for digital nerve loss. J Hand Surg Am 2013;38:1965–71.
9. Millesi H. Bridging defects: autologous nerve grafts. Acta Neurochir Suppl 2007;100:37–8.
10. Gluck T. Ueber Transplantation, Regeneration und entzündliche Neubildung. Berliner Klinische Wochenschrift 1881;18:554–7.
11. Dahlin LB, Lundborg G. Use of tubes in peripheral nerve repair. Neurosurg Clin North Am 2001;12:341–52.
12. Moore AM, Kasukurthi R, Magill CK, et al. Limitations of conduits in peripheral nerve repairs. Hand (N Y) 2009;4:180–6.
13. Isaacs J, Mallu S, Yan W, et al. Consequences of oversizing: nerve-to-nerve tube diameter mismatch. J Bone Joint Surg Am 2014;96:1461–7.
14. Liodaki E, Bos I, Lohmeyer JA, et al. Removal of collagen nerve conduits (NeuraGen) after unsuccessful implantation: focus on histological findings. J Reconstr Microsurg 2013;29:517–22.
15. Schmidhammer R, Zandieh S, Hopf R, et al. Alleviated tension at the repair site enhances functional regeneration: the effect of full range of motion mobilization on the regeneration of peripheral nerves–histologic, electrophysiologic, and functional results in a rat model. J Trauma 2004;56:571–84.
16. Lundborg G, Rosén B, Dahlin L, et al. Tubular repair of the median or ulnar nerve in the human forearm: a 5-year follow-up. J Hand Surg Br 2004;29:100–7.
17. Weber RA, Breidenbach WC, Brown RE, et al. A randomized prospective study of polyglycolic

acid conduits for digital nerve reconstruction in humans. Plast Reconstr Surg 2000;106:1036–45.

18. Lohmeyer JA, Sommer B, Siemers F, et al. Nerve injuries of the upper extremity-expected outcome and clinical examination. Plast Surg Nurs 2009;29:88–93.

19. Taras JS, Jacoby SM, Lincoski CJ. Reconstruction of digital nerves with collagen conduits. J Hand Surg Am 2011;36(9):1441–6.

20. Wangensteen KJ, Kalliainen LK. Collagen tube conduits in peripheral nerve repair: a retrospective analysis. Hand (N Y) 2010;5:273–7.

21. Haug A, Bartels A, Kotas J, et al. Sensory recovery 1 year after bridging digital nerve defects with collagen tubes. J Hand Surg Am 2013;38:90–7.

22. Schmauss D, Finck T, Liodaki E, et al. Is nerve regeneration after reconstruction with collagen nerve conduits terminated after 12 months? The long-term follow-up of two prospective clinical studies. J Reconstr Microsurg 2014;30:561–8.

23. Lohmeyer JA, Kern Y, Schmauss D, et al. Prospective clinical study on digital nerve repair with collagen nerve conduits and review of literature. J Reconstr Microsurg 2014;30(4):227–34.

24. Meek MF, Coert JH. US food and drug administration/Conformit Europe-approved absorbable nerve conduits for clinical repair of peripheral and cranial nerves. Ann Plast Surg 2008;60:110–6.

25. Bertleff MJ, Meek MK, Nicolai JP. A prospective clinical evaluation of biodegradable Neurolac nerve guides for sensory nerve repair in the hand. J Hand Surg Am 2005;30:513–8.

26. Chiriac S, Facca S, Diaconu M, et al. Experience of using the bioresorbable copolyester poly(DL-lactide-epsilon-caprolactone) nerve conduit guide Neurolac for nerve repair in peripheral nerve defects: report on a series of 28 lesions. J Hand Surg Eur 2012;37:342–9.

27. Buncke GM, Rinker B, Safa B, et al. Evaluating nerve repair outcomes in upper extremity nerve injuries utilizing processed nerve allografts, tube conduit, and nerve autograft. J Hand Surg 2015;40(9):e5.

28. Mackinnon SE, Dellon AL. Clinical nerve reconstruction with a bioabsorbable polyglycolic acid tube. Plast Reconstr Surg 1990;85:419–24.

29. Boeckstyns ME, Sørensen AI, Viñeta JF, et al. Collagen conduit versus microsurgical neurorrhaphy: 2-year follow-up of a prospective, blinded clinical and electrophysiological multicenter randomized, controlled trial. J Hand Surg Am 2013;38:2405–11.

30. Evans PJ, Bain JR, Mackinnon SE, et al. Selective reinnervation: a comparison of recovery following microsuture and conduit nerve repair. Brain Res 1991;559:315–21.

31. Hasegawa J, Shibata M, Takahashi H. Nerve coaptation studies with and without a gap in rabbits. J Hand Surg Am 1996;21:259–65.

32. Lee JY, Parisi TJ, Friedrich PF, et al. Does the addition of a nerve wrap to a motor nerve repair affect motor outcomes? Microsurgery 2014;34:562–7.

33. Wolfe SW, Strauss HL, Garg R, et al. Use of bioabsorbable nerve conduits as an adjunct to brachial plexus neurorrhaphy. J Hand Surg Am 2012;37:1980–5.

34. Aberg M, Ljungberg C, Edin E, et al. Clinical evaluation of a resorbable wrap-around implant as an alternative to nerve repair: a prospective, assessor-blinded, randomised clinical study of sensory, motor and functional recovery after peripheral nerve repair. J Plast Reconstr Aesthet Surg 2009;62:1503–9.

35. Leuzzi S, Armenio A, Leone L, et al. Repair of peripheral nerve with vein wrapping. G Chir 2014;35:101–6.

36. Tang P, Kilic A, Konopka G, et al. Histologic and functional outcomes of nerve defects treated with acellular allograft versus cabled autograft in a rat model. Microsurgery 2013;33:460–7.

37. Albert E. Einige operationen an nerven. Wien Med Presse 1885;26:1285–8.

38. Evans PJ, Midha R, Mackinnon SE. The peripheral nerve allograft: a comprehensive review of regeneration and neuroimmunology. Prog Neurobiol 1994;43:187–233.

39. Best TJ, Mackinnon SE, Midha R, et al. Revascularization of peripheral nerve autografts and allografts. Plast Reconstr Surg 1999;104:152–60.

40. Mackinnon SE, Doolabh VB, Novak CB, et al. Clinical outcome following nerve allograft transplantation. Plast Reconstr Surg 2001;107:1419–29.

41. Borschel GH, Kia KF, Kuzon WM Jr, et al. Mechanical properties of acellular peripheral nerve. J Surg Res 2003;114:133–9.

42. Sondell M, Lundborg G, Kanje M. Regeneration of the rat sciatic nerve into allografts made acellular through chemical extraction. Brain Res 1998;795:44–54.

43. Hudson TW, Zawko S, Deister C, et al. Optimized acellular nerve graft is immunologically tolerated and supports regeneration. Tissue Eng 2004;10:1641–51.

44. Wakimura Y, Wang W, Itoh S, et al. An experimental study to bridge a nerve gap with a decellularized allogeneic nerve. Plast Reconstr Surg 2015;136:319e–27e.

45. Hoben G, Yan Y, Iyer N, et al. Comparison of acellular nerve allograft modification with Schwann cells or VEGF. Hand (N Y) 2015;10:396–402.

46. Tajdaran K, Gordon T, Wood MD, et al. A glial cell line-derived neurotrophic factor delivery system enhances nerve regeneration across acellular nerve allografts. Acta Biomater 2015;29:62–70.

47. Muir D. The potentiation of peripheral nerve sheaths in regeneration and repair. Exp Neurol 2010;223:102–11.

48. Gause TM 2nd, Sivak WN, Marra KG. The role of chondroitinase as an adjuvant to peripheral nerve repair. Cells Tissues Organs 2014;200:59–68.

49. Silver J. Inhibitory molecules in development and regeneration. J Neurol 1994;242:S22–4.

50. Zuo J, Neubauer D, Graham J, et al. Regeneration of axons after nerve transection repair is enhanced by degradation of chondroitin sulfate proteoglycan. Exp Neurol 2002;176:221–8.

51. Graham JB, Xue QS, Neubauer D, et al. A chondroitinase-treated, decellularized nerve allograft compares favorably to the cellular isograft in rat peripheral nerve repair. J Neurodegener Regen 2009;2:19–29.

52. Krekoski CA, Neubauer D, Zuo J, et al. Axonal regeneration into acellular nerve grafts is enhanced by degradation of chondroitin sulfate proteoglycan. J Neurosci 2001;21:6206–13.

53. Graham JB, Neubauer D, Xue QS, et al. Chondroitinase applied to peripheral nerve repair averts retrograde axonal regeneration. Exp Neurol 2007;203:185–95.

54. Neubauer D, Graham JB, Muir D. Chondroitinase treatment increases the effective length of acellular nerve grafts. Exp Neurol 2007;207:163–70.

55. Johnson PJ, Newton P, Hunter DA, et al. Nerve endoneurial microstructure facilitates uniform distribution of regenerative fibers: a post hoc comparison of midgraft nerve fiber densities. J Reconstr Microsurg 2011;27:83–90.

56. Saheb-Al-Zamani M, Yan Y, Farber SJ, et al. Limited regeneration in long acellular nerve allografts is associated with increased Schwann cell senescence. Exp Neurol 2013;247:165–77.

57. Karabekmez FE, Duymaz A, Moran SL. Early clinical outcomes with the use of decellularized nerve allograft for repair of sensory defects within the hand. Hand (N Y) 2009;4:245–9.

58. Vögelin E, Juon B. Nerve allografts and vein grafts in nerve reconstructions. In: Dahlin LB, Grűsel Leblebicioğlu, editors. Current treatment of nerve injuries and disorders. Zurich (Switzerland): Palme Publications; 2013. Chapter 7–3, p. 271–8.

59. Guo Y, Chen G, Tian G, et al. Sensory recovery following decellularized nerve allograft transplantation for digital nerve repair. J Plast Surg Hand Surg 2013;47:451–3.

60. Cho MS, Rinker BD, Weber RV, et al. Functional outcome following nerve repair in the upper extremity using processed nerve allograft. J Hand Surg Am 2012;37:2340–9.

61. Brooks D, Weber RV, Chao J, et al. Processed nerve allografts for peripheral nerve reconstruction: a multicenter study of utilization and outcomes in sensory, mixed, and motor nerve reconstructions. Microsurgery 2012;32(1):1–14.

62. Rinker BD, Ingari JV, Greenberg JA, et al. Outcomes of short-gap sensory nerve injuries reconstructed with processed nerve allografts from a multicenter registry study. J Reconstr Microsurg 2015;31:384–90.

63. Berrocal YA, Almeida VW, Levi AD. Limitations of nerve repair of segmental defects using acellular conduits. J Neurosurg 2013;119:733–8.

64. Meek MF, Coert JH, Robinson PH. Poor results after nerve grafting in the upper extremity: Quo vadis? Microsurgery 2005;25:396–402.

65. Safa B, Ko J, Pet MA, et al. Evaluation of outcomes from processed nerve allograft and nerve autograft repairs in upper extremity mixed nerve injuries. J Hand Surg 2015;40(9):e14.

66. Zuniga JR. Sensory outcomes after reconstruction of lingual and inferior alveolar nerve discontinuities using processed nerve allograft–a case series. J Oral Maxillofac Surg 2015;73:734–44.

67. Squintani G, Bonetti B, Paolin A, et al. Nerve regeneration across cryopreserved allografts from cadaveric donors: a novel approach for peripheral nerve reconstruction. J Neurosurg 2013;119:907–13.

68. Yang RG, Zhong HB, Zhu JL, et al. Clinical safety about repairing the peripheral nerve defects with chemically extracted acellular nerve allograft. Zhonghua Wai Ke Za Zhi 2012;50:74–6.

69. He B, Zhu Q, Chai Y, et al. Safety and efficacy evaluation of a human acellular nerve graft as a digital nerve scaffold: a prospective, multicentre controlled clinical trial. J Tissue Eng Regen Med 2015;9:286–95.

70. Li XY, Hu HL, Fei JR, et al. One-stage human acellular nerve allograft reconstruction for digital nerve defects. Neural Regen Res 2015;10:95–8.

71. Ducic I, Fu R, Iorio ML. Innovative treatment of peripheral nerve injuries: combined reconstructive concepts. Ann Plast Surg 2012;68:180–7.

72. Peled ZM. Treatment of a patient with small fiber pathology using nerve biopsy and grafting: a case report. J Reconstr Microsurg 2013;29:551–4.

73. Kale SS, Glaus SW, Yee A, et al. Reverse end-to-side nerve transfer: from animal model to clinical use. J Hand Surg Am 2011;36:1631–9.

74. Center for Medicare and Medicaid Services, Physician Fee Schedule, Regulation # CMS-1590-FC. Federal Register/Vol. 78, No. 155. 2013.

Donor Distal, Recipient Proximal and Other Personal Perspectives on Nerve Transfers

Susan E. Mackinnon, MD

KEYWORDS

- Nerve transfers • Donor distal • Recipient proximal

KEY POINTS

- This article presents a personal overview of nerve transfers and emphasizes the various factors that contribute to outcome following these surgeries.
- There is no "one result" for all nerve transfers. The results will vary depending on factors relating to the donor nerve and the recipient nerve, the degree of the surgical difficulty of the specific procedure, and issues relating to preoperative and postoperative rehabilitation.
- The general issues that influence all nerve injury and recovery, such as age of the patient, comorbidities, and time since injury, pertain to nerve transfers as well.

INTRODUCTION

Surgeons who came of age treating brachial plexus injuries with nerve graft reconstruction in the early 1980s remember bilateral sural nerve harvest and difficult and tedious dissections of the brachial plexus. They remember the very time-consuming nerve grafting procedures, and at best, poor to fair recovery of function several years later. The impetus for the surgical shift from nerve grafts to modern nerve transfers came from the frustration and disappointment with that experience. Indeed, it was the failure of longer nerve grafts that ushered in the era of nerve transfers. This nerve transfer technique translated to clinical practice with the advances of microsurgical techniques, an awareness and then understanding of the specificity of intraneural anatomy and the feasibility of detailed internal neurolysis that permits surgeons to move safely between fascicles and enter the nerve without damage. Nerve transfers effectively eliminated the key factors

associated with poorer functional outcome related to traditional nerve repair and graft (**Box 1**).

In the early 1990s, nerve transfer was extremely controversial. In 1999, an article on nerve transfers in a similar *Hand Clinics* issue was described as "new options" for reconstruction; by 2008, an entire *Hand Clinics* issue was devoted to nerve transfers.[1,2] Today, nerve transfers are options for many nerve and hand surgeons with microsurgical skills. The indications for nerve transfers have been well described and are the subject of this issue of *Hand Clinics*. In this article, the author presents an overview of her current thoughts and new perspectives on nerve transfers based on her experiences with "modern" nerve transfers over the last quarter century.

In the spring of 1991 at the University of Toronto, the author did her first 2 thoughtful nerve transfers. In an upper plexus injury, she transferred medial pectoral nerves to the musculocutaneous nerve, and in a patient with a high ulnar nerve laceration, performed a distal anterior interosseous nerve

Division of Plastic & Reconstructive Surgery, Washington University School of Medicine, 660 South Euclid Avenue, St Louis, MO 63110, USA
E-mail address: mackinnons@wudosis.wustl.edu

Hand Clin 32 (2016) 141–151
http://dx.doi.org/10.1016/j.hcl.2015.12.003
0749-0712/16/$ – see front matter © 2016 Elsevier Inc. All rights reserved.

> **Box 1**
> **Nerve transfer addresses factors associated with poor outcome**
>
> - Proximal injuries
> - Delayed repair
> - Tension at nerve repair site
> - Inappropriate sensory/motor internal topography alignment
> - Injury requiring nerve graft

(AIN) to deep motor ulnar nerve transfer. In general, nerve transfers are indicated for proximal nerve injuries. However, the results of nerve transfers have been remarkable enough that indications are expanding:

- The author now uses nerve transfer technique in combination with nerve grafting in order to achieve specific reinnervation of critical nerve function. For example, a sharp laceration of the median nerve in the midarm will be nerve grafted in conjunction with a specific distal nerve transfer from the extensor carpi radialis brevis (ECRB) nerve to the pronator muscle to ensure recovery of pronation and a tendon transfer for thumb opposition.[3]
- There are several proximal injuries that also have an extensive distal component of injury. In these long injuries, the nerve transfers are more challenging, because they are closer to the zone of injury. A short nerve graft may be needed to facilitate a tension-free nerve transfer between the donor and recipient nerves.
- As surgeons are seeing their results with motor recovery with nerve transfers, they are becoming more interested in the possibility of sensory nerve transfers to recover sensibility—so important to the patient, but not as "obvious" to the surgeon.

This issue of *Hand Clinics* highlights the specifics of common nerve transfer techniques. This article presents a personal overview of nerve transfers and emphasizes the various factors that contribute to outcome following these surgeries. There is no "one result" for all nerve transfers. The results will vary depending on factors relating to the donor nerve and the recipient nerve, the degree of the surgical difficulty of the specific procedure, and issues relating to preoperative and postoperative rehabilitation. The general issues that influence all nerve injury and recovery, such as age of the patient, comorbidities, and time since injury, pertain to nerve transfers as well.

However, the qualities of the donor nerve, recipient functional requirements, difficulty of surgical technique, and the cortical impact of re-education can be considered specific to nerve transfers and explain why there is no one "result" following nerve transfer procedures (**Box 2**).

Donor Nerve Considerations

Synergy and nerve fiber count are key donor considerations impacting functional recovery. The more synergistic the donor is with the recipient, the easier the postoperative re-education is. For example, the donors for the double fascicular nerve transfer (DFT) innervate wrist and finger flexors. Grip and wrist flexion is completely synergistic with the function of the recipient nerves that control elbow flexion. Thus, postoperative motor re-education is essentially intuitive (**Fig. 1**). Similarly, the nerve transfer of the brachialis nerve to the median motor (essentially the opposite of the DFT transfer) is an equally synergistic nerve transfer. These transfers are much easier to re-educate than an AIN transfer to the deep motor branch of the ulnar nerve (**Fig. 2**).

In general, the greater the number of the nerve fibers in the donor nerve, the better the recovery of muscle force.[4] However, fortunately for both the surgeon and the patient, the "bar is set relatively low." Experimental work has shown that muscles will generate normal muscle tension until about 80% of the motor neuron connections are lost, after which there is a precipitous loss of function[5] (**Fig. 3**). This experimental finding is in keeping with clinical experience that tends to show bimodal recovery following nerve injury—either a good result or a poor result. Keeping the number of motor neurons connecting to target above that critical level is the motivation for using as many nerve fibers in the donor nerve as possible. This rationale is the motivation for the DFT nerve transfer for elbow flexion reinnervating elbow flexors, the biceps, and the brachialis.[6,7] It is also the intent

---

> **Box 2**
> **Factors influencing outcome of nerve transfers**
>
> - Synergy between donor and recipient nerves
> - Fiber count match between donor and recipient nerves
> - Recipient functional demands
> - Surgical technical difficulty
> - Quality of rehabilitation protocols/motor re-education

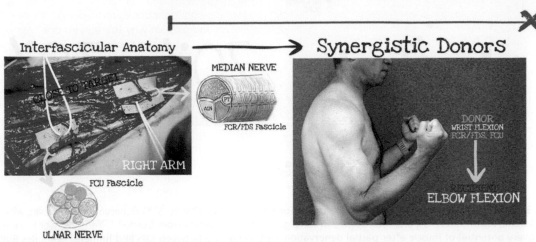

Fig. 1. The results of the DFT are generally excellent (*right panel*). The distance to target is short. The intrafascicular anatomy is known so that the motor donor fascicles on the medial side of the median nerve and the motor donor fascicles on the lateral side of the ulnar nerve can be reliably identified (*left panel*). The recipient and donor nerves are also synergistic. FCU, flexor carpi ulnaris. (*Courtesy of* nervesurgery.wustl.edu. Copyright 2015.)

of innervating the long thoracic nerve at 2 levels, with a pectoral nerve fascicle from the middle trunk at the level of the brachial plexus and a nerve transfer from the thoracodorsal nerve more distally along the course of the long thoracic nerve in the chest.[8] The biceps and brachialis nerves each contain about 3500 nerve fibers,[6] and the fascicles that the author uses for a DFT transfer each contain about 2000 nerve fibers. That is a good donor-recipient fiber match.

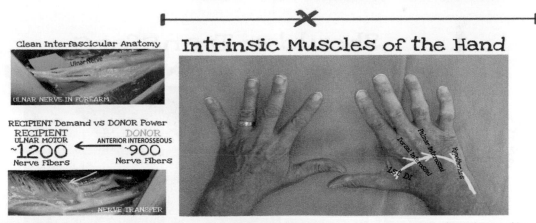

Fig. 2. The AIN to the pronator quadratus (500–900 nerve fibers) provides an adequate number of nerve fibers to satisfy the fiber count of the motor fascicular group of the ulnar nerve (1200 nerve fibers) (*left panel*). However, the demands of the ulnar intrinsic muscles are complex, and the synergy between pronation and ulnar intrinsic function is challenging. Thus, the anticipated result with an ETE AIN to ulnar motor transfer in general is "just good" (*right panel*). However, other options for ulnar nerve intrinsic recovery through tendon transfers are limited, making an AIN (ETE) transfer for complete high ulnar nerve injuries appealing. Similarly, the technical ease of this transfer makes an SETS a procedure to consider for patients with severe ulnar intrinsic atrophy with incontinuity, recoverable, ulnar palsies, and patients with transection injuries in the "gray" zone with a possibility but uncertainty of recovery. DI, dorsal interosseous. (*Courtesy of* nervesurgery.wustl.edu. Copyright 2015.)

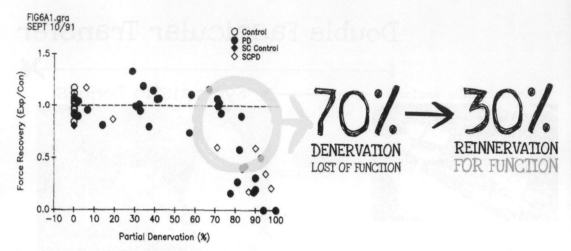

FIG6A1.gra
SEPT 10/91

Fig. 3. The maximum force generated is essentially normal even after 70% to 80% denervation. However, after 80% denervation, there is a dramatic decline in force generated. (*Modified from* Gordon T, Yang JF, Aver K, et al. Recovery potential of muscle after partial denervation—a Comparison between rats and humans. Brain Res Bull 1993;30:477–82; with permission.)

Recipient Nerve Requirements

Results of nerve transfers vary significantly based on the functional demands of the recipient nerve. Other than the facial nerve, there are few motor nerves with more intricate functional demands than the deep motor branch of the ulnar nerve. Although there are appropriate fiber counts from the AIN (500–900) to supply functional strength to the deep motor branch of the ulnar nerve (1200), the functions of the ulnar nerve innervated intrinsic muscles are so complex that it is a challenge for "pronation" to substitute for ulnar intrinsic nerve function. Thus, postoperative motor re-education is imperative for even good recovery of ulnar intrinsic function following an end-to-end (ETE) AIN to deep motor nerve transfer. Similarly, the functional requirement for excellent shoulder movement requires recovery of multiple muscles (**Fig. 4**). Thus, it should not be surprising that results of nerve reconstruction for shoulder function are poorer than for elbow function.

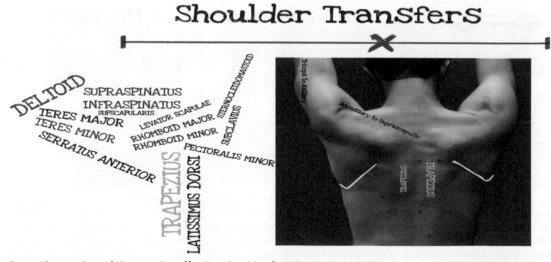

Fig. 4. The number of the muscles affecting shoulder function makes results of nerve transfers to recover shoulder function more challenging for reconstruction (*left panel*). This patient had a nerve transfer of the accessory to left SSN and medial triceps to the entire axillary nerve (*right panel*). (*Courtesy of* nervesurgery.wustl.edu. Copyright 2015.)

Consider that an isolated accessory nerve injury is a devastating injury that greatly impacts shoulder function. The fact that the accessory nerve is used as the donor of choice for suprascapular nerve (SSN) function is contrary to the basic tenant of nerve transfers of using expendable donors. The author modifies the posterior approach described by Bahm of the accessory to SSN to leave a small fascicle of the accessory nerve intact.[9] The author relies on that fascicle to respond to adjacent denervated motor endplates within the middle and lower trapezius muscle with collateral sprouting and reinnervation. Similarly, when doing an anterior approach to reinnervate the SSN with the accessory nerve, she advocates using an end-to-side (ETS) transfer with an essential caveat. The author makes a partial neurectomy in the donor accessory nerve and then "crushes" the more proximal portion of the accessory nerve with microforceps to create a second-degree injury to direct regenerating axons into both the distal accessory and the SSN nerve to recover function back into the donor accessory as well as the SSN.[10] In upper plexus injuries, the author routinely reinnervates the long thoracic nerve either ETE with C5,6,7 injuries or ETS with C5,6 injuries to make every effort to maximize recovery of serratus anterior function. When reinnervating the axillary nerve from a posterior approach, the author uses both branches of the medial triceps nerve as donors to provide maximum motor donor axon counts and innervates the entire axillary nerve, including the nerve to teres minor. The author also innervates the entire axillary nerve, not just the anterior or posterior branches.

Surgical Technique

The author always repeats the mantra, "donor distal, recipient proximal," when doing a nerve transfer to ensure absolutely no tension on the nerve repair and also to avoid doing the transfers "backwards." Absolutely no tension on the repair through full range of extremity movement is critical. When doing a median to radial nerve transfer or radial to median nerve transfer, the overlap between the divided end of the recipient and proximal nerves is 6 to 7 cm (**Fig. 5**, *upper left*). When doing an ECRB to pronator nerve, the author will have a 10-cm overlap between the proximal and distal ends of the nerves to avoid tension on the nerve transfers. With a DFT, the author cuts the recipients first and drapes them across the donor median and ulnar nerves to determine the best location for the neurolysis of the donors. With a median to radial nerve transfer, the author cuts the median donors first and brings them to the recipient radial nerve before cutting the recipients.

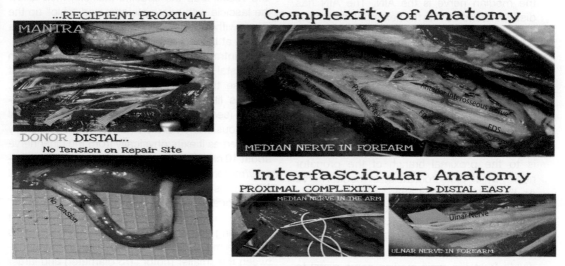

Fig. 5. The complexity of the surgical technique varies with each nerve transfer and the mantra, "donor distal, recipient proximal" (*upper left*), is critical to ensure no tension at the repair site (*lower left*). The branches of the median nerve in the forearm have already separated from the main median nerve, making certainty of the anatomic function easier to determine (*upper right*). By contrast, identifying the specific motor/sensory components of the median nerve in the arm is a more challenging surgical technique requiring detailed knowledge of the intraneural anatomy (*lower right*). In the distal forearm, the ulnar nerve has longer distances between the plexi (*lower right*). The motor component is "sandwiched" between the dorsal cutaneous ulnar sensory and the main sensory to the volar aspect of the ring and small finger. (*Courtesy of* nervesurgery.wustl.edu. Copyright 2015.)

The author is able to move the extremity through a full range of movement on the operating room table with no tension at all. Hanno Millesi spent his entire career teaching the importance of no tension at the nerve repair/graft site, and the author follows this advice religiously.

The complexity of the anatomy varies considerably from one nerve transfer to another. For example, the donor and recipient nerves are "predissected" in the median to radial or radial to median nerve transfers in the proximal forearm. They have already branched from the median and radial nerves. The donor nerves need to be neurolysed free from the main donor nerves proximally for ease of transfer. However, given that they have already branched from the donor nerves, the procedure is technically easier to perform as compared with a DFT, wherein donor fascicles must be safely and accurately identified by the surgeon from within the main trunks of the median and ulnar nerves (see **Fig. 5**, *upper right*). Before nerve transfer technique, there was not a particular need to understand the specific of the location of these branches. Therefore, even in these less complex nerve transfers, there still is a knowledge gap in basic textbooks of the important anatomy and delineations of where the branches separate from the main nerves. The critical points, with respect to the median nerve, are as follows:

- The only branch coming off the radial side of the median nerve is the AIN. The AIN has distinct fascicles with the flexor pollicis longus (FPL) fascicle radial to the flexor profundus to the index finger. These fascicles are easily separable for reconstruction of isolated FPL palsies seen with neuritis.
- The distal pronator branch is on the anterior surface of the median nerve in the proximal forearm below the elbow.
- All of the remaining branches come off the ulnar side of the median nerve. The first branch is to the proximal branch of the pronator nerve, which exits from the main median nerve on the ulnar side just above the elbow. The branch to the flexor carpi radialis (FCR) and palmaris longus (PL) divides from the median nerve on the ulnar side just distal to the elbow. The superficialis (FDS) has 2 branches, which divide from the main median nerve distal to the FCR/PL branch.
- This median nerve branch pattern anatomy is consistent.

Other nerve transfers are more technically challenging. These transfers involve intrafascicular dissection of the main nerve at the trunk level before the branch points. This anatomy is not yet described in standard textbooks. It is reliable and reproducible, but not well recognized. Thus, nerve transfers requiring this anatomic familiarity will be more challenging to perform. The median nerve anatomy in the arm is an excellent example and is the front cover illustration of *Nerve Surgery*.[11] The lateral side of the median nerve is predominantly sensory. The medial side is motor (see **Fig. 1**). The distinct nerve fascicle to the pronator muscle sits on the anterior surface of the median nerve between the lateral/sensory and medial/motor component of the median nerve. There are typically 2 microvessels on either side of this pronator fascicle that help to delineate its location. Open up the epineurium to more easily visualize this pronator fascicle and these vessels. Use microforceps to tap along the surface of the median nerve in the mid/distal arm to delineate the location of this separate, distinct pronator fascicle. In the arm, the AIN is located on the medial posterior quadrant of the median nerve (see **Fig. 1**).[11,12] Between the AIN and the pronator fascicle is the motor component to the wrist and finger flexors (FCR, FDS). When first teaching herself this anatomy, the author identified the AIN and the pronator nerves in the proximal forearm and followed these nerves back proximally using a technique she calls "neurolysis with my eyes" so that she could confirm the location of these fascicles in the arm. She would perform a short length of intraneural dissection and vessel loop the specific fascicle, then follow the fascicle with micro pickups and "skip" up the nerve without physically separating the fascicles except at these short neurolysis points.

The intrafascicular anatomy of the ulnar nerve in the distal forearm is also very specific, but because the dissection is in the distal forearm, there is little plexus formation over longer distances (see **Fig. 5**, *lower right*). As well, the dorsal cutaneous branch of the ulnar nerve (DCU) is easily identified as it exits physically from the ulnar nerve about 10 cm proximal to the wrist crease. The sensory/motor anatomy of the ulnar nerve in the distal forearm is constant with the motor fascicular group located between the DCU sensory group and the main sensory group to the volar aspect of the ring and small finger. Once the DCU exits from the main ulnar nerve, the size difference between the smaller motor (1/3 diameter) and larger sensory (2/3 diameter) is also consistent. As well, there is a small epineural microvessel on the surface of the ulnar nerve that delineates the "split" between the motor and sensory groups. Again, using microinstrumentation, the surgeon can "tap" across the surface of the ulnar nerve and the microforceps will "fall into this cleavage plane" between the motor and sensory groups. With custom-made tenotomy scissors (Fischer Surgical, St Louis, MO, USA), the author gently splits longitudinally between the motor and sensory fascicular groups. These tenotomy scissors are also carefully maintained by the Fischer technicians so that the outer edges are smooth and the inner "cutting" surfaces are sharp. These scissors are terrific! Again, when the author first started to do the AIN to ulnar motor nerve transfer in the distal forearm, she would identify the deep motor branch of the ulnar nerve in the region of the Guyon canal and trace it back using the neurolysis "with my eyes" technique to ensure that she had the appropriate motor versus sensory component of the ulnar nerve. That is something the author no longer needs to do to ensure topography but she certainly does release the deep motor branch entrapment site in all cases.

Decompress Nearby Distal Entrapment Sites

There is great power in understanding the ability of decompression of nearby distal entrapment points to improve functional recovery after any nerve injury. As the nerve regenerates, it is more susceptible to distal areas of nerve entrapment. As well, any extremity that has been injured will have edema associated with that injury, making known areas of nerve entrapment physically more significant because of the edema process itself. This situation is true for any nerve injury, even favorable second- and third-degree, axonotmetic, recovering injuries. Take, for example, radial nerve palsies associated with closed humeral fractures. These injuries routinely recover well over time. However, there are 3 well-known entrapment points along the course of the radial nerve: one at the lateral triceps septum in the spiral groove; the second in the region of the arcade of Frohse; and the third described by Wartenberg, at the junction between the brachioradialis and extensor carpi radialis longus tendons. The edema caused by the humeral fracture and any surgery is compounded by the edema from dependency and lack of normal use of the extremity associated with the radial nerve palsy. Patients with recovering radial nerve palsy may frequently benefit from a distal release to speed up recovery. If patients with radial nerve palsies fail to progress in a timely fashion and clinical examination with provocative maneuvers demonstrate evidence of clinical entrapment at those levels (for example, Tinel sign, pressure provocative testing, and a positive scratch collapse test),[13] then the author decompresses the nerve (typically at the arcade of Frohse). Therefore, with nerve transfers performed in areas near known entrapment points (eg, the arcade of Frohse, the pronator teres in the forearm, and Guyon canal), decompression at those entrapment points will improve functional recovery following nerve transfer procedures.

Your Hand Therapist and Physical Therapist Can Improve Your Results

Without question, the results following nerve transfers can be greatly enhanced with input and guidance from your hand and physical therapists. During the period of time the muscles are denervated, keeping the muscles at normal resting length will facilitate recovery once reinnervation occurs.[14] Surgeons are familiar with this concept in the management of radial nerve palsy with splints to keep the extensor muscles from stretching and lengthening. By contrast, they do not typically extend this concept to other denervated muscles. Splints to keep the interphalangeal joint of the thumb and distal interphalangeal joint of the index finger in a flexed position will enhance ultimate function following nerve transfers for AIN palsies. Shoulder braces to prevent altered muscle length of denervated scapular muscles until reinnervation has occurred will enhance the results of nerve transfers around the shoulder.

Trained physical therapists are also aware of inappropriate muscle substitution patterns and are trained in motor re-education. In the author's practice, the physical therapist sees the patient for a 1-hour visit, 1 month after the nerve transfer surgery to discuss, in detail, the transfers that were performed and begin patient education of anticipated rehabilitation protocols. As soon as there is M1 recovery, motor re-education begins in earnest. Graded motor imagery may be used.[15–17] Lorna C. Kahn, BSPT, CHT has written an article for this issue on rehabilitation and likens the rehabilitation protocol to giving someone the owner's manual for a new car so they can "turn on and drive" the nerve transfers that have been performed. (See Kahn LC, Moore AM: Donor Activation Focused Rehabilitation Approach (DAFRA): Maximizing Outcomes after Nerve Transfers, in this issue.) The patients know their specific donors and recipients. If they have had an AIN to deep motor branch ulnar nerve transfer, they know how to "turn on and drive" the transfer by resisting pronation. They learn the donor/recipient movements in their normal extremity and translate these to the reinnervated extremity. As a surgeon, the author does not supervise the postoperative rehabilitation protocol. Nerve therapists are the experts on that. If you have not yet established a close working relationship with your hand therapist or physical therapist, then you and your patients are missing out on the power of the brain to improve your results following nerve transfers.

The Quality of Results Following Nerve Transfer Varies

The critical factors associated with poor functional recovery after nerve injury include proximal injuries, delay of reconstruction, tension at a primary repair site, injuries requiring nerve grafts, and a lack of knowledge of the sensorimotor topography of the nerve being reconstructed. All of these factors are negated with the use of nerve transfer technique. Thus, it is not surprising that the results associated with nerve transfers in general are significantly superior to many traditional nerve reconstructions. The proximal nerve injuries are treated with distal nerve transfers, thus eliminating months of denervation time. The use of the mantra, "donor distal, recipient proximal," ensures no tension at the nerve repair and obviates a nerve graft. The entire discipline of nerve transfer is predicated on deep understanding of the sensorimotor internal topography of the nerve.

The "results" of nerve transfers are specific to each transfer. **Table 1** outlines the author's personal opinion of the surgical difficulty of various transfers, the time to recovery, and the overall quality that can be anticipated with these nerve transfers. Just as nerve repairs or nerve grafts or tendon transfers will give varying results, so will nerve transfers. Although it is said that the results of nerve transfers are superior to nerve grafts, the results from nerve transfers vary from procedure to procedure, just as would any other type of nerve reconstruction. For example, the DFT for elbow flexion results in excellent recovery and rather quick recovery with some evidence of early reinnervation around 4 months, M3+ by 9 months, and frequently essentially near normal functional recovery by a year. The surgical difficulty of the DFT, however, is high, because an understanding of the complicated but reliable and consistent internal topography of the median nerve is imperative for a good result. Although FCR/FDS is expendable, the pronator and the AIN fascicles certainly are not.

The AIN transfer to the side of the motor component of the ulnar nerve, which the author calls a supercharge end-to-side transfer (SETS), is the easiest transfer she does.[18] SETS transfer is far superior to the ETE ulnar AIN transfer. SETS results will vary depending on how much recovery occurs from the native injured ulnar nerve. Given the complexity of function of the ulnar intrinsic muscles, the overall results with an ETE AIN to deep motor branch transfer are probably the poorest the author acquires with a nerve transfer. However, the results with tendon transfers for the ulnar intrinsic function are also underwhelming, and an ETE AIN nerve transfer does not preclude

Table 1
Quality of results and difficulty of nerve transfers

		SURGICAL DIFFICULTY	TIME TO RESULT	QUALITY OF RESULT
SHOULDER	**SUPRASCAPULAR NERVE** Accessory to Suprascapular Nerve Transfer	+++	14+ mo	
SHOULDER	**AXILLARY NERVE** Triceps to Axillary Nerve Transfer	+++	14+ mo	
SHOULDER	Medial Pectoral to Axillary Nerve Transfer	+++	12+ mo	
ELBOW	**ELBOW FLEXION** Double Fascicular Nerve Transfer	++++	9 mo	
ELBOW	**ELBOW EXTENSION** FCU to Medial Triceps Nerve Transfer	+++	9 mo	
HAND	**FOREARM PRONATION** ECRB to Pronator Teres Nerve Transfer	++	5 mo	
HAND	**FINGER/WRIST EXTENSION** Median to Radial Nerve Transfer	++++	12 mo	
HAND	**FINGER FLEXION** Brachialis to AIN Nerve Transfer	++++	12++ mo	
HAND	ECRB to AIN Nerve Transfer	+++	12 mo	
HAND	FDS to AIN Nerve Transfer	+++	12 mo	
HAND	**HAND INTRINSICS** AIN to Ulnar Motor (End-to-end) Nerve Transfer	++	12 mo	
HAND	AIN to Ulnar Motor (End-to-side) Nerve Transfer	+	9 mo	

additional tendon transfers. The accessory to SSN transfer is problematic given the accessory nerve itself is not an "expendable nerve." The author has previously discussed her strategies to mitigate against that.

Are There Other Options and Alternatives for Reconstruction?

Another factor that will determine when patients will opt for a nerve transfer depends on what other options are available for reconstruction. As noted, the results with ETE AIN to motor branch of ulnar are not terrific, but the tendon transfers are not either. By contrast, tendon transfers for radial nerve palsy are tried and true; recovery is relatively quick, within several months, and routinely delivers very good results. Median to radial nerve transfer is a more challenging procedure to perform, and although the results with independent extension of fingers and thumb can be spectacular, it takes a year to recover that function. In her practice, the author does about 5 median to radial nerve tendon transfers for every one median to radial nerve transfer, predominantly because of the speed of recovery with tendon transfers. However, some patients are extraordinarily stiff, and tendon transfers are not an option. Some have jobs that require a lot of finger dexterity and will wait the year to get that function with a nerve transfer. In complex cases, the author will frequently combine nerve and tendon procedures for best results.[3]

FUTURE AREAS TO CONSIDER FOR NERVE TRANSFER TECHNIQUES
A Few Comments on End-to-Side Transfers

If ETS SETS nerve transfers are a part of your surgical technique, then it is important to understand the difference between the traditional ETS nerve transfer as reintroduced by Viterbo as compared with the SETS supercharge nerve transfer. In a traditional ETS transfer, a denervated nerve is transferred to the side of a normal nerve. That facilitates collateral spontaneous sensory sprouting and reinnervation into the denervated nerve. The more the perineurium is opened, the more spontaneous collateral sprouting will occur.[18] The traditional ETS will not result in spontaneous motor reinnervation.[19] There must be an actual injury to the motor nerve to facilitate motor axonal sprouting. Thus, you do not need to injure the donor nerve to get collateral sensory sprouting, but you do need to injure the donor nerve if you want motor sprouting.[19] The SETS (reverse traditional ETS) is a nerve transfer where the normal donor nerve is completely transected. There will obviously be

motor and sensory axonal sprouting from that transection. Opening the epineurium and perineurium of the recipient nerve will encourage more sprouting from the transected end of the donor nerve into the side of the recipient denervated nerve, resulting in both sensory and motor axons reinnervating the target end organs.

In the authors' practice, SETS nerve transfers have greatly improved ulnar intrinsic function with recoverable axonotmetic injuries typically cubital tunnel cases. The ulnar intrinsic muscles are extraordinarily important for hand function, and the SETS procedure is such a simple operation to do with very little morbidity that in the author's practice the ulnar AIN SETS has found an important role.[18] Understanding the indications for this procedure requires an understanding of the status of the motor endplates and clear understanding of how to interpret and use electrodiagnostic tests. For example, an SETS motor nerve transfer will not be successful if performed after the denervated motor endplates are unreceptive to reinnervation. Thus, for patients with ulnar intrinsic atrophy and weakness with severe cubital tunnel, if the electromyogram shows no fibrillations and just chronic motor units, the author would not perform SETS transfers, because receptive end plates are less likely available.

The ulnar SETS is also useful in complete high ulnar nerve injuries if a Martin-Gruber connection is present and in complete ulnar nerve injuries in the "gray" zone, where there is a possibility but not a certainty of recovery. SETS is a simple procedure to increase the likelihood of intrinsic recovery. The utility of the SETS procedure in other nerve injuries has yet to be determined. In general, if motor unit potentials are present at 3 months, the recovery of function is typically excellent. An SETS transfer, in the author's opinion, is not needed in those situations. By contrast, if it takes a longer period of time for collateral sprouting to occur (ie, motor unit potential present at ≥4 months), an SETS transfer may prove to be the operation of choice to protect the reinnervation that has occurred in second- and third-degree injuries and add to it with the SETS transfer.

Technical points are key:

- Harvest the donor nerve distally as far as its branch points so you can "fan" the donor fascicles across each recipient fascicle.
- Open the perineurium of the recipient widely to facilitate sprouting into the recipient.[20]
- Remember the mantra, "donor distal" remains, but the mantra, "recipient proximal" does not. The recipient will not move; you may need a short graft. Prepare for that.

The author has seen several cases in which there is evidence of reinnervation across the posterior axillary nerve, but not the anterior axillary nerve; this likely relates to the more acute route that the anterior axillary nerve takes around the humerus. In these situations, one branch of the medial triceps nerve can be transferred ETE to the anterior axillary nerve and a second branch ETS can be transferred to the posterior axillary nerve to enhance recovery. If the author "SETS" the axillary nerve in the third-degree injuries, she always releases the potential entrapment point at the quadrangular space by doing a tenotomy of the long head of the triceps.

"Long" nerve injuries

With satisfactory results with nerve transfers in proximal injuries, the author has moved toward using nerve transfers for proximal injuries that also have long, distal extensions. In these cases, the mantra of "donor distal/recipient proximal" may not be feasible because the recipient proximal length is not available (recipient proximal). A short nerve graft may be needed between the donor, which can be followed distally, and the recipient, which cannot be followed as far proximally as is typically done with a localized proximal injury. Plan for that and try to keep the graft less than 6 cm.

Sensory nerve transfers

Once the author developed her experience with nerve transfers for motor recovery, she expanded the potential for sensory nerve transfers to improve sensibility. When an ETE sensory nerve transfer is performed, you must be assured that there is not going to be any proximal regeneration along the course of the proximal native nerve. Otherwise, there is a distinct possibility for neuromatous pain if the proximal nerve fibers reach the distal divided nerve stump. In these situations, the proximal portion of that sensory nerve needs to be treated as a potential source of neuroma pain. The technique that the author uses is a "proximal crush" of the nerve to create a second-degree injury to move the regeneration front proximally.[21] The author then turns the nerve proximally and deep into a muscle environment, typically between the superficial and deep forearm flexors.[21] Thus, she is confident that if there is ever any regeneration along the course of that sensory nerve, it will not cause a painful neuroma. In general, the sensory nerve transfers are more challenging to do than motor transfers. With motor transfers, you will always be able to stimulate the donor nerve and assure topography with intraoperative electrical stimulation. Obviously, with sensory transfers,

neither the donor nor the recipient will stimulate. In her operating room, the author uses drawings of the sensory transfers to be absolutely certain that the correct sensory transfer is done, given that they cannot stimulate the nerves.[11]

The author has recently used cross-cross grafts to bridge between the median and ulnar nerve to provide reinnervation into the ulnar nerve sensory territory in patients with severe ulnar neuropathy. This procedure essentially combines the traditional ETS with the SETS. These grafts are done from the side of the normal nerve (ETS transfer) to the side of the denervated ulnar nerve (SETS transfer). These short (2.5 cm) grafts are done in the carpal tunnel and Guyon canal to bring reinnervation very close to the sensory territories of the ulnar nerve in the ring and small finger. Early results with this technique are very encouraging.

FUTURE DIRECTIONS

As with any new technique, once the initial results are found to be satisfactory, the indications of the original technique expand; this is occurring with nerve transfers as well. Nerve transfers are now being used for the treatment of spinal cord injury, and there is early consideration for its use in stroke patients. In both of these central nervous system injuries, the lower motor neuron is intact to the muscle target mitigating the issues of denervation. There is also early interest in its role in treating patients with transverse myelitis. Similarly, an understanding of specific intraneural topography facilitates selective neurectomy for treatment of recalcitrant muscle spasticity, These areas are all hugely exciting to explore.

REFERENCES

1. Mackinnon SE, Novak CB. Nerve transfers—new option for reconstruction following nerve injury. Hand Clin 1999;15:643–66.
2. Mackinnon SE, Novak CB. Nerve transfers. Hand Clin 2008;24. Saunders, Philadelphia.
3. Poppler LH, Davidge K, Lu JC, et al. Alternatives to sural nerve grafts in the upper extremity. Hand (N Y) 2015;10(1):68–75.
4. Mackinnon SE, Dellon AL, O'Brien JP. Selection of optimal axon ratio for nerve regeneration. Ann Plast Surg 1989;23:129–34.
5. Gordon T, Yang JF, Aver K, et al. Recovery potential of muscle after partial denervation—a Comparison between rats and humans. Brain Res Bull 1993;30: 477–82.
6. Brandt KE, Mackinnon SE. A technique for maximizing biceps recovery in brachial plexus. J Hand Surg Am 1993;18:726–33.

7. Mackinnon SE, Novak CB, Myckatyn TM, et al. Results of reinnervation of the biceps and brachialis muscles with a double fascicular transfer for elbow flexion. J Hand Surg Am 2005;30(5):978–85.

8. Ray WZ, Pet MA, Nicoson MC, et al. Two-level motor nerve transfer for the treatment of long thoracic nerve palsy. J Neurosurg 2011;115:858–64.

9. Colbert SH, Mackinnon SE. Posterior approach for double nerve transfer for restoration of shoulder function in upper brachial plexus palsy. Hand (N Y) 2006;1(2):71–7.

10. Ray WZ, Kasukurthi R, Yee A, et al. Functional recovery following an end to side neurorrhaphy of the accessory nerve to the suprascapular nerve: case report. Hand (N Y) 2010;5(3):313–7.

11. Mackinnon SE. Nerve surgery. New York: Thieme; 2015.

12. Dunn AJ, Salonen DC, Anastakis DJ. MR imaging findings of anterior interosseous nerve lesions. Skeletal Radiol 2007;36(12):1155–62.

13. Davidge KM, Gontre G, Tang D, et al. The "hierarchical" scratch collapse test for identifying multilevel ulnar nerve compression. Hand (N Y) 2015; 10(3):388–95.

14. Gordon AM, Huxley AF, Julian FJ. The variation in isometric tension with sarcomere length. J Physiol 1966;184:170–92.

15. Ramachandran VS, Rogers-Ramachandran D. Synaesthesia in phantom limbs induced with mirrors. Proc Biol Sci 1996;263:377–86.

16. Walsh NE, Jones L, McCabe CS. The mechanisms and actions of motor imagery within the clinical setting. Textbook of Neuromodulation. New York: Springer; 2015. p. 151–8.

17. Priganc VW, Stralka SW. Graded motor imagery. J Hand Ther 2011;24(2):164–9.

18. Davidge KM, Yee A, Moore AM, et al. The supercharge end-to-side anterior interosseous to ulnar motor nerve transfer for restoring intrinsic function: clinical experience. Plast Reconstr Surg 2015;136: 344e–52e.

19. Hayashi A, Pannucchi C, Moradzadeh A, et al. Axotomy or compression is required for axonal sprouting following end-to-side neurorrhaphy. Exp Neurol 2008;211(2):539–50.

20. Walker JC, Brenner MJ, Mackinnon SE, et al. Effect of perineural window on nerve regeneration, blood-nerve barrier integrity and functional recovery. J Neurotrauma 2004;21(2):217–27.

21. Watson CP, Mackinnon SE, Dostrovsky JO, et al. Nerve resection, crush and re-location relieve complex regional pain syndrome type II: a case report. Pain 2014;155(6):1168–73.

Nerve Transfers to Restore Shoulder Function

Somsak Leechavengvongs, MD[a],*, Kanchai Malungpaishorpe, MD[a],
Chairoj Uerpairojkit, MD[a], Chye Yew Ng, FRCS(Tr&Orth), BDHS, EBHSD[b],
Kiat Witoonchart, MD[a]

KEYWORDS

- Brachial plexus injuries • Nerve injury • Nerve transfer • Shoulder function

KEY POINTS

- Spinal accessory nerve to suprascapular nerve transfer could restore some abduction, forward flexion, and possibly external rotation of the shoulder.
- Double nerve transfers to both suprascapular and axillary nerves, when adequate donors are available, provide better shoulder abduction than single nerve transfer does.
- The long head of the triceps branch to the anterior branch of the axillary nerve transfer via the posterior approach could restore good shoulder function.
- Serratus anterior is a major muscle stabilizer of the shoulder and should be reconstructed to achieve optimal shoulder function.
- Intercostal nerves could be used as donor nerves for transfer to the axillary nerve via a posterior approach or to the long thoracic nerve via an anterior approach.

INTRODUCTION

The shoulder girdle consists of 5 articulations, namely the glenohumeral, acromioclavicular, sternoclavicular, subacromial, and scapulothoracic. Complex movements of these articulations, as coordinated by the girdle musculature, allow accurate placement of the hand in time and space. Normal shoulder function is thus fundamental to normal prehensile function. Apart from the initial 30°, full shoulder abduction in the coronal plane is effected by simultaneous motion of both the glenohumeral joint and scapular rotation in the ratio of 2:1.[1] Normal scapular motion is controlled by 17 muscles that receive innervations from some 12 named peripheral nerves. Different injuries of the

nerve supply to the musculature may thus result in a spectrum of functional deficits.

Paralysis of the deltoid and rotator cuff muscles is encountered commonly in patients with upper roots brachial plexus injury. In this group of patients, restoration of shoulder function is generally regarded as the second reconstructive priority after restoration of elbow flexion. To achieve better shoulder abduction, most surgeons now would recommend double nerve transfers to both suprascapular and axillary nerves when adequate donors are available.[2–4]

Serratus anterior is an essential scapular stabilizer. Injury to the long thoracic nerve or the upper brachial plexus roots may result in scapular winging and limitation of shoulder movement.

Disclosure Statement: Nil of note.
[a] Department of Medical Services, Institute of Orthopaedics, Lerdsin General Hospital, 190 Silom Road, Bangrak, Bangkok 10500, Thailand; [b] Upper Limb Unit, Wrightington Hospital, Hall Lane, Appley Bridge, Wigan WN6 9EP, UK
* Corresponding author.
E-mail address: somsakortho@gmail.com

Hand Clin 32 (2016) 153–164
http://dx.doi.org/10.1016/j.hcl.2015.12.004
0749-0712/16/$ – see front matter © 2016 Elsevier Inc. All rights reserved.

As the stability of the scapula is fundamental for optimal shoulder function, reanimation of the paralyzed serratus anterior muscle is recommended.[5]

Isolated axillary nerve injury may occur after shoulder trauma or surgery.[6–8] In some patients with the nerve injury, normal shoulder range of motion is still possible provided the rotator cuff tendons and the suprascapular nerve are intact.[9] On clinical examination, these patients can be deceptively functional. However, without a functioning deltoid, the shoulder would fatigue easily.[10] With advancing age, there is a significant increase in the incidence of asymptomatic and symptomatic rotator cuff tears in those without deltoid function compared with those with functional deltoids.[11,12] It is thus generally accepted that isolated axillary nerve injury should be treated to avoid the potential risk of a future rotator cuff tear.[10]

In this article, we outline the various surgical techniques of nerve transfers to restore shoulder function and summarize the clinical results.

SURGICAL TECHNIQUES
Spinal Accessory Nerve to Suprascapular Nerve Transfer (Anterior Approach)

The spinal accessory nerve is a pure motor nerve, which innervates the sternocleidomastoid and trapezius muscles. When it is used as a donor nerve, it is important to isolate the distal branch while preserving the branches to the upper and middle trapezius to preserve some trapezius function. Interposition nerve graft is best avoided, because that would require 2 neurorrhaphy sites for a single transfer, thereby compromising the potential outcome.

The functional aim of this nerve transfer is to regain some abduction and forward flexion of the arm. External rotation of the shoulder may be restored to variable degrees and this can only be achieved when the scapula is stable.

Preoperative planning
Contraindications to this nerve transfer include trapezius muscle power of less than M4 or extensive injury of the supraclavicular area.

Preparation and patient positioning
The patient is placed in a supine position with a sandbag beneath the affected upper extremity. The head is turned to the contralateral side and the upper part of the body is elevated slightly to reduce venous congestion (relaxed beach chair position). Long-acting paralytic agents and muscle relaxants are avoided to allow intraoperative electrical stimulation.

Surgical approach and procedure
Our preferred exposure of the supraclavicular plexus is through a V-shaped incision. We use the lateral portion of the transverse limb, which lies 1 cm above and parallel to the clavicle, for exploration of the spinal accessory nerve. The lateral part of the trapezius is detached from the distal clavicle for 1 to 2 cm. Dissection is then performed on the anterior surface of the trapezius muscle several centimeters above the clavicle. The landmark for detecting the nerve is the transverse cervical vessels that accompany the nerve. An electrical stimulator can be used around the vessels to identify the distal part of the spinal accessory nerve. This nerve should not be confused with the small branches from the cervical plexus, which will not elicit any muscle response when stimulated. The spinal accessory nerve should be dissected as far distally as possible.

The suprascapular nerve is normally found arising from the upper trunk 2 to 3 cm above the clavicle. However, the nerve can be difficult to find after traction injury to the plexus. A technical tip is to ask the assistant to pull the patient's affected arm downward while the operator palpates with a finger for a tented structure on the most lateral aspect of the brachial plexus. This is then followed with further blunt finger dissection down to the scapular notch, where the integrity of the nerve is confirmed. The suprascapular nerve is then traced from distal to proximal and disconnected from the upper trunk before coaptation with the donor spinal accessory nerve (**Fig. 1**).

Postoperative care and rehabilitation
The patient's arm is placed in a sling for 3 weeks. Gentle passive mobilization is then performed to

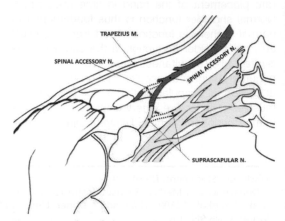

Fig. 1. Transfer of the spinal accessory nerve to the suprascapular nerve by anterior approach. M., muscle; N., nerve. (*Courtesy of* Kunakorn Lohagard, FA, Bangkok, Thailand.)

prevent joint stiffness. Cortical retraining focuses on learning how to effect abduction by shrugging the affected shoulder.

Clinical results

The outcome is influenced by multiple factors, including the type of injury and the number of nerve transfers performed. The more extensive the injury, the worse outcome of the shoulder function, with reported mean shoulder abduction ranging between 45° and 122°.[5,13–16] The outcome of external rotation is more inconsistent with reported motion, which varied from 0° to 118°.[5,15,16]

Spinal Accessory Nerve to Suprascapular Nerve Transfer (Posterior Approach)

Guan and colleagues[17] first described the posterior approach to the spinal accessory nerve to fully utilize the dispensable nerve axons while preserving the function of the upper trapezius. A number of anatomic studies have shown that, at the level of the superior margin of the scapular spine, the locations of the suprascapular and the spinal accessory nerves are relatively constant.[18,19] After mobilization, the 2 nerve ends can be easily coapted without any tension. We would recommend the posterior approach when there is extensive scarring at the supraclavicular area.

The advantages of the posterior approach (over the anterior approach) include that:

1. A greater part of the upper trapezius is potentially preserved[20];
2. The neurorrhaphy site is more distal and hence closer to the target muscles; and
3. The second lesion of the suprascapular nerve beyond the suprascapular notch, if present, could be identified and managed accordingly.[21]

The disadvantages, compared with the anterior approach, include that:

1. The incision and exposure required tend to be more extensive;
2. Some of the trapezius muscle insertion has to be cut to expose the nerve adequately, resulting in some degree of collateral damage to the muscle; and
3. The donor motor nerve axonal count decreases as the more distal portion of the nerve is used, although the number of myelinated axons may still be sufficient for neurotization of the suprascapular nerve.[22]

Preoperative planning

Trapezius muscle power has to be at least M4.

Preparation and patient positioning

The patient is placed in the prone or lateral decubitus position with the operative side upward.

Surgical approach and procedure

The spinal accessory nerve can be located along a line parallel to the superior border of the scapula at a point two-fifths of the distance from the midline of the cervicothoracic spine to the acromion or at the cross-point of the scapular spine and the medial border of the scapula. The suprascapular nerve is also located along this line, at the midpoint between the superior angle of the scapula and the acromion.[23]

A transverse incision (12–15 cm) is made parallel to the scapular spine. The trapezius muscle is elevated from the scapular spine and a plane is developed between the trapezius and the supraspinatus muscles. In some cases, a thin fatty layer can be seen between the 2 muscles. The trapezius is gently lifted, revealing the spinal accessory nerve on its anterior surface. The nerve is then dissected as far distally as possible before the nerve is cut.

The suprascapular notch is approached next by retracting the supraspinatus muscle caudally. Use a finger to palpate for a firm fibrous structure that is, the superior transverse ligament. Suprascapular artery and vein, which are located superficial to the ligament, are then ligated. Next the ligament is sectioned while protecting the underlying suprascapular nerve. The nerve is dissected as far proximally as possible before division (**Fig. 2**). The 2 nerve ends are then coapted without any tension. The trapezius is reattached to the scapular spine.

Postoperative care and rehabilitation

Same as the anterior approach.

Clinical results

The outcomes of the spinal accessory nerve transfer to the suprascapular nerve done through the posterior approach are mixed for restoration of shoulder abduction.[24–27] Souza and colleagues[27] reported better results in terms of external rotation, but not shoulder abduction when compared with anterior approach in those with late traumatic brachial plexus injuries. In contrast, Rui and colleagues[26] did not identify any difference between the posterior and anterior approaches. They recommended the posterior approach only if the anterior approach was not feasible.

Radial Nerve (Long Head of Triceps Branch) to Axillary Nerve Transfer (Posterior Approach)

Different treatment options are available in isolated injury of the axillary nerve. Nerve grafting,

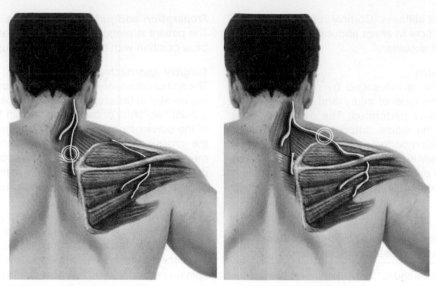

Fig. 2. Transfer of the spinal accessory nerve to the suprascapular nerve by the posterior approach. (*Courtesy of* Kunakorn Lohagard, FA, Bangkok, Thailand.)

traditionally the preferred surgical treatment for isolated axillary lesions distal to its origin from the posterior cord, potentially restores both the anterior and posterior branches of the axillary nerve. In 1948, Lurje[28] described the technique of transferring the triceps fascicles of the radial nerve to the axillary nerve without nerve grafting in a patient with Erb's palsy. Nath and Mackinnon[29] subsequently reported satisfactory results in 5 patients using Lurje's technique. In 2003, we reported nerve transfer to the anterior branch of the axillary nerve using the nerve to the long head of triceps.[30,31] Okazaki and colleagues[32] stated that the posterior deltoid is usually supplied by the posterior branch of the axillary nerve and would not be reinnervated by nerve transfer to the anterior branch alone. However, our cadaveric study demonstrated that, in most cases (91.5%), the anterior branch of the axillary nerve also supplies the posterior part of the deltoid.[33] Therefore, nerve transfer to the anterior branch of the axillary nerve not only restores the anterior and middle parts, but also the posterior part in most cases. We deliberately avoid the posterior branch of the axillary nerve that contain axons to teres minor and the superior lateral brachial cutaneous nerve. Teres minor is an external rotator of the shoulder, but it is also a strong adductor, which is antagonistic to what we intend to restore. We believe that external rotation in our patients result partly from the suprascapular nerve transfer to reanimate the infraspinatus and partly from reinnervation of the posterior part of the deltoid muscle.

Subsequently, the nerve to the lateral head and the nerve to the medial head of the triceps have

both been promoted as the donor nerve.[10,23,34,35] We prefer the nerve to the long head because of its constant branching point, proximity to the recipient and the largest diameter offering the best size match to the recipient nerve.[36] In addition, the long head branch is the most dispensable branch, because it plays the least important role in elbow extension among the 3 heads of triceps.[37]

Preoperative planning
Triceps muscle power has to be at least M4.

Preparation and patient positioning
The patient is placed in the supine position with a sandbag beneath the affected upper extremity. The affected arm is placed across the chest thus exposing the posterior aspect of the shoulder.

Surgical approach and procedure
A 12-cm, curved incision is made along the border of the posterior deltoid. Because the deltoid is atrophic, the posterior border can be elevated easily without having to detach its origin from the scapular spine. The interval between the long and the lateral heads of the triceps is then developed to expose the quadrilateral space and the triangular interval. Teres major is the key structure, which divides the space from the interval. Next, the radial nerve at the triangular interval is isolated and the first branch of the nerve, which usually comes off at about 1 cm proximal to the inferior edge of teres major, is the nerve to the long head of the triceps.

The axillary nerve is accompanied by the posterior circumflex humeral artery and vein at the quadrilateral space. After emerging from the space, the axillary nerve gives off a branch to the teres minor and then divides into 1 to 3 anterior branch(es) and 1 posterior branch. The anterior branch(es), which are the major motor branch to deltoid muscle, are dissected as proximally as possible. Electrical stimulation of the nerves is used to confirm paralysis of the deltoid and strong contractions of the triceps. The long head of the triceps nerve (donor) is cut as distally as possible just before it enters the muscle and the anterior branch of the axillary nerve (recipient) is transected as proximally as possible. In our experience, this would always provide sufficient length for a tension-free, direct neurorrhaphy (**Figs. 3** and **4**). A technical tip to increase mobility of the donor nerve, which is rarely required, is to incise the inferior edge of teres major for approximately 1 cm.

Postoperative care and rehabilitation

The patient's arm is placed in a sling for 3 weeks. Gentle passive mobilization is then performed to prevent joint stiffness. No specific motor reeducation is necessary.

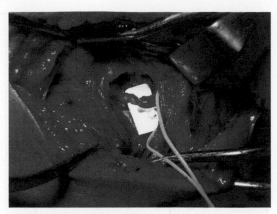

Fig. 4. Intraoperative view of a transfer to the anterior branch of the axillary nerve from the nerve to the long head of triceps.

Clinical results

In our first series of 7 patients who had dual nerve transfers of spinal accessory nerve to suprascapular nerve and the long head of triceps branch to the axillary nerve, all patients achieved M4 deltoid function with mean abduction of 124°.[31] Bertelli and Ghizoni[34] reported their results of dual nerve transfers in 10 patients with C5 and C5 to C6 injuries. Three patients achieved M4 and 7 achieved M3 shoulder abduction. The mean abduction was 92° and the mean external rotation was 93°. In 2006, we reported another series of 15 patients with C5 and C6 injures; 13 patients achieved M4 deltoid function and 2 patients regained M3. The mean shoulder abduction was 115° and the mean external rotation was 97°.[38]

A recent review of 21 patients with an isolated axillary nerve injury treated with a nerve to the long head of triceps transfer resulted in an average deltoid power of M3.5 ± 1.1.[9] A few studies have also demonstrated that isolated axillary nerve injury can be treated successfully with triceps motor nerve transfer.[39–41] Additional case[42–46] series are summarized in **Table 1**.

Thoracodorsal Nerve to Long Thoracic Nerve Transfer

Palsy of the serratus anterior muscle causes pain, weakness, limitation of shoulder movements, and winging of the scapula (**Fig. 5**).[47] The muscle is innervated by the long thoracic nerve, which usually receives nerve fibers from C5 to C7 roots. However, some patients with C5 and C6 brachial plexus injury in whom there is no C7 contribution to the serratus anterior muscle or in those who have sustained partial injury to C7 root can present with paralysis or weakness of the muscle. In these situations, the thoracodorsal nerve, which is a pure

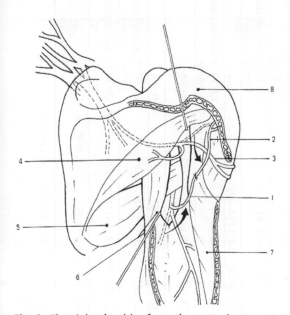

Fig. 3. The right shoulder from the posterior aspect. Nerve transfer to the anterior branch of the axillary nerve using the nerve to the long head of the triceps. (*1*) The nerve to the long head of the triceps. (*2*) The anterior branch of the axillary nerve. (*3*) The posterior branch of the axillary nerve. (*4*) Teres minor muscle. (*5*) Teres major muscle. (*6*) The long head of the triceps. (*7*) The lateral head of the triceps. (*8*) Deltoid muscle (*cut*). (*From* Leechavengvongs S, Witoonchart K, Uerpairojkit C. Combined nerve transfers for C5 and C6 brachial plexus avulsion injury. J Hand Surg Am 2006;31(2):185; with permission.)

Table 1
Published case series of radial to axillary nerve neurotization

Authors and Year	No. of Cases	Average Patient Age, y (Range)	Average Time to Operation, mo (Range)	Average Preoperative Deltoid Abduction	Concomitant Nerve Transfers	Donor Nerve	Average FU (mo)	Median Postoperative Deltoid Strength	Mean Postoperative Shoulder Abduction
Leechavengvongs et al,[31] 2003	7	25 (13–35)	6.3 (3–10)	0/5	CN XI to suprascapular nerve, Oberlin	Long HTB	20	4/5	124°
Bertelli & Ghizoni,[34] 2004	10	28 (19–32)	6.0 (5–7)	0/5	CN XI to suprascapular nerve, Oberlin	7 long HTB, 3 lateral HTB	24	4/5	92°
Kawai & Akitia,[55] 2004	6	20 (15–27)	2.3 (1.3–3)	0/5	5/6 cases: CN XI to suprascapular nerve, Oberlin	Radial	39	—	90° elevation in 5/6; 45° in 1/6
Leechavengvongs et al,[38] 2006	15	27 (13–62)	6.0 (3–10)	0/5	CN XI to suprascapular nerve, Oberlin	Long HTB	32	4/5	115°
Bertelli et al,[13] 2007	3	23 (19–27)	9.0 (8–10)	0/5	None	2 long HTB, 1 medial HTB	18	4/5	Abduction, improved strength by 50%
Bhandari et al,[54] 2008	23	26 (8–38)	5.3 (3–9)	0/5	CN XI to suprascapular, Oberlin	Long HTB	32	4/5	123
Jerome,[44] 2011	5	27 (—)	— (1–6)	—	CN XI to suprascapular nerve	Long HTB	26	5/5	120°
Dahlin et al,[42] 2012	3	12 (9–24)	18.3 (14–22)	3/5	None	Radial	12	4/5	—
Jerome,[43] 2012	6	28 (20–52)	4.2 (3–5)	0/5	CN XI to suprascapular nerve	Long HTB	26	5/5	133°
Jerome & Rajmohan,[45] 2012	9	26 (20–52)	3.8 (3–5)	0/5	None	Long HTB	35	5/5	134°
Lee et al,[9] 2012	21	38 (16–79)	7.6 (4–14)	0/5	None	Long HTB	21	4/5	119°
Lu et al,[46] 2012	9	27 (21–39)	7.0 (3–11)	0/5	CN XI to suprascapular nerve, Oberlin	Long HTB and medial HTB	33	3/5–4/5	Full abduction in 6/9, 50°–130° in 3/9
Kostas-Agnantis et al,[35] 2013	9	27 (21–35)	7.2 (4–11)	0/5	CN XI to suprascapular nerve	Long HTB and medial HTB	18	4/5	112°
Zuckerman et al,[40] 2014	7	6 (0.6–17)	7.0 (5–9)	0/5, 0/4[a]	Oberlin	Long HTB and medial HTB	15	3/4[a], 4/5	>90° in 3/7, = 90° in 3/7, <90° in 1/7

Abbreviations: CN, cranial nerve; FU, follow-up; HTB, head of triceps brachii.
[a] Infant motor scores are on a scale of 0 to 4.
Data from Refs.[9,13,31,34,35,38,40,42–46,54,55]

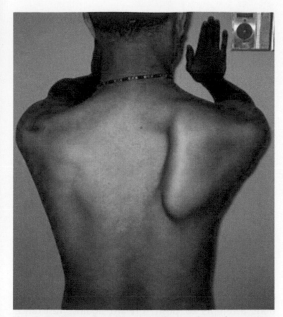

Fig. 5. Prominent, right-winged scapula as the patient attempted to push forward against resistance. (*From* Uerpairojkit C, Leechavengvongs S, Witoonchart K, et al. Nerve transfer to the serratus anterior muscle using the thoracodorsal nerve for winged scapula in C5 and C6 brachial plexus root avulsions. J Hand Surg Am 2009;34:75; with permission.)

motor nerve and receives nerve fibers from C7 and C8 roots, is still preserved and may be used as a donor nerve for transfer.

Preoperative planning

The patient must have at least M4 power of the latissimus dorsi muscle.

Preparation and patient positioning

The patient is placed in the supine position with a sandbag underneath the affected scapula. The arm is placed across the chest.

Surgical approach and procedure

A 12-cm longitudinal incision is made along the posterior axillary fold, which represents the anterior margin of latissimus dorsi. We use fingers to develop the plane between the latissimus dorsi and the pectoralis major. The latissimus dorsi is then retracted posteriorly to expose the thoracodorsal and long thoracic nerves. Dissection around the anterior border of latissimus dorsi will reveal the thoracodorsal nerve and vessels. There are 2 main branches of the nerve, namely, the medial and the lateral. The lateral branch runs parallel to the lateral border of the muscle and the medial branch parallels the upper muscle border and separates from the lateral branch at the neurovascular hilum at an angle of 45°. Use the nerve

stimulator to select the branch that causes the stronger contraction. The selected branch, usually the lateral, is then cut as distally as possible.

The long thoracic nerve appears as a fine silvery white structure situated slightly anterior to the mid-axillary line on the lateral chest wall (**Fig. 6**). In some instances, the fatty tissue around this area may obscure the nerve and make dissection difficult. Again, blunt dissection using fingers is useful in this situation. Release the overlying fascia and take care not to damage the accompanying fine vessels, which bleed easily. Once the paralysis of serratus anterior is confirmed, the nerve is transected as proximally as possible to maximize the amount of muscle that can be reinnervated and to facilitate a tension-free neurorrhaphy with the thoracodorsal nerve (**Fig. 7**).

Immediate postoperative care

The patient's arm is placed in an arm sling for 3 weeks. Rehabilitation aims to prevent shoulder stiffness, but there is no specific motor reeducation program necessary.

Clinical results in the literature

Novak and Mackinnon[48] transferred the medial branch of the thoracodorsal nerve to the long thoracic nerve in a patient with idiopathic serratus anterior muscle weakness. At the 7-year follow-up,

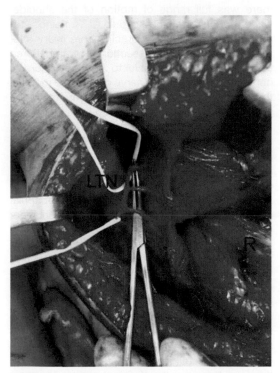

Fig. 6. The long thoracic nerve innervates the serratus anterior muscle. LTN, Long thoracic nerve; R, rib.

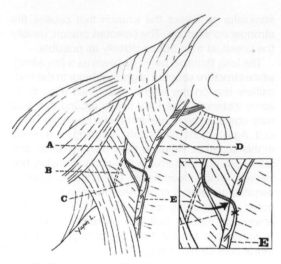

Fig. 7. The right shoulder showing nerve transfer to the long thoracic nerve from the lateral branch of the thoracodorsal nerve. (*A*) The thoracodorsal nerve. (*B*) The lateral branch of the thoracodorsal nerve. (*C*) The medial branch of the thoracodorsal nerve. (*D*) The proximal part of the long thoracic nerve. (*E*) The distal part of the long thoracic nerve. (*From* Uerpairojkit C, Leechavengvongs S, Witoonchart K, et al. Nerve transfer to the serratus anterior muscle using the thoracodorsal nerve for winged scapula in C5 and C6 brachial plexus root avulsions. J Hand Surg Am 2009;34:76; with permission.)

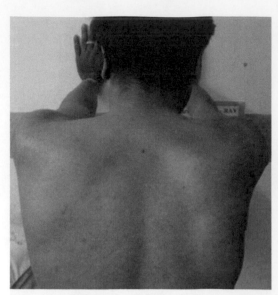

Fig. 8. No winged scapula of the right arm as the patient attempts to push forward against resistance. (*From* Uerpairojkit C, Leechavengvongs S, Witoonchart K, et al. Nerve transfer to the serratus anterior muscle using the thoracodorsal nerve for winged scapula in C5 and C6 brachial plexus root avulsions. J Hand Surg Am 2009;34:77; with permission.)

there was full range of motion of the shoulder without winging of the scapula.[48] Tomaino[49] reported a case of long thoracic nerve injury after axillary lymph node dissection. He transferred the medial pectoral nerve to the long thoracic nerve via an 11-cm sural nerve graft. At 18 months, the scapular winging improved. In our series of 5 patients with C5 to C6 brachial plexus injury who underwent the thoracodorsal nerve transfer to the long thoracic nerve, preoperatively all patients had winged scapula owing to paralysis of the serratus anterior, which was confirmed clinically and electromyographically. At a mean follow-up of 28 months, 2 patients had no winged scapula, and 3 had mild winging. The mean arc of shoulder abduction was 134°. The mean arc of external rotation from full internal rotation was 124°. No patient complained of any functional deficit from harvesting a branch of the thoracodorsal nerve. The overall results were excellent in 2 patients, good in 2 patients, and fair in 1 patient (**Fig. 8**).[50] The outcomes seem to be better than our previous patients with similar injuries but who did not have the additional thoracodorsal nerve transfer.[38] This is echoed by Suzuki and colleagues,[5] who reported the long-term results of spinal accessory nerve transfer to suprascapular nerve in upper brachial

plexus injury. They noted that shoulder flexion and abduction were better among the patients without concomitant paralysis of serratus anterior than those with the paralysis. They thus recommended neurotization of the long thoracic nerve to achieve optimal shoulder function in this group of patients.

Intercostal Nerves to Axillary Nerve Transfer (Posterior Approach)

In C5 to C7 roots avulsion injuries, the triceps is weakened or paralyzed and the radial nerve is thus not suitable as a donor nerve. In this situation, intercostal nerves are potential donor nerves for neurotization of the axillary nerves (**Fig. 9**).

Preoperative planning
Associated rib fracture is a contraindication of using the intercostal nerve as donor nerve.

Preparation and patient positioning
The patient is placed in a supine position with a sandbag beneath the scapula of the affected upper extremity.

Surgical approach and procedure
For exposure of the intercostal nerve, a curvilinear incision extending from the parasternal border to the midaxillary line is made along the inferior border of the fifth rib. The pectoralis major and

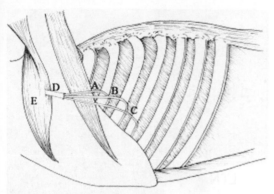

Fig. 9. Nerve transfer to the anterior axillary branch of the axillary nerve using the third, fourth, and fifth intercostal nerves: third intercostal (*A*), fourth intercostal (*B*), fifth intercostal nerve (*C*), the anterior axillary branch of the axillary nerve (*D*), and deltoid muscle (*E*). (*From* Malungpaishrope K, Leechavengvongs S, Uerpairojkit C, et al. Nerve transfer to deltoid muscle using the intercostal nerves through the posterior approach: an anatomic study and two case reports. J Hand Surg 2007;32(A):219; with permission.)

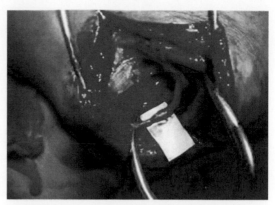

Fig. 10. The fourth and the fifth intercostal nerves transferred directly to the anterior axillary nerve through the posterior approach. (*From* Malungpaishrope K, Leechavengvongs S, Uerpairojkit C, et al. Nerve transfer to deltoid muscle using the intercostal nerves through the posterior approach: an anatomic study and two case reports. J Hand Surg 2007;32(A):221; with permission.)

minor are elevated to expose the fourth to sixth ribs. We usually use 2 intercostal nerves from the fourth to the fifth ribs as donor. Anterior fascia of each rib is incised. The rib periosteal elevator is used to dissect and elevate each rib from the external and internal intercostal muscles. The internal intercostal membrane is then incised along the inferior border of each rib. Each intercostal nerve is identified underneath the internal intercostal muscle. Dissection starts from the parasternal border to the midaxillary line. Great care is needed not to damage the delicate intercostal nerve, vessels, or the pleura. Just anterior to the midaxillary line, the sensory branch of each intercostal nerve is identified and cut to enhance the mobility of the intercostal nerve.

The exposure of the axillary nerve through a posterior approach has been described in previous section. The intercostal nerves are passed through a subcutaneous tunnel in the axilla to reach the axillary nerve. After performing the transfer, full passive shoulder abduction is confirmed intraoperatively to ensure that there is no undue tension on the neurorrhaphy (**Fig. 10**).

Postoperative care and rehabilitation

The patient's arm is immobilized with a sling for 3 weeks. After that, the patient is advised to exercise in the supine position. Cortical retraining involves shrugging the shoulder (spinal accessory nerve) and attempting trunk flexion and deep inspiration (intercostal nerves) to effect shoulder

abduction.[51] This is continued until abduction can be achieved with the gravity eliminated. Then, the same exercises are performed in the upright position.

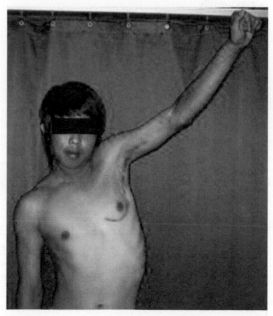

Fig. 11. Patient showing good abduction of left shoulder 2 years after surgery. (*From* Malungpaishrope K, Leechavengvongs S, Uerpairojkit C, et al. Nerve transfer to deltoid muscle using the intercostal nerves through the posterior approach: an anatomic study and two case reports. J Hand Surg 2007;32(A):222; with permission.)

Clinical results

Chuang and colleagues[4] reported less than 20° of shoulder abduction using either the phrenic or spinal accessory nerve transfer to neurotize the axillary nerve. Samardzić and colleagues[52] reported 33% excellent and good results from using the intercostal nerve transfer to the axillary nerve. In contrast, Malungpaishrope and colleagues[53] reported an average shoulder abduction of 69° in 10 patients who underwent combined spinal accessory nerve transfer to the suprascapular nerve and 2 intercostal nerves transfer to the anterior axillary nerve (**Fig. 11**).

Intercostal Nerves to Long Thoracic Nerve Transfer

If the thoracodorsal nerve is not available and there is paralysis of serratus anterior, we would recommend using the intercostal nerves to neurotize the long thoracic nerve (**Fig. 12**).

Preoperative planning

A history of severe blunt chest trauma or rib fracture is contraindication to using the intercostal nerves.

Preparation and patient positioning

The patient is placed in a supine position with a sandbag beneath the scapula of the affected upper extremity.

Surgical approach and procedure

The exposures of the intercostal nerve and the long thoracic nerve have already been described. We prefer to use the sixth and seventh intercostal nerves to neurotize the long thoracic nerve.

Postoperative care and rehabilitation

Postoperative care and rehabilitation are similar to intercostal nerve to axillary nerve transfer.

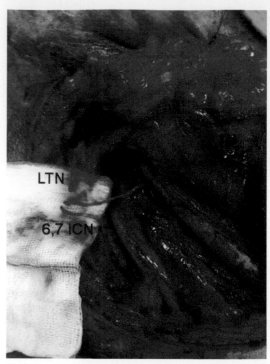

Fig. 12. The sixth and the seventh intercostal nerve and the long thoracic nerve. 6,7 ICN, sixth and seventh intercostal nerve; LTN, long thoracic nerve.

Clinical results

In upper brachial plexus avulsion injuries, we recommend using 2 intercostal nerves to neurotize the long thoracic nerve combined with spinal accessory nerve transfer to the suprascapular nerve for shoulder reconstruction. In addition, we would recommend simultaneous reanimation of the triceps brachii muscle by transferring 3 intercostal nerves (third to fifth ribs) to the radial nerve. We have used this strategy in 3 of our patients. At a

---

Table 2
Our current treatment algorithm for nerve transfers to restore the shoulder function in different situations

Extent of Nerve Injuries	Our Preferred Nerve Transfers
Isolated axillary nerve injury	Long head of triceps nerve to anterior branch of axillary nerve
C5 root injury or combined suprascapular and axillary nerve injuries	Spinal accessory nerve to suprascapular nerve Long head of triceps nerve to anterior branch of axillary nerve
C5 and C6 roots injury	Spinal accessory nerve to suprascapular nerve Long head of triceps nerve to anterior branch of axillary nerve Thoracodorsal nerve to long thoracic nerve (in case of winged scapula)
C5, C6 and C7 roots injury	Spinal accessory nerve to suprascapular nerve Two intercostal nerves to the anterior branch of axillary nerve or to the long thoracic nerve
Panplexus injury	Spinal accessory nerve to suprascapular nerve

mean 2 years of follow-up, 2 patients achieved M4 and 1 M3 shoulder abduction. The average shoulder abduction was 93° (Malungpaishrope and colleagues, unpublished data, 2015).

SUMMARY

The restoration of shoulder function after brachial plexus injury represents a significant challenge facing the peripheral nerve surgeons. This is owing to a combination of the complex biomechanics of the shoulder girdle, the multitude of muscles and nerves that could be potentially injured, and a limited number of donor options. In general, nerve transfer is favored over tendon transfer, because the biomechanics of the musculotendinous units are not altered. Our current preferred options of nerve transfers to restore the shoulder function in different situations are presented in **Table 2**.

REFERENCES

1. Sinnatamby CS. Last's anatomy. Regional and applied. 10th edition. London: Churchill Livingstone; 1999.
2. Samardzic M, Grujicic D, Antunovic V. Nerve transfer in brachial plexus traction injuries. J Neurosurg 1992;76(2):191–7.
3. Merrell GA, Barrie KA, Katz DL, et al. Results of nerve transfer techniques for restoration of shoulder and elbow function in the context of a meta-analysis of the English literature. J Hand Surg Am 2001;26(2):303–14.
4. Chuang DC, Lee GW, Hashem F, et al. Restoration of shoulder abduction by nerve transfer in avulsed brachial plexus injury: evaluation of 99 patients with various nerve transfers. Plast Reconstr Surg 1995;96(1):122–8.
5. Suzuki K, Doi K, Hattori Y, et al. Long-term results of spinal accessory nerve transfer to the suprascapular nerve in upper-type paralysis of brachial plexus injury. J Reconstr Microsurg 2007;23(6):295–9.
6. Perlmutter GS. Axillary nerve injury. Clin Orthop Relat Res 1999;(368):28–36.
7. Steinmann SP, Moran EA. Axillary nerve injury: diagnosis and treatment. J Am Acad Orthop Surg 2001; 9(5):328–35.
8. Narakas AO. Paralytic disorders of the shoulder girdle. Hand Clin 1988;4(4):619–32.
9. Lee JY, Kircher MF, Spinner RJ, et al. Factors affecting outcome of triceps motor branch transfer for isolated axillary nerve injury. J Hand Surg Am 2012;37(11):2350–6.
10. Bertelli JA, Ghizoni MF. Nerve transfer from triceps medial head and anconeus to deltoid for axillary nerve palsy. J Hand Surg Am 2014;39(5):940–7.
11. Sher JS, Uribe JW, Posada A, et al. Abnormal findings on magnetic resonance images of asymptomatic shoulders. J Bone Joint Surg Am 1995;77(1):10–5.
12. Tempelhof S, Rupp S, Seil R. Age-related prevalence of rotator cuff tears in asymptomatic shoulders. J Shoulder Elbow Surg 1999;8(4):296–9.
13. Bertelli JA, Ghizoni MF. Transfer of the accessory nerve to the suprascapular nerve in brachial plexus reconstruction. J Hand Surg Am 2007; 32(7):989–98.
14. Cardenas-Mejia A, O'Boyle CP, Chen KT, et al. Evaluation of single-, double-, and triple-nerve transfers for shoulder abduction in 90 patients with supraclavicular brachial plexus injury. Plast Reconstr Surg 2008;122(5):1470–8.
15. Malessy MJ, de Ruiter GC, de Boer KS, et al. Evaluation of suprascapular nerve neurotization after nerve graft or transfer in the treatment of brachial plexus traction lesions. J Neurosurg 2004;101(3): 377–89.
16. Soncharoen P, Wongtrakul S, Spinner RJ. Brachial plexus injuries in the adult nerve transfers: the Siriraj Hospital experience. Hand Clin 2005;21(1):83–9.
17. Guan SB, Chen DS, Fang YS, et al. An anatomic study of the descending branch of the spinal accessory nerve transfer for the repair of suprascapular nerve to restore the abduction function of the shoulder through the dorsal-approach. Chin J Hand Surg (Chin) 2004;20:55–7.
18. Ozer Y, Grossman JA, Gilbert A. Anatomic observations on the suprascapular nerve. Hand Clin 1995; 11(4):539–44.
19. Pereira MT, Williams WW. The spinal accessory nerve distal to the posterior triangle. J Hand Surg Br 1999;24(3):368–9.
20. Dailiana ZH, Mehdian H, Gilbert A. Surgical anatomy of spinal accessory nerve: is trapezius functional deficit inevitable after division of the nerve? J Hand Surg Br 2001;26(2):137–41.
21. Alnot JY. Traumatic brachial plexus lesions in the adult. Indications and results. Hand Clin 1995; 11(4):623–31.
22. Pruksakorn D, Sananpanich K, Khunamornpong S, et al. Posterior approach technique for accessory-suprascapular nerve transfer: a cadaveric study of the anatomical landmarks and number of myelinated axons. Clin Anat 2007;20(2):140–3.
23. Colbert SH, Mackinnon S. Posterior approach for double nerve transfer for restoration of shoulder function in upper brachial plexus palsy. Hand (N Y) 2006;1(2):71–7.
24. Guan SB, Hou CL, Chen DS, et al. Restoration of shoulder abduction by transfer of the spinal accessory nerve to suprascapular nerve through dorsal approach. a clinical study. Chin Med J (Engl) 2006;119(9):707–12.
25. Bhandari PS, Sadhotra LP, Bhargava P, et al. Dorsal approach in spinal accessory to suprascapular nerve transfer in brachial plexus injuries: technique details. IJNT 2010;7(1):71–4.

26. Rui J, Zhao X, Zhu Y, et al. Posterior approach for accessory-suprascapular nerve transfer: an electrophysiological outcomes study. J Hand Surg Eur Vol 2013;38(3):242–7.

27. Souza FH, Bernardino SN, Filho HC, et al. Comparison between the anterior and posterior approach for transfer of the spinal accessory nerve to the suprascapular nerve in late traumatic brachial plexus injuries. Acta Neurochir (Wien) 2014;156(12):2345–9.

28. Lurje A. Concerning surgical treatment of traumatic injury of the upper division of the brachial plexus (Erb's-type). Ann Surg 1948;127(2):317–26.

29. Nath RK, Mackinnon SE. Nerve transfers in the upper extremity. Hand Clin 2000;16(1):131–9.

30. Witoonchart K, Leechavengvongs S, Uerpairojkit C, et al. Nerve transfer to deltoid muscle using the nerve to the long head of the triceps, part I: an anatomic feasibility study. J Hand Surg Am 2003;28(4):628–32.

31. Leechavengvongs S, Witoonchart K, Uerpairojkit C, et al. Nerve transfer to deltoid muscle using the nerve to the long head of the triceps, part II: a report of 7 cases. J Hand Surg Am 2003;28(4):633–8.

32. Okazaki M, Al-Shawi A, Gschwind CR, et al. Outcome of axillary nerve injuries treated with nerve grafts. J Hand Surg Eur Vol 2011;36(7):535–40.

33. Leechavengvongs S, Teerawutthichaikit T, Witoonchart K, et al. Surgical anatomy of the axillary nerve branches to the deltoid muscle. Clin Anat 2015;28(1):118–22.

34. Bertelli JA, Ghizoni MF. Reconstruction of C5 and C6 brachial plexus avulsion injury by multiple nerve transfers: spinal accessory to suprascapular, ulnar fascicles to biceps branch, and triceps long or lateral head branch to axillary nerve. J Hand Surg Am 2004;29(1):131–9.

35. Kostas-Agnantis I, Korompilias A, Vekris M, et al. Shoulder abduction and external rotation restoration with nerve transfer. Injury 2013;44(3):299–304.

36. Uerpairojkit C, Ketwongwiriya S, Leechavengvongs S, et al. Surgical anatomy of the radial nerve branches to triceps muscle. Clin Anat 2013;26(3):386–91.

37. Travill AA. Electromyographic study of the extensor apparatus of the forearm. Anat Rec 1962;144(4):373–6.

38. Leechavengvongs S, Witoonchart K, Uerpairojkit C, et al. Combined nerve transfers for C5 and C6 brachial plexus avulsion injury. J Hand Surg Am 2006;31(2):183–9.

39. Wheelock M, Clark TA, Giuffre JL. Nerve transfers for treatment of isolated axillary nerve injuries. Plast Surg (Oakv) 2015;23(2):77–80.

40. Zuckerman SL, Eli IM, Shah MN, et al. Radial to axillary nerve neurotization for brachial plexus injury in children: a combined case series. J Neurosurg Pediatr 2014;14(5):518–26.

41. Chim H, Kircher MF, Spinner RJ, et al. Triceps motor branch transfer for isolated traumatic pediatric axillary nerve injuries. J Neurosurg Pediatr 2015; 15(1):107–11.

42. Dahlin LB, Cöster M, Björkman A, et al. Axillary nerve injury in young adults–an overlooked diagnosis? Early results of nerve reconstruction and nerve transfers. J Plast Surg Hand Surg 2012; 46(3–4):257–61.

43. Jerome JT. Anterior deltopectoral approach for axillary nerve neurotisation. J Orthop Surg (Hong Kong) 2012;20(1):66–70.

44. Jerome JT. Long head of the triceps branch transfer to axillary nerve in C5, C6 brachial plexus injuries: anterior approach. Plast Reconstr Surg 2011; 128(3):740–1.

45. Jerome JT, Rajmohan B. Axillary nerve neurotization with the anterior deltopectoral approach in brachial plexus injuries. Microsurgery 2012;32(6):445–51.

46. Lu J, Xu J, Xu W, et al. Combined nerve transfers for repair of the upper brachial plexus injuries through a posterior approach. Microsurgery 2012; 32(2):111–7.

47. Warner JJ, Navarro RA. Serratus anterior dysfunction. Recognition and treatment. Clin Orthop Relat Res 1998;(349):139–48.

48. Novak CB, Mackinnon SE. Surgical treatment of a long thoracic nerve palsy. Ann Thorac Surg 2002; 73(5):1643–5.

49. Tomaino MM. Neurophysiologic and clinical outcome following medial pectoral to long thoracic nerve transfer for scapular winging: a case report. Microsurgery 2002;22(6):254–7.

50. Uerpairojkit C, Leechavengvongs S, Witoonchart K, et al. Nerve transfer to serratus anterior muscle using the thoracodorsal nerve for winged scapula in C5 and C6 brachial plexus root avulsions. J Hand Surg Am 2009;34(1):74–8.

51. Chalidapong P, Sananpanich K, Klaphajone J. Electromyographic comparison of various exercises to improve elbow flexion following intercostal nerve transfer. J Bone Joint Surg Br 2006;88(5):620–2.

52. Samardzić M, Rasulić L, Grujicić D, et al. Results of nerve transfers to the musculocutaneous and axillary nerves. Neurosurgery 2000;46(1):93–101.

53. Malungpaishrope K, Leechavengvongs S, Witoonchart K, et al. Simultaneous intercostal nerve transfers to deltoid and triceps muscle through the posterior approach. J Hand Surg Am 2012;37(4):677–82.

54. Bhandari PS, Sadhotra LP, Bhargava P, et al. Multiple nerve transfers for the reanimation of shoulder and elbow functions in irreparable C5, C6 and upper truncal lesions of the brachial plexus. IJNT 2008; 5(2):95–104.

55. Kawai H, Akitia S. Shoulder muscle reconstruction in the upper type of the brachial plexus injury by partial radial nerve transfer to the axillary nerve. Tech Hand Up Extrem Surg 2004;8:51–5.

Nerve Transfers to Restore Elbow Function

Liselotte F. Bulstra, BS[a,b], Alexander Y. Shin, MD[a,*]

KEYWORDS

- Nerve transfers • Elbow flexion • Elbow extension • Proximal nerve injury • Nerve root avulsion
- Brachial plexus injury

KEY POINTS

- Elbow flexion is considered the most important function of the upper limb.
- Nerve transfers allow for conversion of a proximal nerve injury to a more distal injury.
- The functional gain of the recipient nerve should be greater than the expected functional loss from the donor nerve.
- The use of interpositional nerve grafts to bridge gaps in transferred nerves should be avoided.
- Nerve transfers can also be used for innervation of free-functioning muscle transfers.

INTRODUCTION

Elbow flexion is considered the most important function to restore in the paralyzed upper extremity as it provides positioning of the hand in a useful position for daily activities. Elbow extension is necessary to stabilize the elbow, to achieve a stable grasp, and for any activity that requires the arm to be lifted above horizontal position. Moreover, in cases of insufficient (M0 to M2) recovery of elbow flexion with primary surgery, the reinnervated triceps could be transferred to provide this function.[1]

Causes of loss of elbow function include traumatic brachial plexus injury, spinal cord injuries, and injury to the nerves innervating the elbow flexors and/or extensors such as stab wounds, gunshot injuries, radiation-induced neuropathies, and brachial plexus birth palsy.[2,3] When direct nerve repair is not possible, and nerve grafting is not expected to provide satisfactory results, nerve transfers are a viable option. The role of nerve transfers has expanded drastically in the past 15 years, providing a commonly used treatment strategy for the restoration of elbow function, being used for direct neurotization of target muscles as well as neurotization of free-functioning muscle transfers (FFMTs).[4,5]

HISTORICAL PERSPECTIVE

Nerve transfers were described in the early 20th century by Harris[6] and Tuttle,[7] who in 1913 reported coaptation of the anterior terminal branch of C4 to the split upper trunk. Unfortunately, results were not well recorded in these early cases.

A seminal advancement was the application of intercostal nerves for the neurotization of the musculocutaneous nerve described by Seddon[8] in 1961. The unsatisfactory results were secondary to the interposition nerve grafts, and subsequently Tsuyama and Hara[9] modified the technique such that direct intercostal to motor biceps branch could be performed. The use of intercostal nerves to innervate the musculocutaneous nerve was further popularized by Narakas,[10] and good results have been reported by multiple groups.[11–15] The challenge of restoration

No conflicts of interest are declared by any author on this study.
Source of Funding: No disclosures of funding were received for this work.
[a] Department of Orthopedic Surgery, Mayo Clinic, 200 First Street Southwest, Rochester, MN 55905, USA;
[b] Department of Plastic, Reconstructive and Hand Surgery, Erasmus Medical Center, 's-Gravendijkwal 230, 3015 CE Rotterdam, The Netherlands
* Corresponding author.
E-mail address: shin.alexander@mayo.edu

of elbow flexion worldwide resulted in many groups exploring the potential of different donor nerves, expanding the options that were already described by Lurje[16] in 1948, including the long thoracic nerve, medial and lateral pectoral nerve, radial nerve, and thoracodorsal and subscapular nerve.[17–19] More recent developments in nerve transfers for elbow function, the ulnar nerve fascicle transfer as described by Oberlin,[20] and transfer of fascicles of the median nerve as described by Mackinnon and colleagues[21] successfully moved the coaptation site more distal, further improving functional outcome. Over the past decade, many of these options have been modified and refined resulting in more reliable restoration of elbow function.

INDICATIONS AND CONTRAINDICATIONS

Nerve transfers are indicated in patients with no hope for spontaneous recovery or improvement of their nerve injury. Possible indications and contraindications are described in **Table 1**.[22,23] It is important to note that strategies of reconstruction have evolved and changed and will continue to do so. Some authors prefer not to explore the brachial plexus, stating that the surgery is difficult, especially in a scarred bed, and proceed to nerve transfers, while others always explore the brachial plexus to evaluate for viable nerve roots that can be used with nerve grafts to critical targets in lieu of nerve transfers. Although this controversy will remain until better outcome studies are performed, it is the authors' philosophy to explore every acute (<6–7 months after injury) brachial plexus injury and evaluate the nerve roots. If a viable root exists, it will be used with nerve grafts to target shoulder girdle musculature. If a second viable root exists, it will be used with nerve grafts to target elbow flexion or extension.

PRINCIPLES OF NERVE TRANSFERS

The principle of nerve transfers is the coaptation of one or more healthy (Medical Research Council [MRC]>4) but expandable nerves or nerve fascicles to an injured more important nerve, distal to the site of injury (**Box 1**).

TIMING

The timing of the surgery should be carefully considered based on multiple factors including mechanism of injury, physical examination, and imaging results, as well as the surgeon's preference. Because of the degeneration of motor endplates that becomes mostly irreversible after approximately 12 to 18 months in adult patients, the observation period prior to surgery should be limited, and nerve transfers should be performed within 6 to 9 months after injury.[5,12,18,24–28] Some authors have expanded the time to surgery up to 12 months. Ideally, nerve surgery should be performed prior to 6 months when and if possible.

DESCRIPTION OF NERVE TRANSFER OPTIONS

For elbow flexion, the goal is to innervate the musculocutaneous nerve (MCN), or specifically the biceps (and/or brachialis) branch.[29] For elbow extension, either the whole radial nerve or branches to the long head of the triceps (BLHT) can be targeted.[30] Intraplexal donors are preferred when available.[31] Different nerve transfers may be combined to yield best functional outcome. In selecting the most appropriate donor, the number of motor axons, the distance between donor and recipient nerve and the size match with the recipient nerve should be considered. Different neurotization techniques for restoration of both elbow flexion and extension will be described in more detail.

Table 1	
Indications and contraindications for nerve transfers	
Indications	**Contraindications**
<ul><li>Preganglionic injury (ie, nerve root avulsions)</li><li>High peripheral nerve injuries</li><li>Multiple level nerve injuries</li><li>Delayed presentation (between 6–12 mo)</li><li>Large neuromas in continuity</li><li>Innervation for free functioning muscle transfer</li></ul>	<ul><li>Absolute contraindications<ul><li>Less invasive options possible</li><li>Spontaneous recovery expected</li><li>Irreversible damage of atrophy of recipient muscles (>12 mo from injury)</li><li>Unmotivated patient for invasive procedure and intensive rehabilitation</li></ul></li><li>Relative contraindications<ul><li>Joint stiffness and contractures, patient age, comorbidities, traumatic brain injury, or spinal cord injury</li></ul></li></ul>

<table>
<tr><td>

Box 1
General principles of nerve transfers

- Nerve transfers allow for conversion of a proximal nerve injury to a more distal injury, decreased time to reinnervation, preventing motor end-plate degeneration.

- A large number of "pure motor" axons can be delivered

- Extensive dissection in a scarred wound bed can be avoided

- Aim to avoid the use of nerve grafts and therefore an extra anastomosis, considering the better functional outcomes.

- The use of donor nerves with a synergistic function as the recipient is preferred but not necessary.

</td></tr>
</table>

Ulnar Fascicular Transfer (Oberlin)

Since its description by Oberlin and colleagues,[20] this technique has become widely accepted. A fascicle of the ulnar nerve to the Flexor Carpi Ulnaris (FCU) is divided and transferred to the biceps motor branch, as shown in **Fig. 1**.[20,32] This technique is only suitable for patients with preserved C8-T1 function and is most frequently used for

C5-6 injury, but success for C5-7 injuries has also been reported.[33] Important advantages of this technique are the relative technical ease and quick reinnervation, as the nerve coaptation site is close to the motor endplates. The first recovery of biceps contraction usually begins several months after the procedure. Adequate grip strength (more than 10 kg) should be present prior to considering this technique.[32]

The Oberlin procedure is one of the most successful techniques to restore useful elbow flexion in adult upper trunk brachial plexus injury, achieving MRC grade 3 strength or better in the vast majority of patients with no evidence of donor site morbidity.[20,34–37] Although early reinnervation is preferred, Sedain and colleagues[38] performed this procedure in 9 patients with brachial plexus injury 7 to 24 months after injury and found useful biceps recovery (MRC≥3) in almost 80%.

Flores[30] and Pet and colleagues[39] transferred a motor fascicle of the ulnar nerve to the BLHT, obtaining M4 or better elbow extension in 4 cases.

Double Fascicular Transfer

As described by Tung and colleagues[40] and Ray and colleagues,[41] in addition to neurotization of

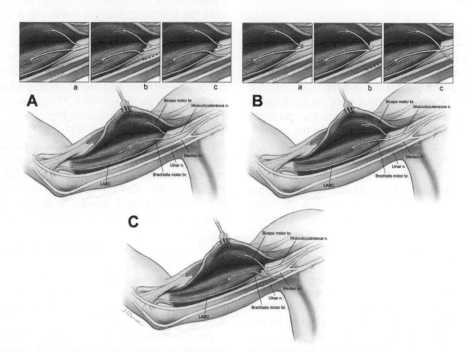

Fig. 1. Schematic overview of the double fascicular nerve transfer. (*A*) The brachialis motor branch and suitable median nerve fascicle are identified (details in left upper panes). (*B*) The biceps motor branch and ulnar nerve fascicle to the FCU are identified (details in right upper panes). (*C*) The median nerve fascicle is coapted to the brachialis motor branch and the ulnar nerve fascicle to the biceps motor branch. (*Courtesy of* Mayo Foundation, Rochester, MN; with permission.)

the biceps, the brachialis muscle can be neurotized to improve functional outcome. Local donor nerve options are provided by median nerve fascicles to the flexor carpi radialis (FCR), flexor digitorum superficialis (FDS), or palmaris longus.[40] A schematic overview of this technique is shown in **Fig. 1**. For patients with weakness and sensory deficit in the median or ulnar nerve distribution regions preoperatively, other strategies should be considered.

This combined nerve transfer has shown an over 80% recovery of ≥M4 elbow flexion strength with minimal donor morbidity in the outcomes from Tung and Ray.[5,21,40–42] In contradistinction, Carlsen and colleagues[33] found that there was not a statistical improvement in elbow flexion strength using the double versus the single nerve transfer and recommended sparing the median nerve for another use. Martins and colleagues[43] prospectively compared outcomes and morbidity of the single and double fascicular nerve transfer. This study showed no significant differences between the 2 procedures regarding elbow flexion strength. Donor site morbidity including detoriation of grip strength and sensibility were observed in a small number of patients and resolved during follow-up. No differences were observed between the groups, supporting the findings of Carlsen and colleagues.[33]

Medial Pectoral Nerve

In patients with upper (C5-6) or upper extended (C5-7) brachial plexus palsy, collateral motor branches of the plexus are available as regional donor.[44,45] When using the medial pectoral nerve (MPN), selecting only one of its multiple branches can preserve innervation of the pectoralis sternal head.[46] The number of motor fibers in the MPN ranges from 1170 to 2140 in the main trunk and 400 to 600 fibers in a muscular branch.[45] An important disadvantage of this nerve is the large discrepancy in nerve diameter with the MCN and the limited length of most MPNs.[40]

Multiple series have been published regarding MPN to MCN transfer reporting variable but encouraging results with useful recovery (≥M3) in 60% to 100% of the cases. Of the studies reporting M4 recovery, the average M4 recovery was 71%.[40,44–50] The variability in outcome may be explained by the different solutions chosen by different groups to overcome the diameter mismatch, including combination with other nerve transfers (intercostals, spinal accessory).

As shown by Flores,[51] the MPN can also be used for triceps reinnervation in patients sustaining C5-7 brachial plexus palsies. Targeting either the radial nerve or the BLHT, M3 was found in 5 and M4 in 7 of 12 cases (58%).

Thoracodorsal Nerve

The thoracodorsal nerve (TDN) receives nerve fibers from C7 (more than 52%), C8, and sometimes C6 nerve roots and innervates the latissimus dorsi muscle.[45,52] The mean surgically useable length of the nerve is 12.3 cm, with an average of 2409 myelinated fibers.[53,54] An important advantage of the TDN in comparison to the MPN is its sufficient length for direct coaptation to the biceps nerve.

Different studies found consistently good MRC grade 3 or higher biceps recovery in 85% to 100% of patients, with an average reported grade 4 or higher in 50% of patients.[45,48,50,55–59] Using the thoracodorsal nerve, Soldado and colleagues[60] found MRC 4 triceps recovery in 7 out of their 8 patients and MRC 3 in 1 patient. None of the studies found serious adverse effects of the (partial) denervation of the latissimus dorsi muscle.

Intercostal Nerves

If donor nerves from within the brachial plexus are not available, extraplexal nerves such as intercostal nerves (ICNs) can be transferred to reinnervate the biceps or triceps. Generally 3 to 4 ICNs provide a good size match for musculocutaneous nerve innervation or 2 to 3 ICNs for biceps motor branch or triceps reinnervation.[61–63] The third to sixth ICN often allows for direct coaptation to the MCN. The sensory and motor components, which contain 1300 axons, of the ICN can be separated for the delivery of more pure motor axons.[64] ICN to MCN transfer is shown in **Fig. 2**. The lateral antebrachial cutaneous nerve can be separated from the biceps branch of the MCN to allow a maximum number of motor axons to reach the target muscle. Pulmonary function can be temporarily impaired but normalizes by 3 months.[65] When chest wall trauma is present, ICN may be damaged, although this is rare.

ICNs are also used for the innervation of free functioning muscle transfers (FFMT) for late brachial (pan)plexus injuries (presenting 7–8 months or later after injury). This procedure can be combined with innervation of the native biceps with ICN, as shown in **Fig. 3**.[66,67]

For biceps flexion, it takes at least 12 months for patients to learn to flex the joint voluntarily.[61] Coughing and sneezing may continue to cause involuntary muscle contractions.[68]

The influence of interposition nerve grafts for ICN transfers is controversial in the literature.

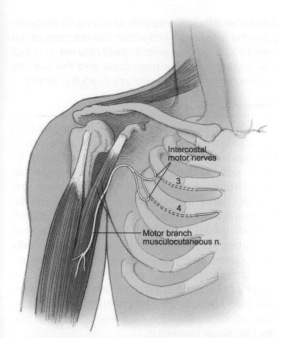

Fig. 2. Transfer of the third and fourth Intercostal motor nerves to the musculocutaneous nerve for restoration of elbow flexion. (*Courtesy of* Mayo Foundation, Rochester, MN; with permission.)

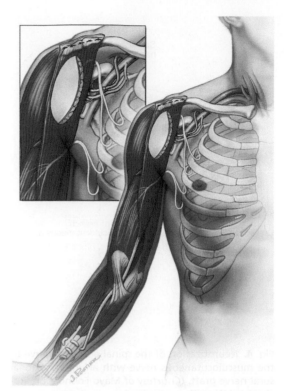

Fig. 3. Combined neurotization of both the native biceps muscle and free functioning muscle transfers (FFMT) with intercostal nerves. A skin paddle is used for monitoring of the FFMT. (*Courtesy of* Mayo Foundation, Rochester, MN; with permission.)

Although nerve grafts allow for the use of more proximal parts of the ICN to avoid loss of motor axons, having an extra coaptation site could impair recovery.[62] A meta-analysis by Merrell and colleagues[5] describes restoration of elbow flexion MRC grade 3 strength or better in 72% of patients when a direct coaptation was performed compared to 47% of the patients with an interposition nerve graft. This significant difference advocates avoiding interposition grafts when possible. More recent studies show more variable results of elbow flexion after ICN to MCN transfer, ranging from 33% to 89% of patients reaching functional recovery.[50,69–72]

For elbow extension, an advantage is that the radial nerve is spared, which gives a chance of spontaneous triceps recovery by reinnervation from the C8 root. Results of triceps reinnervation with ICN are strongly variable.[30,73–76]

One of the main drawbacks of intercostal nerve transfer is the need to prevent abduction and external rotation of the shoulder greater than 90° and 90° respectively. Such motion can potentially disrupt the nerve coaptation. Thus in patients who have good potential for shoulder function recovery, an alternative nerve transfer should be considered. Intercostal nerve transfers are typically used in patients with panplexus avulsive injuries when no other options exist.

Spinal Accessory Nerve (Cranial Nerve XI)

When using the spinal accessory nerve for neurotization, a distal branch of this nerve is used to spare the innervation of the trapezius muscle. In brachial plexus injury, the spinal accessory nerve (with approximately 1700 axons) is frequently preferred for neurotization of the suprascapular nerve but is also successfully used to restore elbow flexion.[5,28,64,77] If used for elbow flexion, an intervening nerve graft is typically necessary as shown in **Fig. 4.** Similar to the ICN, the spinal accessory can also be used for the innervation of FFMT.[4]

The first signs of recovery of biceps function may be seen after 6 to 15 months.[50] A meta-analysis described a recovery rate of 77% ≥ M3 and 29% ≥ M4 for biceps strength.[5] Later series confirmed the effectiveness of the spinal accessory to MCN transfer, reporting a functional recovery rate of 65% and 66%.[50,69] Grafts less than 12 cm and operation within 6 months after injury show significantly better results.[78] When compared, ICN transfers show a better ability to achieve ≥ M4 elbow strength than the spinal accessory nerve (41% vs 29%, $P<.001$).[5]

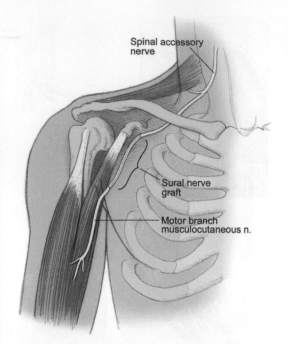

Fig. 4. Neurotization of the spinal accessory nerve to the musculocutaneous nerve with an interpositional sural nerve graft. (*Courtesy of* Mayo Foundation, Rochester, MN; with permission.)

Reports on the use of the spinal accessory nerve for triceps reinnervation (with an interpositional graft) are not sufficient to draw any conclusions about the usefulness of this transfer for elbow extension.[30]

Contralateral C7

The use of the contralateral C7 (cC7) was first described by Gu and colleagues[64] in 1991, providing a new extraplexal donor. Either the complete cC7 or partial C7 can be used, providing a sufficient amount of nerve fibers (approx. 24,000 for the whole C7).[9,64,79]

During the past 15 years, several groups implemented cC7 transfer for reconstruction of elbow function. Functional (≥M3) biceps recovery varies strongly among groups, ranging from 33% to 85%.[9,79–82] Functional triceps recovery is achieved in only 20% to 66% of patients.[79,81,82]

Immediately after surgery, temporary motor and sensory deficits always occur, usually recovering within 6 months due to cross-innervation by other spinal nerves. An important disadvantage is the need for extremely long nerve grafts despite alternative proposed techniques.[83,84] Regarding functional outcome, the most important issue is that independent function after this transfer is often not achieved. This means that patients need to activate muscles previously innervated by the C7 in their normal

arm to bend their injured arm, which significantly impairs the function.[19] Altogether, the outcome of the (hemi-)cC7 does not seem to justify the risk of donor site morbidity of this procedure, and the authors have abandoned the procedure in adult patients.

Phrenic Nerve

The phrenic nerve (approximately 800 myelinated axons) is often functioning in cases of complete brachial plexus avulsion injuries as a result of its major contributions from C3 and C4, providing an extraplexal nerve donor.[66,85,86] When the phrenic nerve is harvested in a supraclavicular fashion, it always needs an intervening nerve graft to reach the MCN; to reach the anterior division of the upper trunk (ADUT) nerve grafts are typically not required, yielding similar results.[87] An alternative harvesting route using video-assisted thoracic surgery (VATS) has been proposed by Xu and colleagues,[88] providing direct coaptation to the MCN and significantly faster recovery compared with the traditional technique.

Biceps contractions can be expected 8 to 9 months after surgery, initiated by a deep breath.[89] Functional biceps recovery is by most groups achieved in 70% to 85% of the patients.[65,75,87–93] Phrenic and intercostal nerve transfers provide similar results in global brachial plexus injury.[94] A drawback of the phrenic nerve transfer is that long-term effects on pulmonary function remain unknown.[65,75,93]

Flores[30] used the phrenic nerve for triceps recovery. Out of 7 patients, 5 showed meaningful recovery. It seems that coaptation to the BLHT may be more successful than coaptation to the whole radial nerve, but larger numbers need to be studied.

Hypoglossal Nerve

Two studies report a case of biceps neurotization using part of the hypoglossal nerve. Although both Bertelli and colleagues[95] and Malessy and colleagues[96] report good functional recovery of M4 and M5 respectively, significant adverse effects have been reported. Even after 5 years follow-up, tongue movement still provoked biceps contraction, and patients did not become able to regain volitional control over the target muscle.[95,96] Therefore, the hypoglossal nerve does not seem to provide a suitable nerve for reconstruction of elbow function.

Posterior Branch of the Axillary Nerve

For restoration of elbow extension, a nerve transfer to the triceps using the posterior branch of the axillary nerve was recently described.[97] **Fig. 5** describes the technique that was used.

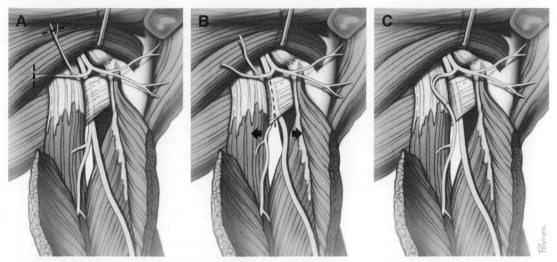

Fig. 5. Transfer of the posterior branch of the axillary nerve branches to the triceps branch. (*A*) The posterior axillary nerve branches to the teres minor and posterior deltoid are identified and separated. (*B*) The branch to the triceps is separated from the posterior cord to obtain additional length (*black arrows*). (*C*) Both posterior axillary nerve branches are coapted to the triceps branch. (*Courtesy of* Mayo Foundation, Rochester, MN; with permission.)

The authors report improvement of elbow extension from M0 to M4 in an 18-year-old woman with C7-T1 injury who was operated 6 months after injury. Triceps contraction was first noted 6 months after surgery, recovering up to M4 by 12 months. Good deltoid function is imperative when considering this technique.

Although the number of cases is still limited, this so called "reversed Leechavengvong procedure" seems a promising technique to restore triceps function without significant donor site morbidity in lower brachial plexus injuries.

SUMMARY

Depending on the extent of the injury, different nerve transfer options are available for reconstruction of elbow function in the flail arm. If hand function is preserved, the double fascicular has proven good and consistent results. In total brachial plexus injuries, where only extraplexal donors are available, ICNs are most widely used for both direct target muscle neurotization and innervation of a free-functioning muscle transfer. Although outcomes using the contralateral C7 nerve root seem promising in some hands, independent function is often not achieved.

REFERENCES

1. Haninec P, Szeder V. Reconstruction of elbow flexion by transposition of pedicled long head of triceps brachii muscle. Acta Chir Plast 1999;41(3):82–6.

2. Ruhmann O, Schmolke S, Gosse F, et al. Transposition of local muscles to restore elbow flexion in brachial plexus palsy. Injury 2002;33(7):597–609.

3. Tung TH, Liu DZ, Mackinnon SE. Nerve transfer for elbow flexion in radiation-induced brachial plexopathy: a case report. Hand 2009;4(2):123–8.

4. Chim H, Kircher MF, Spinner RJ, et al. Free functioning gracilis transfer for traumatic brachial plexus injuries in children. J Hand Surg 2014; 39(10):1959–66.

5. Merrell GA, Barrie KA, Katz DL, et al. Results of nerve transfer techniques for restoration of shoulder and elbow function in the context of a meta-analysis of the English literature. J Hand Surg Am 2001;26(2): 303–14.

6. Harris W, Low VW. On the Importance of accurate muscular analysis in lesions of the brachial plexus; and the treatment of erb's palsy and infantile paralysis of the upper extremity by cross-union of the nerve roots. Br Med J 1903;2(2234):1035–8.

7. Tuttle HK. Exposure of the brachial plexus with nerve-transplantation. JAMA 1913;61(1):15–7.

8. Seddon HJ. Nerve grafting. J Bone Joint Surg Br 1963;45:447–61.

9. Tsuyama N, Hara T. Intercostal nerve transfer in the treatment of brachial plexus injury of root avulsion type. Exerpta Medica 1972;29(1):35 l.

10. Narakas A. Surgical treatment of traction injuries of the brachial plexus. Clin Orthop Relat Res 1978;(133):71–90.

11. Nagano A, Ochiai N, Okinaga S. Restoration of elbow flexion in root lesions of brachial plexus injuries. J Hand Surg Am 1992;17(5):815–21.

12. Krakauer JD, Wood MB. Intercostal nerve transfer for brachial plexopathy. J Hand Surg Am 1994; 19(5):829–35.

13. Nagano A, Yamamoto S, Mikami Y. Intercostal nerve transfer to restore upper extremity functions after brachial plexus injury. Ann Acad Med Singapore 1995;24(4 Suppl):42–5.

14. Ogino T, Naito T. Intercostal nerve crossing to restore elbow flexion and sensibility of the hand for a root avulsion type of brachial plexus injury. Microsurgery 1995;16(8):571–7.

15. Kotani PT, Matsuda H, Suzuki T. Trial surgical procedures of nerve transfers to avulsion injuries of plexus brachialis. Exerpta Medica 1972;29(1):348.

16. Lurje A. Concerning surgical treatment of traumatic injury to the upper division of the brachial plexus (Erb's type). Ann Surg 1948;127(2):317–26.

17. Allieu Y, Privat JM, Bonnel F. Paralysis in root avulsion of the brachial plexus. Neurotization by the spinal accessory nerve. Clin Plast Surg 1984;11(1): 133–6.

18. Allieu Y, Cenac P. Neurotization via the spinal accessory nerve in complete paralysis due to multiple avulsion injuries of the brachial plexus. Clin Orthop Relat Res 1988;(237):67–74.

19. Sammer DM, Kircher MF, Bishop AT, et al. Hemicontralateral C7 transfer in traumatic brachial plexus injuries: outcomes and complications. J Bone Joint Surg Am 2012;94(2):131–7.

20. Oberlin C, Beal D, Leechavengvongs S, et al. Nerve transfer to biceps muscle using a part of ulnar nerve for C5-C6 avulsion of the brachial plexus: anatomical study and report of four cases. J Hand Surg Am 1994;19(2):232–7.

21. Mackinnon SE, Novak CB, Myckatyn TM, et al. Results of reinnervation of the biceps and brachialis muscles with a double fascicular transfer for elbow flexion. J Hand Surg Am 2005;30(5):978–85.

22. Tung TH, Mackinnon SE. Nerve transfers: indications, techniques, and outcomes. J Hand Surg Am 2010;35(2):332–41.

23. Boyd KU, Nimigan AS, Mackinnon SE. Nerve reconstruction in the hand and upper extremity. Clin Plast Surg 2011;38(4):643–60.

24. Gorio A, Carmignoto G. Reformation, maturation and stabilization of neuromuscular junctions in peripheral nerve regeneration. In: Gorio A, Millesi H, Mingrino S, editors. Posttraumatic peripheral nerve regeneration. New York: Raven Press; 1981. p. 481–92.

25. Bishop AT. Functioning free-muscle transfer for brachial plexus injury. Hand Clin 2005;21(1):91–102.

26. Narakas AO, Hentz VR. Neurotization in brachial plexus injuries. Indication and results. Clin Orthop Relat Res 1988;(237):43–56.

27. Ruch DS, Friedman A, Nunley JA. The restoration of elbow flexion with intercostal nerve transfers. Clin Orthop Relat Res 1995;(314):95–103.

28. Songcharoen P, Mahaisavariya B, Chotigavanich C. Spinal accessory neurotization for restoration of elbow flexion in avulsion injuries of the brachial plexus. J Hand Surg Am 1996;21(3):387–90.

29. Terzis JK, Kostopoulos VK. The surgical treatment of brachial plexus injuries in adults. Plast Reconstr Surg 2007;119(4):73e–92e.

30. Flores LP. Triceps brachii reinnervation in primary reconstruction of the adult brachial plexus: experience in 25 cases. Acta Neurochir (Wien) 2011; 153(10):1999–2007.

31. Samardzic M, Grujicic D, Antunovic V. Nerve transfer in brachial plexus traction injuries. J Neurosurg 1992;76(2):191–7.

32. Oberlin C, Ameur NE, Teboul F, et al. Restoration of elbow flexion in brachial plexus injury by transfer of ulnar nerve fascicles to the nerve to the biceps muscle. Tech Hand Up Extrem Surg 2002;6(2):86–90.

33. Carlsen BT, Kircher MF, Spinner RJ, et al. Comparison of single versus double nerve transfers for elbow flexion after brachial plexus injury. Plast Reconstr Surg 2011;127(1):269–76.

34. Leechavengvongs S, Witoonchart K, Uerpairojkit C, et al. Combined nerve transfers for C5 and C6 brachial plexus avulsion injury. J Hand Surg Am 2006;31(2):183–9.

35. Leechavengvongs S, Witoonchart K, Uerpairojkit C, et al. Nerve transfer to biceps muscle using a part of the ulnar nerve in brachial plexus injury (upper arm type): a report of 32 cases. J Hand Surg Am 1998;23(4):711–6.

36. Teboul F, Kakkar R, Ameur N, et al. Transfer of fascicles from the ulnar nerve to the nerve to the biceps in the treatment of upper brachial plexus palsy. J Bone Joint Surg Am 2004;86–A(7):1485–90.

37. Ali ZS, Heuer GG, Faught RW, et al. Upper brachial plexus injury in adults: comparative effectiveness of different repair techniques. J Neurosurg 2015; 122(1):195–201.

38. Sedain G, Sharma MS, Sharma BS, et al. Outcome after delayed oberlin transfer in brachial plexus injury. Neurosurgery 2011;69(4):822–7.

39. Pet MA, Ray WZ, Yee A, et al. Nerve transfer to the triceps after brachial plexus injury: report of four cases. J Hand Surg Am 2011;36(3):398–405.

40. Tung TH, Novak CB, Mackinnon SE. Nerve transfers to the biceps and brachialis branches to improve elbow flexion strength after brachial plexus injuries. J Neurosurg 2003;98(2):313–8.

41. Ray WZ, Pet MA, Yee A, et al. Double fascicular nerve transfer to the biceps and brachialis muscles after brachial plexus injury: clinical outcomes in a series of 29 cases. J Neurosurg 2011;114(6):1520–8.

42. Liverneaux PA, Diaz LC, Beaulieu JY, et al. Preliminary results of double nerve transfer to restore elbow flexion in upper type brachial plexus palsies. Plast Reconstr Surg 2006;117(3):915–9.

43. Martins RS, Siqueira MG, Heise CO, et al. A prospective study comparing single and double fascicular transfer to restore elbow flexion after brachial plexus injury. Neurosurgery 2013;72(5):709–14 [discussion: 714–5; quiz: 715].

44. Samardzic M, Grujicic D, Rasulic L, et al. Transfer of the medial pectoral nerve: myth or reality? Neurosurgery 2002;50(6):1277–82.

45. Samardzic M, Rasulic LG, Grujicic DM, et al. Nerve transfers using collateral branches of the brachial plexus as donors in patients with upper palsy–thirty years' experience. Acta Neurochir (Wien) 2011;153(10):2009–19 [discussion: 2019].

46. Chuang D. Neurotization procedures for brachial plexus injuries. Hand Clin 1995;11(4):633–45.

47. Hems T. Nerve transfers for traumatic brachial plexus injury: advantages and problems. J Hand Microsurg 2011;3(1):6–10.

48. Haninec P, Samal F, Tomas R, et al. Direct repair (nerve grafting), neurotization, and end-to-side neurorrhaphy in the treatment of brachial plexus injury. J Neurosurg 2007;106(3):391–9.

49. Sulaiman OA, Kim DD, Burkett C, et al. Nerve transfer surgery for adult brachial plexus injury: a 10-year experience at Louisiana State University. Neurosurgery 2009;65(4 Suppl):A55–62.

50. Samardzic M, Rasulic L, Grujicic D, et al. Results of nerve transfers to the musculocutaneous and axillary nerves. Neurosurgery 2000;46(1):93–101 [discussion: 101–3].

51. Flores LP. Reanimation of elbow extension with medial pectoral nerve transfer in partial injuries to the brachial plexus. J Neurosurg 2013;118(3):588–93.

52. Lu W, Xu JG, Wang DP, et al. Microanatomical study on the functional origin and direction of the thoracodorsal nerve from the trunks of brachial plexus. Clin Anat 2008;21(6):509–13.

53. Shin AY, Spinner RJ, Steinmann SP, et al. Adult traumatic brachial plexus injuries. J Am Acad Orthop Surg 2005;13(6):382–96.

54. Schreiber JJ, Byun DJ, Khair MM, et al. Optimal axon counts for brachial plexus nerve transfers to restore elbow flexion. Plast Reconstr Surg 2015;135(1):135e–41e.

55. Soldado F, Ghizoni MF, Bertelli J. Thoracodorsal nerve transfer for elbow flexion reconstruction in infraclavicular brachial plexus injuries. J Hand Surg Am 2014;39(9):1766–70.

56. Samardzic M, Rasulic L, Lakicevic N, et al. Collateral branches of the brachial plexus as donors in nerve transfers. Vojnosanit Pregl 2012;69(7):594–603.

57. Samardzic MM, Grujicic DM, Rasulic LG, et al. The use of thoracodorsal nerve transfer in restoration of irreparable C5 and C6 spinal nerve lesions. Br J Plast Surg 2005;58(4):541–6.

58. Novak CB, Mackinnon SE, Tung TH. Patient outcome following a thoracodorsal to musculocutaneous nerve transfer for reconstruction of elbow flexion. Br J Plast Surg 2002;55(5):416–9.

59. Richardson PM. Recovery of biceps function after delayed repair for brachial plexus injury. J Trauma 1997;42(5):791–2.

60. Soldado F, Ghizoni MF, Bertelli J. Thoracodorsal nerve transfer for triceps reinnervation in partial brachial plexus injuries. Microsurgery 2015 [Epub ahead of print].

61. Chuang DC, Yeh MC, Wei FC. Intercostal nerve transfer of the musculocutaneous nerve in avulsed brachial plexus injuries: evaluation of 66 patients. J Hand Surg Am 1992;17(5):822–8.

62. Malessy MJ, Thomeer RT. Evaluation of intercostal to musculocutaneous nerve transfer in reconstructive brachial plexus surgery. J Neurosurg 1998;88(2):266–71.

63. Xiao C, Lao J, Wang T, et al. Intercostal nerve transfer to neurotize the musculocutaneous nerve after traumatic brachial plexus avulsion: a comparison of two, three, and four nerve transfers. J Reconstr Microsurg 2014;30(5):297–304.

64. Gu YD, Zhang GM, Chen DS, et al. Cervical nerve root transfer from contralateral normal side for treatment of brachial plexus root avulsions. Chin Med J (Engl) 1991;104(3):208–11.

65. Chalidapong P, Sananpanich K, Kraisarin J, et al. Pulmonary and biceps function after intercostal and phrenic nerve transfer for brachial plexus injuries. J Hand Surg Br 2004;29(1):8–11.

66. Brandt KE, Mackinnon SE. A technique for maximizing biceps recovery in brachial plexus reconstruction. J Hand Surg Am 1993;18(4):726–33.

67. Carlsen BT, Bishop AT, Shin AY. Late reconstruction for brachial plexus injury. Neurosurg Clin N Am 2009;20(1):51–64, vi.

68. Nagano A, Tsuyama N, Ochiai N, et al. Direct nerve crossing with the intercostal nerve to treat avulsion injuries of the brachial plexus. J Hand Surg Am 1989;14(6):980–5.

69. Bhatia A, Shyam AK, Doshi P, et al. Nerve reconstruction: a cohort study of 93 cases of global brachial plexus palsy. Indian J Orthop 2011;45(2):153–60.

70. Moiyadi AV, Devi BI, Nair KP. Brachial plexus injuries: outcome following neurotization with intercostal nerve. J Neurosurg 2007;107(2):308–13.

71. Terzis JK, Barbitsioti A. Primary restoration of elbow flexion in adult post-traumatic plexopathy patients. J Plast Reconstr Aesthet Surg 2012;65(1):72–84.

72. El-Gammal TA, Fathi NA. Outcomes of surgical treatment of brachial plexus injuries using nerve grafting and nerve transfers. J Reconstr Microsurg 2002;18(1):7–15.

73. Goubier JN, Teboul F, Khalifa H. Reanimation of elbow extension with intercostal nerves transfers in total brachial plexus palsies. Microsurgery 2011;31(1):7–11.

74. Gao K, Lao J, Zhao X, et al. Outcome after transfer of intercostal nerves to the nerve of triceps long head in 25 adult patients with total brachial plexus root avulsion injury. J Neurosurg 2013; 118(3):606–10.

75. Zheng MX, Xu WD, Qiu YQ, et al. Phrenic nerve transfer for elbow flexion and intercostal nerve transfer for elbow extension. J Hand Surg Am 2010;35(8): 1304–9.

76. Terzis JK, Barmpitsioti A. Our experience with triceps nerve reconstruction in patients with brachial plexus injury. J Plast Reconstr Aesthet Surg 2012; 65(5):590–600.

77. Giuffre JL, Kakar S, Bishop AT, et al. Current concepts of the treatment of adult brachial plexus injuries. J Hand Surg 2010;35(4):678–88.

78. Samii A, Carvalho GA, Samii M. Brachial plexus injury: factors affecting functional outcome in spinal accessory nerve transfer for the restoration of elbow flexion. J Neurosurg 2003;98(2):307–12.

79. Gao K, Lao J, Zhao X, et al. Outcome of contralateral C7 transfer to two recipient nerves in 22 patients with the total brachial plexus avulsion injury. Microsurgery 2013;33(8):605–11.

80. Chuang DC, Hernon C. Minimum 4-year follow-up on contralateral C7 nerve transfers for brachial plexus injuries. J Hand Surg Am 2012;37(2):270–6.

81. Terzis JK, Kokkalis ZT. Selective contralateral C7 transfer in posttraumatic brachial plexus injuries: a report of 56 cases. Plast Reconstr Surg 2009; 123(3):927–38.

82. Gu Y, Xu J, Chen L, et al. Long term outcome of contralateral C7 transfer: a report of 32 cases. Chin Med J (Engl) 2002;115(6):866–8.

83. Xu L, Gu Y, Xu J, et al. Contralateral C7 transfer via the prespinal and retropharyngeal route to repair brachial plexus root avulsion: a preliminary report. Neurosurgery 2008;63(3):553–8 [discussion: 558–9].

84. Wang S, Yiu HW, Li P, et al. Contralateral C7 nerve root transfer to neurotize the upper trunk via a modified prespinal route in repair of brachial plexus avulsion injury. Microsurgery 2012;32(3):183–8.

85. Gu YD, Wu MM, Zhen YL, et al. Phrenic nerve transfer for treatment of root avulsion of the brachial plexus. Chin Med J (Engl) 1990;103(4):267–70.

86. Gu YD, Wu MM, Zhen YL, et al. Phrenic nerve transfer for brachial plexus motor neurotization. Microsurgery 1989;10(4):287–9.

87. Liu Y, Lao J, Gao K, et al. Comparative study of phrenic nerve transfers with and without nerve graft for elbow flexion after global brachial plexus injury. Injury 2014;45(1):227–31.

88. Xu WD, Gu YD, Xu JG, et al. Full-length phrenic nerve transfer by means of video-assisted thoracic surgery in treating brachial plexus avulsion injury. Plast Reconstr Surg 2002;110(1):104–9 [discussion: 110–1].

89. Dong Z, Zhang CG, Gu YD. Surgical outcome of phrenic nerve transfer to the anterior division of the upper trunk in treating brachial plexus avulsion. J Neurosurg 2010;112(2):383–5.

90. Bertelli JA, Ghizoni MF. Contralateral motor rootlets and ipsilateral nerve transfers in brachial plexus reconstruction. J Neurosurg 2004;101(5):770–8.

91. Gu YD, Ma MK. Use of the phrenic nerve for brachial plexus reconstruction. Clin Orthop Relat Res 1996;(323):119–21.

92. Monreal R. Restoration of elbow flexion by transfer of the phrenic nerve to musculocutaneous nerve after brachial plexus injuries. Hand 2007;2(4):206–11.

93. Siqueira MG, Martins RS. Phrenic nerve transfer in the restoration of elbow flexion in brachial plexus avulsion injuries: how effective and safe is it? Neurosurgery 2009;65(4 Suppl):A125–31.

94. Liu Y, Lao J, Zhao X. Comparative study of phrenic and intercostal nerve transfers for elbow flexion after global brachial plexus injury. Injury 2015;46(4):671–5.

95. Bertelli JA. Platysma motor branch transfer in brachial plexus repair: report of the first case. J Brachial Plex Peripher Nerve Inj 2007;2:12.

96. Malessy MJ, Hoffmann CF, Thomeer RT. Initial report on the limited value of hypoglossal nerve transfer to treat brachial plexus root avulsions. Journal of Neurosurgery 1999;91(4):601–4.

97. Klika BJ, Spinner RJ, Bishop AT, et al. Posterior branch of the axillary nerve transfer to the lateral triceps branch for restoration of elbow extension: case report. J Hand Surg Am 2013;38(6):1145–9.

Nerve Transfers in Birth Related Brachial Plexus Injuries: Where Do We Stand?

Kristen M. Davidge, MD, MSc[a,b,*],
Howard M. Clarke, MD, PhD[a,b], Gregory H. Borschel, MD[a,b]

KEYWORDS

- Obstetrical brachial plexus palsy • Erb's palsy • Nerve graft • Nerve transfer • Neurotization

KEY POINTS

- Birth-related or obstetrical brachial plexus palsy (OBPP) differs from adult brachial plexus palsy in important ways.
- Interpositional nerve grafting remains the mainstay of operative treatment for OBPP.
- Unlike in adults, outcomes after nerve grafting in infants are very good.
- Good indications for distal nerve transfers in OBPP include late presentation (>12 months of age), isolated nerve deficits, and absence of proximal roots for grafting.
- The role of distal nerve transfers as a primary reconstructive strategy for Erb's palsy (C5-C6 injuries) remains unknown.

INTRODUCTION

Birth-related, or obstetrical, brachial plexus palsies (OBPP) occur in approximately 1 in 1000 live births.[1] Risk factors associated with OBPP include greater fetal weight, maternal diabetes, shoulder dystocia, and difficult delivery requiring forceps or vacuum suction.[2–5] The most common mechanism involves a traction injury to the brachial plexus during the last stage of a vaginal vertex delivery, when the infant's head is laterally displaced away from the shoulder.[2–5] Less commonly, OBPP is seen after breech delivery and cesarean section.[6,7] Patterns of birth-related brachial plexus injury include the upper (Erb's) palsy (C5, C6 ± C7), total palsy (C5, C6, C7, C8 ± T1), and intermediate palsy (C7, ±C8, T1).[8] Isolated injury to the lower plexus roots (C8-T1), traditionally known as Klumpke's paralysis, is exceedingly rare.[9]

There is a wide spectrum of severity in OBPP, and many infants with a birth-related brachial plexus injury recover satisfactory function spontaneously without need for operative intervention.[7,10–12] However, only those children with the mildest neurologic injury, who demonstrate complete neurologic recovery before 1 month of age, go on to develop a truly normal limb.[13] When visible differences in the movement between the upper limbs persist beyond this time frame, long-term differences in appearance and function of the affected limb are expected. Such differences can include limb length discrepancy, joint contractures, glenohumeral dysplasia, and subtle differences in upper limb coordination, even when functional recovery is otherwise excellent.[14–16]

Approximately 10% to 30% of infants with OBPP require surgical intervention owing to unsatisfactory motor recovery.[13,17–19] However,

Disclosures: The authors have no conflicts of interest to declare.
[a] Division of Plastic & Reconstructive Surgery, The Hospital for Sick Children, 555 University Avenue, Toronto, Ontario M5G 1X8, Canada; [b] Department of Surgery, University of Toronto, Toronto, Ontario, Canada
* Corresponding author. Division of Plastic and Reconstructive Surgery, Hospital for Sick Children, 555 University Avenue, 5th floor Black Wing, Room 5421, Toronto, Ontario M5G 1X8, Canada.
E-mail address: kristen.davidge@sickkids.ca

Hand Clin 32 (2016) 175–190
http://dx.doi.org/10.1016/j.hcl.2015.12.006
0749-0712/16/$ – see front matter © 2016 Elsevier Inc. All rights reserved.

indications for surgical intervention and specific reconstructive approaches in OBPP remain controversial and vary widely by institution. Furthermore, the assessment and management of OBPP differs fundamentally from brachial plexus injuries in adults and older children owing to several factors, such as greater neuroregenerative capacity and cortical plasticity, shorter limb length, and differing therapy approaches in infants.[20] The traditional approach to brachial plexus reconstruction in OBPP entails neuroma resection and interpositional nerve grafting, which may be combined with extraplexal nerve transfers depending on the severity of the lesion and availability of proximal cervical roots for grafting.[13,18,21–26] Intraplexal distal nerve transfers, now widely used as a primary surgical approach for adult brachial plexus injuries, have only recently been applied as a primary approach to reconstruction in OBPP. The purpose of this article is to review the available evidence for use of distal nerve transfers in infants with birth-related brachial plexus injuries in the broader context of OBPP management.

PRIMARY SURGICAL MANAGEMENT USING INTERPOSITIONAL NERVE GRAFTING ± NERVE TRANSFERS (CONVENTIONAL APPROACH)
Surgical Indications and Timing

Total plexus palsy
Most surgeons agree that infants with T1 involvement who fail to show rapid recovery, and/or presence of Horner's syndrome, are indications for early surgical intervention at 3 months of age or younger.[4,13,27–29] Unlike in adults, recovery of T1 function can reliably occur after early interpositional nerve grafting and/or extraplexal transfers, and is the first priority in the surgical reconstruction of OBPP.

Upper plexus palsy
More debate exists as to the timing and indications for surgical intervention in infants where T1 is intact. Absence of elbow flexion at defined time points, such as 3 months[30] or 5 months,[13] and the Hospital for Sick Children algorithm[29,31] (Fig. 1), are commonly used indications. The Hospital for Sick Children algorithm was developed to identify those children who are likely to develop poor functional recovery, while minimizing the false-positive and false-negative predictions. In this approach, children who fail the "test score" at 3 months of age, who fail to progress in their motor recovery between 3 and 6 months of age, who fail the "cookie test" at 9 months of age, or demonstrate poor shoulder recovery by 9 months of age are offered a primary nerve operation.[7,29,31] The "test score" is calculated at 3 months of age based on 5 movements (elbow flexion, and elbow, wrist, finger, and thumb extension) that together were found to statistically limit the false prediction rate for poor recovery to 5.3%.[7] The "cookie test" evaluates the ability of the infant to bring their hand to their mouth against gravity, with the shoulder held in adduction and with less than 45° of neck flexion.[29,31]

Preoperative Evaluation

Once the decision to proceed with a primary nerve operation has been made, preoperative computed tomography or magnetic resonance myelography is performed to screen for cervical root avulsion.[1,32–35] In the setting of OBPP after a vaginal vertex delivery, ruptures (postganglionic injuries) are frequently seen in the upper plexus, whereas root avulsions (preganglionic injuries) are more common in the lower plexus.[4,36,37] The presence or absence of root avulsion has implications for reconstruction, because avulsed roots have no capacity for spontaneous regeneration and cannot serve as donors for interpositional nerve grafting.[37] Root avulsions in the upper plexus are more frequently seen in the setting of OBPP after a breech delivery.[38,39]

A preoperative diaphragmatic ultrasound examination may also be obtained to evaluate the integrity and function of the phrenic nerve.[18] We routinely obtain this study in our center.

Surgical Techniques

The mainstay of brachial plexus reconstruction in OBPP is neuroma excision and interpositional nerve grafting.[13,18,21–26] Extraplexal nerve transfers may also be performed if there are insufficient cervical roots to act as donors for nerve grafting or if there is insufficient graft material available to accomplish the desired reconstruction. Specific reconstructive algorithms vary between surgeons and institutions, but there is overall consensus that the primary target for reinnervation in a total plexus injury is the lower trunk, and that the reconstruction should be anatomic when possible.[18,27,40,41] Detailed descriptions of the surgical approaches for interpositional nerve grafting and extraplexal transfers in OBPP have been published elsewhere,[18,27,40–44] and are not the focus of this article. A brief overview is provided here to set the broader context of OBPP management for later discussion of nerve transfers.

Interpositional nerve grafting
Sural nerve harvest The sural nerves are the primary source for nerve graft, and can be

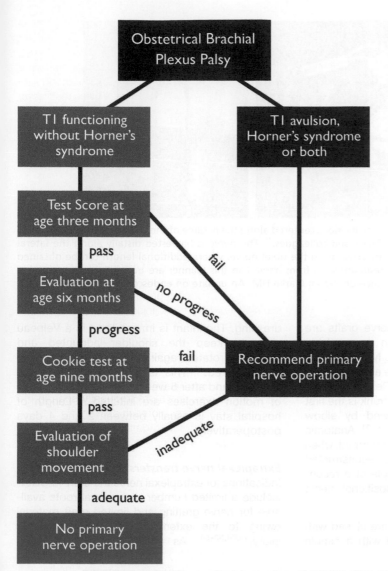

Fig. 1. Extended indications for primary nerve surgery in obstetrical brachial plexus palsy in our center (revised Hospital for Sick Children algorithm). (*From* Bade SA, Lin JC, Curtis CG, et al. Extending the indications for primary nerve surgery in obstetric brachial plexus palsy. Biomed Res Int 2014;2014:627067.)

harvested using small transverse incisions in an open or endoscopic fashion to minimize donor site scars **(Fig. 2)**.[45,46] This can be performed in the prone or supine position. The supraclavicular branches of the cervical plexus can be used as additional nerve graft material.[41]

Exposure of the brachial plexus The infant is positioned supine, with the head turned away from the affected extremity and the neck slightly extended **(Fig. 3)**.[18,40,41,47] Exposure of the supraclavicular brachial plexus is performed using a V-shaped (our preferred approach) or transverse incision. Dissection proceeds in a standard fashion with division of the omohyoid muscle, transverse cervical vessels, and supraclavicular vessels, and retraction of the adipolymphatic pad of Brown to expose

the underlying brachial plexus. Division of the clavicle and infraclavicular exposure may be necessary in rare cases, although our routine is to avoid clavicular osteotomy where possible. Dissection should continue until healthy nerves are seen proximal and distal to the neuroma.

Neuroma resection Intraoperative stimulation of proximal nerve roots to evaluate motor response is performed to provide further confirmation of root avulsion versus rupture before neuroma resection.[18,40,41] After resection, proximal nerve roots are examined histologically for neural architecture to ensure the roots are suitable for nerve grafting.[48] It is critical that nerve roots are cut proximal enough to the injury to allow for axonal sprouting into the coapted nerve grafts.

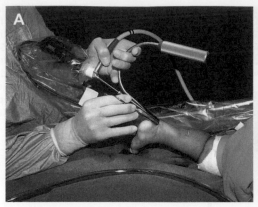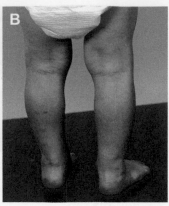

Fig. 2. (*A*) A series of three 2-cm transverse incisions centered along the midline of the calf are used in endoscopic sural nerve harvest, as described by Capek and colleagues.[45] The nerve is harvested distally along the lateral aspect of the foot and proximally to its origin from the tibial nerve, where additional length can be obtained by intrafascicular dissection. (*B*) The resultant scars from harvest in this manner are generally very acceptable and avoids the long "stocking seam" incision. (*From* Clarke HM. An update on endoscopic sural nerve harvest. Plast Reconstr Surg 1998;102:1304.)

Nerve grafting Reversed sural nerve grafts are used to bridge the gap between the available nerve roots and the distal targets. Nerve coaptations are performed with fibrin glue and/or sutures under the operating microscope. Reinnervation of the hand via grafting to the lower trunk is the first priority for reconstruction, followed by elbow flexion and shoulder motion.[18,27,40,41] Anatomic reconstruction of the plexus is performed when possible (ie, the upper trunk is reconstructed from both C5 and C6). An example of a reconstructive approach using interpositional nerve grafts is shown in **Fig. 4.**

Postoperative care The incisions are closed with dissolving sutures, and covered with a simple dressing. The infant is immobilized in a Velpeau sling to keep the shoulder adducted and internally rotated against the chest, and the elbow flexed.[49] This is worn continuously for 3 weeks, and after 5 weeks gentle passive range of motion exercises are initiated.[18] Length of hospital stay is usually between 2 and 4 days postoperatively.

Extraplexal nerve transfers
Indications for extraplexal nerve transfers in OBPP include a limited number of proximal roots available for nerve grafting and limited graft material owing to the extent of the brachial plexus injury.[43,44,50–54] As such, extraplexal nerve

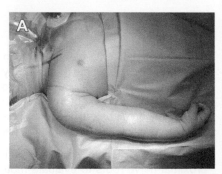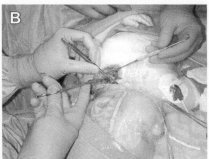

Fig. 3. (*A*) The infant is positioned in such a way that the surgeon may work above, beside, and below the field. The neck is extended slightly, and the head faces away from the field. The hand and arm are accessible for observation of stimulated movements. A clear plastic head drape is used so that the patient's face and the nasotracheal tube are always visible to the anesthetist and the other members of the surgical team. (*B*) A V-shaped flap is created and reflected posterolaterally by an incision along the posterior border of the sternocleidomastoid and the clavicle. Through this exposure, the entire posterior triangle is visible. For longer lesions the incision may be extended along the deltopectoral groove, if necessary. (*From* Marcus JR, Clarke HM. Management of obstetric brachial plexus palsy. In: Bentz ML, Bauer BS, Zuker RM, editors. Principles and practice of pediatric plastic surgery. St Louis (MO): Quality Medical Publishing Inc; 2007. p. 1427–53; with permission.)

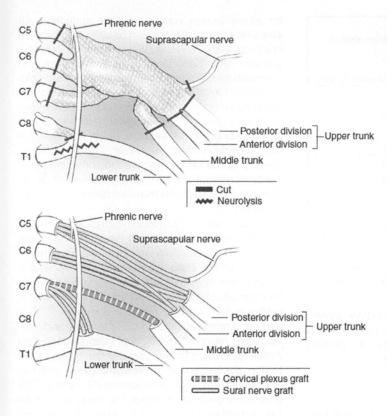

Fig. 4. An example of neuroma resection and interpositional nerve grafting in birth-related or obstetrical brachial plexus palsies. This patient presented with an upper plexus palsy and was found to have an avulsion of C8, demonstrated unequivocally by the presence of a dorsal root ganglion. C5-C7 was involved in a dense neuroma, and T1 was found to have a normal fascicular pattern with minimal involvement in the neuroma. Anatomic grafting was performed to the suprascapular nerve, anterior and posterior divisions of the upper trunk, and the middle trunk. Intraplexal neurotization to the lower trunk was performed from C7. T1 was treated with neurolysis. The phrenic nerve is shown traversing longitudinally over the plexus. (*From* Marcus JR, Clarke HM. Management of obstetric brachial plexus palsy. In: Bentz ML, Bauer BS, Zuker RM, editors. Principles and practice of pediatric plastic surgery. St Louis (MO): Quality Medical Publishing Inc; 2007. p. 1427–53; with permission.)

transfers are performed more frequently in total plexus palsies. Commonly performed extraplexal transfers in OBPP include the spinal accessory nerve (SAN) to suprascapular nerve (SSN) transfer for restoration of shoulder external rotation and abduction,[42,50,51] the intercostal nerve to musculocutaneous nerve transfer for restoration of elbow flexion,[43,52,55,56] and the contralateral C7 transfer for reconstruction of the lower trunk.[44,53,54] The technical nuances of these transfers have been described in detail elsewhere, and do not differ substantially from adults. It deserves mentioning that the SAN to SSN transfer is often performed from an anterior approach in OBPP,[42,50,51] because the brachial plexus is already exposed for interpositional nerve grafting. More recently, the posterior approach to the SAN to SSN, as described by Mackinnon and others,[57–59] has been used in infants with OBPP.[60] Generally speaking, the posterior approach is used when anterior exposure of the brachial plexus is not being performed, for example, when the sole indication for surgery is to restore shoulder external rotation, when the infant presents late and a transfer closer to the target muscle is desired, or in the newer context of primary OBPP reconstruction with nerve transfers alone.

Surgical Outcomes

Outcome assessment

Assessment of motor recovery in infants with OBPP both preoperatively and postoperatively is challenging, and there is a lack of consistency in how surgeons assess and report functional outcomes. The most commonly used outcome measures for motor function include the Hospital for Sick Children Active Movement Scale (AMS)[4,29,61] (**Table 1**), the Mallet score[62,63] (**Fig. 5**), and the Medical Research Council grading system[64] (**Table 2**). A recent publication by Tse and colleagues[20] compared the Active Movement Scale and various modified Medical Research Council scales in use, yet it remains challenging to directly contrast outcomes in the published literature. Furthermore, the Mallet score requires voluntary participation from the child and therefore can only be used postoperatively in children older than 4 years of age.[20,41,65] Indeed, lack of direct preoperatively and postoperative comparisons of motor function is a major limitation of many studies in OBPP. Finally, most of the outcome literature in OBPP focuses on motor recovery with little or no attention paid to sensory outcomes. All of these factors will be critical as we move forward in trying

Table 1
Hospital for Sick Children Active Movement Scale

Observation	Muscle Grade
Gravity eliminated	
No contraction	0
Contraction, no motion	1
Motion $\leq\frac{1}{2}$ range	2
Motion $>\frac{1}{2}$ range	3
Full motion	4
Against gravity	
Motion $\leq\frac{1}{2}$ range	5
Motion $>\frac{1}{2}$ range	6
Full motion	7

From Clarke HM, Curtis CG. An approach to obstetric brachial plexus injuries. Hand Clin 1995;11:563–80. [discussion: 580-1]; with permission.

to understand and compare the relative advantages and disadvantages of nerve transfers versus interpositional nerve grafting as a primary approach for OBPP reconstruction.

Clinical results in the literature

In the early 1990s, there was a general shift in the surgical approach to OBPP away from neurolysis toward neuroma resection and grafting. Many past studies evaluating outcomes of interpositional nerve grafting were directed toward demonstrating superior outcomes over neurolysis, a concept that is now generally accepted by OBPP surgeons around the world.[22,25,40,66–70] Often, results are presented for a combination of interpositional nerve grafting and extraplexal nerve transfers, or use composite movements as outcomes.

For the purposes of comparing outcomes to distal nerve transfers, only those studies evaluating pure movements after interpositional nerve grafting[13,25,43,71,72] and extraplexal transfers[43,44,52–56] are shown in **Tables 3** and **4**, respectively. Additionally, because distal nerve transfers are targeted primarily toward reconstruction of upper trunk functions (elbow flexion, shoulder abduction, shoulder external rotation) in the context of upper plexus injuries, we have excluded data on outcomes of lower plexus reconstruction in OBPP.

Putting aside individual study limitations and between-study variability, general conclusions that can be made from the literature in regard to upper plexus functional outcomes after interpositional nerve grafting, with or without extraplexal nerve transfers are the following: (1) outcomes for elbow flexion and shoulder abduction are good, with better results reported in upper plexus palsy versus total plexus palsy, (2) superior results tend to be seen

for elbow flexion versus shoulder abduction, (3) shoulder external rotation can be difficult to achieve in infants with OBPP, and (4) donor morbidity is a concern after harvest of intercostal nerves and contralateral C7 in infants. Potential long-term risks associated with intercostal nerve harvest include chest wall deformity and abnormal breast development with growth.[20] The long-term consequences of harvesting the contralateral C7 in an infant are not well-delineated; however, most children develop some form of synchronous movement of the contralateral upper limb with movement of the affected extremity, and transient donor deficits are common.[44,53,54]

We also have limited data directly comparing extraplexal nerve transfers with interpositional nerve grafting. The best data are for shoulder external rotation, where 2 studies have failed to show any difference in motor outcomes or donor morbidity after reconstruction of the SSN using a graft from C5 versus a SAN transfer (anterior approach).[50,51] In another comparative study, El-Gammal and colleagues[71] reported that 92% of infants attained an Active Movement Scale score 6 or greater for elbow flexion after extraplexal neurotization using a variety of donors (SAN, ICB, contralateral C7) versus 72% after nerve grafting. However, there was no statistical analysis performed and the indications for each approach were not fully explained.[20]

PRIMARY SURGICAL MANAGEMENT USING DISTAL NERVE TRANSFERS
Why Has the Application of Distal Nerve Transfers in Obstetric Brachial Plexus Palsy Lagged Behind Adults?

There are several important reasons why distal nerve transfers have not been adopted at the same rate in infants as in adults. First, functional outcomes after neuroma excision and nerve grafting in adults with upper brachial plexus lesions were suboptimal owing to several factors that include the long distance between the proximal nerve roots and the target motor endplates, and reduced axonal regeneration in the presence of comorbidities and increased age. There was a strong impetus to look for alternative reconstructive strategies to find donor axons in closer proximity to their target muscle, and distal nerve transfers have provided such solutions with improved functional outcomes.[59,73–78] For total and near-total plexus injuries in adults, reinnervation of the hand and wrist is not yet a realistic goal and the focus of reconstruction is on the upper plexus. By contrast, good functional outcomes can be achieved from interpositional nerve grafting in infants owing to shorter limb length and the

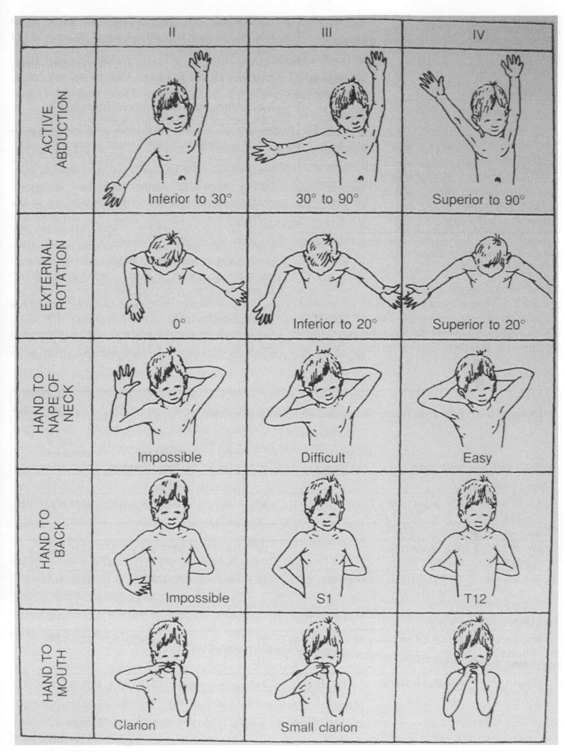

Fig. 5. The classification system of Mallet evaluates global movement of the extremity to identify functional or maladaptive patterns. It requires cooperation from the patient to perform voluntary movements on command. (*From* Gilbert A. Obstetric brachial plexus palsy. In: Tubiana R, editor. The hand. Philadelphia: Saunders; 1993. p. 579; with permission.)

Table 2
Medical Research Council muscle grading system

Observation	Muscle Grade
No contraction	0
Flicker or trace of contraction	1
Active movement, with gravity eliminated	2
Active movement, against gravity	3
Active movement against gravity and resistance	4
Normal power	5

From British Medical Research Council. Aids to the investigation of peripheral nerve injuries. London: Her Majesty's Stationery Office; 1943.

robust axonal regeneration seen in young age groups.[20,79] Furthermore, pure C5 to C6 injuries are less commonly encountered than C5 to C7 or C5 to C8 injuries, where interpositional nerve grafting remains the best chance to reconstruct all affected motions beyond elbow flexion, shoulder abduction, and shoulder external rotation.[20] For these reasons, the necessity to search for alternatives to interpositional nerve grafting in Erb's palsy and total plexus palsy is limited.

Indications for Distal Nerve Transfers in Obstetrical Brachial Plexus Palsy

There are select circumstances when distal nerve transfers are clearly advantageous in OBPP. Late presentation is one such indication, where minimizing time to reinnervation is important. Al-Qattan provided the first report of using the Oberlin transfer for restoration of elbow flexion in 2002, for 2 infants with Erb's palsy presenting later than 12 months of age.[80,81] Subsequently, other small case series were published using the flexor carpi ulnaris (FCU) or flexor carpi radialis (FCR) branches of the ulnar and median nerves, respectively, to neurotize the biceps nerve for late elbow reconstruction up to 24 months of age.[82–86] Along the same lines, nerve transfers have been reported for late salvage of a failed primary nerve graft

Table 3
Functional outcomes after neuroma excision and grafting in OBPP

Publication	Indication	n	Mean FU (y)	Outcome: Elbow Flexion	Outcome: Shoulder Abduction
Upper plexus palsy					
Lin et al,[25] 2009	HSC algorithm	48	4	AMS 6.6 ± 0.5	AMS 5.6 ± 1.6
Total plexus palsy					
Lin et al,[25] 2009	HSC algorithm	44	4	AMS 6.0 ± 1.3	AMS 4.2 ± 1.7
El-Gammal et al,[71] 2010	C5-T1 injury at 3 mo of age	18	4.2	72% AMS ≥6	36% AMS ≥6
All OBPP					
Boome and Kaye,[72] 1988	No C5-C6 recovery at 3 mo of age	22	—	78% MRC ≥3	94% MRC ≥3
Gilbert,[22] 1995	No elbow flexion at 3 mo of age	241	—	—	81% MRC ≥3 (C5-6) 76% MRC ≥3 (C5-7) 64% MRC ≥3 (C5-T1)
Waters,[13] 1999	No biceps recovery at 6 mo of age	6	3.8	33% Mallet 2 33% Mallet 3 33% Mallet 4	50% Mallet 3 50% Mallet 4

Abbreviations: AMS, Active Movement Scale score; FU, follow-up; HSC, hospital for sick children; MRC, medical research council grade.
Data from Refs.[13,22,25,71,72]

Table 4
Functional outcomes after extraplexal nerve transfers in OBPP

Publication	Indication	n	Donor	Recipient	Mean FU (y)	Outcome: Elbow Flexion	Donor Morbidity
Upper plexus palsy							
Kawabata et al,[43] 2001	No biceps function at 3 mo of age and root avulsion	30	ICN	MCN	5.2	93% MRC ≥3	None identified
Lin et al,[53] 2011	Root avulsions	15	cC7	Upper trunk or lateral cord	3.9	60% MRC ≥3	80% contralateral movement
Total plexus palsy							
Chen et al,[54] 2007	4 or 5 root avulsions	4	cC7	Variable	3.8	75% MRC ≥3	100% contralateral movement; 25% transient loss of shoulder abduction
Lin et al,[44] 2010	4 or 5 root avulsions	9	cC7	MCN + median nerve	4.2	78% MRC ≥3	66% contralateral movement; 11% transient loss of shoulder abduction
All CBPP							
El-Gammal et al,[55] 2008	Not specified	31	ICN	MCN	4	93.5% AMS ≥6	100% atelectasis, 4.3% pneumonia
Luc et al,[56] 2011	Root avulsion or dissociative recovery	12	ICN	MCN	4.3	100% MRC ≥3	—
Pondaag et al,[52] 2013	C5-T1 at 3 mo of age or poor shoulder and biceps function at 4-6 mo of age; and no proximal root C5/C6	17	ICN	MCN	3.7	82% MRC ≥3	None identified

Abbreviations: AMS, Active Movement Scale score; cC7, contralateral C7; FU, follow-up; ICN, intercostal nerve; MCN, musculocutaneous nerve; MRC, medical research council grade.
Data from Refs.[43,44,52–56]

reconstruction.[84,86] A third clear indication for distal nerve transfers in OBPP is a rare C5 to C6 injury where both C5 and C6 are avulsed and thus no proximal roots are available for grafting.[86,87] In this situation, the so-called triple nerve transfer can be performed, using the SAN to SSN transfer for external rotation, a triceps branch to axillary nerve transfer for shoulder abduction, and the single[81] or double fascicular transfer[74] for elbow flexion.[60,73] There are other uncommon situations where select reinnervation of an isolated functional deficit is required, such as an Oberlin[81] or double fascicular transfer[74] for poor elbow flexion in the context of otherwise excellent shoulder recovery, or an SAN to SSN transfer for absent shoulder external rotation in the context of otherwise excellent shoulder and elbow recovery.[31,80,82,86]

More recently, triple nerve transfers (FCU and/or FCR branches to biceps and/or brachialis branches, triceps branch to axillary nerve, SAN to SSN) have been performed as a complete primary reconstructive strategy for Erb's palsy.[60,88]

Surgical Techniques

The surgical techniques and principles for distal nerve transfers in OBPP are the same as that in adults, and are detailed elsewhere in this issue. Nerve coaptations are made with fibrin glue and/or sutures. Postoperative care in infants ranges from short-term use of a Velpeau sling to no immobilization at all.[86,88] Gentle passive range of motion exercises are initiated once immobilization is discontinued.

Elbow flexion
Reported approaches in Erb's palsy include the medial pectoral nerve to musculocutaneous nerve transfer,[52,89,90] a single fascicular transfer using the FCU or FCR branches to the biceps or brachialis nerves,[60,80,82–85] and a double fascicular transfer using the FCU and FCR branches to neurotize both the biceps and brachialis nerves.[86,87]

Shoulder abduction
A triceps branch to axillary nerve transfer has been performed in Erb's palsy, using either the lateral[60] or medial[88] heads of the triceps as the donor nerve branch. As in adults, this transfer is usually performed in conjunction with the SAN to SSN transfer from a posterior approach for additional restoration of shoulder abduction and external rotation.[60,88] The posterior approach to the SAN to SSN is thought to be advantageous by some surgeons, because it provides access to decompress the suprascapular notch, a site of potential secondary injury to, or compression of, the SSN.

Surgical Outcomes: Review of the Literature

There are few studies reporting functional outcomes after distal nerve transfers as the complete treatment in OBPP, most of which are small case series and have limited follow-up (**Table 5**).[52,60,80,82–90] Seeing as many of these studies also used distal nerve transfers for late presentation of OBPP, their results are not directly comparable to results of neuroma resection and grafting for infants younger than 1 year of age. From the data we have, it does seem that good recovery of elbow flexion can be achieved after an Oberlin or double fascicular transfer in situations of late presentation, C5 to C6 avulsions and failed nerve graft reconstruction in Erb's palsy.[80,82–87] As such, these seem to be excellent indications for distal nerve transfers in OBPP. Furthermore, donor morbidity remains minimal after distal nerve transfers as is seen in adults. Little and colleagues[86] did report a transient AIN palsy in 3% of infants after harvest of the FCR branch, which is a rare event in adults. This is something to be conscious of in the preoperative discussion with the family, as well as during the interfascicular dissection of the very small nerves seen in infants.

To date, there remains no direct comparison of nerve grafting versus distal nerve transfers in OBPP as a primary surgical approach. The study of Ladak and colleagues[60] suggested that outcomes for elbow flexion, shoulder abduction, and shoulder external rotation after triple nerve transfers were comparable with those reported for neurolysis and grafting. However, the sample size was small, the follow-up was short, and future work is needed to determine if this is truly a viable alternative to interpositional nerve grafting for complete primary treatment of C5 to C6 injuries in OBPP.

Advantages and Disadvantages of Nerve Transfers in Obstetrical Brachial Plexus Palsy

There are several advantages to distal nerve transfers, which include decreased time to reinnervation of target muscles, lack of separate donor site scars for sural nerve harvest, shorter operative time, and reduced technical complexity relative to grafting of the brachial plexus in the neck. It may also bring more specificity to the reinnervation, with less risk of cocontraction postoperatively, and may avoid an extra general anesthetic because preoperative myelography would be obviated.

However, there are also disadvantages to nerve transfers. One of the greatest disadvantages of nerve transfers as a complete treatment for OBPP is that thousands of motor fibers are left without an opportunity to reinnervate the limb. Additionally,

Table 5
Functional outcomes after intraplexal distal nerve transfers in OBPP

Publication	n	Donor	Recipient	Mean FU (y)	Outcome: Elbow Flexion	Outcome: Shoulder Abduction	Donor Morbidity	Indication
Upper plexus palsy								
Blaauw and Slooff,[89] 2003	25	MPN	MCN	5.8	68% MRC ≥3	—	—	Not specified
Wellons et al,[90] 2009	20	MPN	MCN	1.8	80% Mallet hand-to-mouth	—	None	Not specified
Pondaag and Malessy,[52] 2013	25	MPN	MCN	3.7	92% MRC ≥3	—	None	C5-T1 at 3 mo of age or poor shoulder and biceps function at 4-6 mo of age; and no proximal root C5/C6
Al-Qattan,[80] 2002	2	FCU	Biceps	0.4	100% AMS 7 100% MRC 5	—	—	Late presentation (16–18 mo) Stable shoulder
Noaman et al,[82] 2004	7	FCU	Biceps	1.6	71% MRC ≥3	—	—	Late presentation (11–24 mo)
Shigematsu et al,[83] 2006	1	FCU SAN	Biceps SSN (ant.)	3.3	MRC 5	MRC 4	None	Late presentation (8 mo)
Siqueira et al,[84] 2012	17	FCU	Biceps	2.6	82% MRC ≥3	—	None	Late presentation, no proximal root, failed prior reconstruction
Estrella and Mella,[87] 2013	1	FCR FCU SAN	Brachialis Biceps SAN	5	MRC 5	MRC 4	None	No proximal root
Al-Qattan and Al-Kharfy,[85] 2014	10	FCR	Biceps	1.5	90% AMS ≥6	—	None	Late presentation (13–19 mo)

(continued on next page)

Table 5
(continued)

Publication	Indication	n	Donor	Recipient	Mean FU (y)	Outcome: Elbow Flexion	Outcome: Shoulder Abduction	Donor Morbidity
Little et al,[86] 2014	Late presentation, no proximal root, failed prior reconstruction, dissociative recovery	37	FCR FCU	Brachialis Biceps	1.5	87% AMS ≥6	—	3% transient AIN palsy
McRae and Borschel,[88] 2012	HSC algorithm	2	Triceps (medial) FCR SAN	Axillary Biceps SSN (post)	1	—	100% AMS 6	None
Ladak et al,[60] 2013	Failed cookie test	10	FCU/FCR Triceps (lateral) SAN	Biceps Axillary SSN (post)	2	AMS 6.3 ± 0.2	AMS 5.0 ± 0.5	None

Abbreviations: AMS, Active Movement Scale score; FCR, flexor carpi radialis branch; FCU, flexor carpi ulnaris branch; FU, follow-up; MCN, musculocutaneous nerve; MPN, medial pectoral nerve; MRC, medical research council grade; SAN, spinal accessory nerve; SSN, suprascapular nerve.
Data from Refs.[52,60,80,82–90]

they do not provide sensory reinnervation. The impact of these disadvantages on the developing infant, particularly as it relates to limb growth and long-term function, are unknown. Specific to OBPP, there are also concerns about appropriate patient selection for distal nerve transfers. Patients with C5 to C7, intermediate plexus palsy, and total plexus palsy, are not good candidates for distal nerve transfers as there are insufficient normal donors to restore all the affected motions. Serial preoperative assessments are critical to ensure the pattern of injury is well understood. It is also unclear if an infant with extended Erb's palsy who recovers their C7 and/or C8 functions rapidly, such that only C5 and C6 deficits remain at the 9-month assessment, would be a candidate for nerve transfers. This would entail using recovering axons as donors, which at least in adults tends not to provide the same functional outcomes. Finally, it remains unknown at this time as to whether motor recovery after distal nerve transfers for primary OBPP reconstruction in a C5 to C6 injury is equivalent to neuroma resection and interpositional grafting. This must be investigated further before widespread adoption of this technique.

SUMMARY

Birth-related brachial plexus palsy is a unique entity that differs from adult traumatic brachial plexus palsy in many important ways. Distal nerve transfers have revolutionized the treatment of adult brachial plexus injuries, and now offer a new strategy for dealing with complex problems in OBPP such as late presentation, lack of available donor nerve roots, and isolated functional deficits. Available data suggest that nerve transfers can successfully restore function in these scenarios that are not as well served by traditional nerve grafting in OBPP. Currently, the role of distal nerve transfers as a complete primary reconstructive strategy in OBPP is unknown and the mainstay of surgical treatment remains neuroma resection and interpositional nerve grafting, with or without combined nerve transfers. Owing to unique considerations in OBPP such as growth, caution must be exercised in rapidly adopting distal nerve transfers as a first-line approach in Erb's palsy. We await further outcomes from centers using this approach to help ensure equivalency of motor and limb development outcomes, as well as to refine indications for this potentially useful technique in the OBPP population.

REFERENCES

1. Pondaag W, Malessy MJ, van Dijk JG, et al. Natural history of obstetric brachial plexus palsy: a systematic review. Dev Med Child Neurol 2004; 46(2):138–44.
2. Eng GD, Binder H, Getson P, et al. Obstetrical brachial plexus palsy (OBPP) outcome with conservative management. Muscle Nerve 1996;19:884–91.
3. O'Leary JA. Shoulder dystocia and birth injury: prevention and treatment. New York: McGraw-Hill; 1992.
4. Clarke HM, Curtis CG. An approach to obstetrical brachial plexus injuries. Hand Clin 1995;11:563–80 [discussion: 580–1].
5. Metaizeau JP, Gayet C, Plenat F. Brachial plexus birth injuries. An experimental study. Chir Pediatr 1979;20:159–63 [in French].
6. Al-Qattan MM. Obstetric brachial plexus palsy associated with breech delivery. Ann Plast Surg 2003;51: 257–64 [discussion: 265].
7. Michelow BJ, Clarke HM, Curtis CG, et al. The natural history of obstetrical brachial plexus palsy. Plast Reconstr Surg 1994;93:675–80 [discussion: 681].
8. Al-Qattan MM, Clarke HM. A historical note on the intermediate type of obstetrical brachial plexus palsy. J Hand Surg Br 1994;19:673.
9. Al-Qattan MM, Clarke HM, Curtis CG. Klumpke's birth palsy. Does it really exist? J Hand Surg Br 1995;20(1):19–23.
10. Piatt JH Jr. Birth injuries of the brachial plexus. Pediatr Clin North Am 2004;51:421–40.
11. Jackson ST, Hoffer MM, Parrish N. Brachial-plexus palsy in the newborn. J Bone Joint Surg Am 1988; 70:1217–20.
12. Greenwald AG, Schute PC, Shiveley JL. Brachial plexus birth palsy: a 10-year report on the incidence and prognosis. J Pediatr Orthop 1984;4:689–92.
13. Waters PM. Comparison of the natural history, the outcome of microsurgical repair, and the outcome of operative reconstruction in brachial plexus birth palsy. J Bone Joint Surg Am 1999;81:649–59.
14. van der Sluijs JA, van Ouwerkerk WJ, Manoliu RA, et al. Secondary deformities of the shoulder in infants with an obstetrical brachial plexus lesions considered for neurosurgical treatment. Neurosurg Focus 2004;16:E9.
15. Waters PM, Smith GR, Jaramillo D. Glenohumeral deformity secondary to brachial plexus birth palsy. J Bone Joint Surg Am 1998;80:668–77.
16. Hoeksma AF, Ter Steeg AM, Dijkstra P, et al. Shoulder contracture and osseous deformity in obstetrical brachial plexus injuries. J Bone Joint Surg Am 2003; 85:316–22.
17. Hentz VR. Congenital brachial plexus exploration. Tech Hand Up Extrem Surg 2004;8(2):58–69.
18. Borschel GH, Clarke HM. Obstetrical brachial plexus palsy. Plast Reconstr Surg 2009; 124(1 Suppl):144e–55e.
19. Malessy MJA, Pondaag W. Obstetric brachial plexus injuries. Neurosurg Clin N Am 2009;20(1):1–14.

20. Tse R, Kozin SH, Malessy MJ, et al. International federation of societies for surgery of the hand committee report: the role of nerve transfers in the treatment of neonatal brachial plexus palsy. J Hand Surg Am 2015;40(6):1246–59.

21. Hentz VR, Meyer RD. Brachial plexus microsurgery in children. Microsurgery 1991;12(3):175–85.

22. Gilbert A. Long-term evaluation of brachial plexus surgery in obstetrical palsy. Hand Clin 1995;11:583–94 [discussion: 594–5].

23. Birch R. Obstetric brachial plexus palsy. J Hand Surg Br 2002;27:3–8.

24. Gilbert A, Pivato G, Kheiralla T. Long-term results of primary repair of brachial plexus lesions in children. Microsurgery 2006;26(4):334–42.

25. Lin JC, Schwentker-Colizza A, Curtis CG, et al. Final results of grafting versus neurolysis in obstetrical brachial plexus palsy. Plast Reconstr Surg 2009;123:939–48.

26. Malessy MJA, Pondaag W. Nerve surgery for neonatal brachial plexus palsy. J Pediatr Rehabil Med 2011;4(2):141–8.

27. Gilbert A. Indications and strategy. In: Gilbert A, editor. Brachial plexus injuries. London: Martin Dunitz; 2001. p. 205–10.

28. Al-Qattan MM, Clarke HM, Curtis CG. The prognostic value of concurrent Horner's syndrome in total obstetric brachial plexus injury. J Hand Surg Br 2000;25:166–7.

29. Curtis C, Stephens D, Clarke HM, et al. The Active Movement Scale: an evaluative tool for infants with obstetrical brachial plexus palsy. J Hand Surg Am 2002;7:470–8.

30. Tassin JL. Paralysies obstetrices du plexus brachial. Evolution spontanee, resultats des interventions reparatrices precoses. Paris: Universite Paris; 1984.

31. Bade SA, Lin JC, Curtis CG, et al. Extending the indications for primary nerve surgery in obstetrical brachial plexus palsy. Biomed Res Int 2014;2014:627067.

32. Steens SC, Pondaag W, Malessy MJA, et al. Obstetric brachial plexus lesions: CT myelography. Radiology 2011;259(2):508–15.

33. Chow BC, Blaser S, Clarke HM. Predictive value of computed tomographic myelography in obstetrical brachial plexus palsy. Plast Reconstr Surg 2000;106(5):971–7.

34. Abbott R, Abbott M, Alzate J, et al. Magnetic resonance imaging of obstetrical brachial plexus injuries. Childs Nerv Syst 2004;20:720–5.

35. Tse R, Nixon JN, Iyer RS, et al. The diagnostic value of CT myelography, MR myelography, and both in neonatal brachial plexus palsy. AJNR Am J Neuroradiol 2014;35(7):1425–32.

36. Hale HB, Bae DS, Waters PM. Current concepts in the management of brachial plexus birth palsy. J Hand Surg Am 2010;35(2):322–31.

37. Benjamin K. Part 1. Injuries to the brachial plexus: mechanisms of injury and identification of risk factors. Adv Neonatal Care 2005;5(4):181–9.

38. Geutjens G, Gilbert A, Helsen K. Obstetric brachial plexus palsy associated with breech delivery. A different pattern of injury. J Bone Joint Surg Br 1996;78(2):303–6.

39. Blaauw G. Results of surgery after breech delivery. In: Gilbert A, editor. Brachial plexus injuries. London: Martin Dunitz; 2001. p. 217–24.

40. Borrero JL. Surgical technique. In: Gilbert A, editor. Brachial plexus injuries. London: Martin Dunitz; 2001. p. 189–204.

41. Marcus JR, Clarke HM. Management of obstetrical brachial plexus palsy. In: Bentz ML, Bauer BS, Zuker RM, editors. Principles and practice of pediatric plastic surgery. St Louis (MO): Quality Medical Publishing Inc; 2007. p. 1427–53.

42. Allieu Y, Privat JM, Bonnel F. Neurotization with the spinal nerve (nervus accessorius) in avulsions of roots of the brachial plexus. Neurochirurgie 1982;28:115–20.

43. Kawabata H, Shibata T, Matsui Y, et al. Use of intercostal nerves for neurotization of the musculocutaneous nerve in infants with birth-related brachial plexus palsy. J Neurosurg 2001;94:386–91.

44. Lin H, Hou C, Chen D. Modified C7 neurotization for the treatment of obstetrical brachial plexus palsy. Muscle Nerve 2010;42(5):764–8.

45. Capek L, Clarke HM, Zuker RM. Endoscopic sural nerve harvest in the pediatric patient. Plast Reconstr Surg 1996;98:884–8.

46. Clarke HM. An update on endoscopic sural nerve harvest. Plast Reconstr Surg 1998;102(4):1304.

47. Al-Qattan MM. Identification of the phrenic nerve in surgical exploration of the brachial plexus in obstetric palsy. J Hand Surg Am 2004;29:391–2.

48. Redett R, Hawkins C, Murji A, et al. The value of intraoperative frozen section histology during obstetrical brachial plexus reconstruction. In: Renner A, editor. Proceedings of the Ninth International Federation of Societies for Surgery of the Hand. Budapest (Hungary): Medimond; 2004. p. 493.

49. Gilchrist DK. A stockinette-Velpeau for immobilization of the shoulder-girdle. J Bone Joint Surg Am 1967;49:750–1.

50. Pondaag W, de Boer R, van Wijlen-Hempel MS, et al. External rotation as a result of suprascapular nerve neurotization in obstetric brachial plexus lesions. Neurosurgery 2005;57(3):530–7.

51. Tse R, Marcus JR, Curtis CG, et al. Suprascapular nerve reconstruction in obstetrical brachial plexus palsy: spinal accessory nerve transfer versus C5 root grafting. Plast Reconstr Surg 2011;127:2391–6.

52. Pondaag W, Malessy MJA. Intercostal and pectoral nerve transfers to re-innervate the biceps muscle

in obstetric brachial plexus lesions. J Hand Surg Eur 2013;39(6):647–52.

53. Lin H, Hou C, Chen D. Contralateral C7 transfer for the treatment of upper obstetrical brachial plexus palsy. Pediatr Surg Int 2011;27(9):997–1001.

54. Chen L, Gu Y-D, Hu S-N, et al. Contralateral C7 transfer for the treatment of brachial plexus root avulsions in children - a report of 12 cases. J Hand Surg Am 2007;32(1):96–103.

55. El-Gammal TA, Abdel-Latif MM, Kotb MM, et al. Intercostal nerve transfer in infants with obstetric brachial plexus palsy. Microsurgery 2008;28(7): 499–504.

56. Luo PB, Chen L, Zhou CH, et al. Results of intercostal nerve transfer to the musculocutaneous nerve in brachial plexus birth palsy. J Pediatr Orthop 2011; 31(8):884–8.

57. Bahm J, Naoman H, Becker M. The dorsal approach to the suprascapular nerve in neuromuscular reanimation for obstetric brachial plexus lesions. Plast Reconstr Surg 2005;115:240–4.

58. Bertelli JA, Ghizoni MF. Improved technique for harvesting the accessory nerve for transfer in brachial plexus injuries. Neurosurgery 2006;58(4 Suppl 2): 366–70 [discussion: 370].

59. Colbert SH, Mackinnon S. Posterior approach for double nerve transfer for restoration of shoulder function in upper brachial plexus palsy. Hand (N Y) 2006;1(2):71–7.

60. Ladak A, Morhart M, O'Grady K, et al. Distal nerve transfers are effective in treating patients with upper trunk obstetrical brachial plexus injuries. Plast Reconstr Surg 2013;132(6):985e–92e.

61. Clarke HM, Curtis GG. Examination and prognosis. In: Gilbert A, editor. Brachial plexus injuries. London: Martin Dunitz; 1995. p. 159–72.

62. Mallet J. Obstetric paralysis of the brachial plexus. II. Therapeutics. Treatment of sequelae. Results of different therapeutic technics and indications. Rev Chir Orthop Reparatrice Appar Mot 1972;58(Suppl 1):192–6 [in French].

63. Mallet J. Obstetric paralysis of the brachial plexus. III. Conclusions. Rev Chir Orthop Reparatrice Appar Mot 1972;58(Suppl 1):201–4 [in French].

64. Medical Research Council, Nerve Injuries Committee. Aids to the investigation of peripheral nerve injuries. London: His Majesty's Stationery Office; 1942.

65. Bae DS, Waters PM, Zurakowski D. Reliability of three classification systems measuring active motion in brachial plexus birth palsy. J Bone Joint Surg Am 2003;85(9):1733–8.

66. Kawabata H, Masada K, Isuyuguchi T, et al. Early microsurgical reconstruction in birth palsy. Clin Orthop 1987;215:233–42.

67. Gilbert A, Brockman R, Carlioz H. Surgical treatment of brachial plexus birth injury. Clin Orthop 1991;264: 39–47.

68. Clarke HM, Al-Qattan MM, Curtis CG, et al. Obstetrical brachial plexus palsy: results following neurolysis of conducting neuromas-in-continuity. Plast Reconstr Surg 1996;97:974–82 [discussion 983–4].

69. Capek L, Clarke HM, Curtis CG. Neuroma-in-continuity resection: early outcome in obstetrical brachial plexus palsy. Plast Reconstr Surg 1998; 102:1555–62 [discussion: 1563–4].

70. Aydin A, Mersa B, Erer M, et al. Early results of nerve surgery in obstetrical brachial plexus palsy. Acta Orthop Traumatol Turc 2004;38:170–7 [in Turkish].

71. El-Gammal TA, El-Sayed A, Kotb MM, et al. Total obstetric brachial plexus palsy: results and strategy of microsurgical reconstruction. Microsurgery 2010; 30(3):169–78.

72. Boome RS, Kaye JC. Obstetric traction injuries of the brachial plexus. Natural history, indications for surgical repair and results. J Bone Joint Surg Br 1988; 70(4):571–6.

73. Bertelli JA, Ghizoni MF. Reconstruction of C5 and C6 brachial plexus avulsion injury by multiple nerve transfers: spinal accessory to suprascapular, ulnar fascicles to biceps branch, and triceps long or lateral head branch to axillary nerve. J Hand Surg Am 2004;29(1):131–9.

74. Mackinnon SE, Novak CB, Myckatyn TM, et al. Results of reinnervation of the biceps and brachialis muscles with a double fascicular transfer for elbow flexion. J Hand Surg Am 2005;30(5):978–85.

75. Leechavengvongs S, Witoonchart K, Uerpairojkit C, et al. Combined nerve transfers for C5 and C6 brachial plexus avulsion injury. J Hand Surg Am 2006;31(2):183–9.

76. Colbert SH, Mackinnon SE. Nerve transfers for brachial plexus reconstruction. Hand Clin 2008; 24(4):341–61.

77. Tung TH, Mackinnon SE. Nerve transfers: indications, techniques, and outcomes. J Hand Surg Am 2010;35(2):332–41.

78. Garg R, Merrell GA, Hillstrom HJ, et al. Comparison of nerve transfers and nerve grafting for traumatic upper plexus palsy: a systematic review and analysis. J Bone Joint Surg Am 2011;93(9):819–29.

79. Painter MW, Brosius Lutz A, Cheng YC, et al. Diminished Schwann cell repair responses underlie age-associated impaired axonal regeneration. Neuron 2014;83(2):331–43.

80. Al-Qattan MM. Oberlin's ulnar nerve transfer to the biceps nerve in Erb's birth palsy. Plast Reconstr Surg 2002;109:405–7.

81. Oberlin C, Beal D, Leechavengvongs S, et al. Nerve transfer to biceps muscle using a part of ulnar nerve for C5-C6 avulsion of the brachial plexus: anatomical study and report of four cases. J Hand Surg Am 1994;19:232–7.

82. Noaman HH, Shiha AE, Bahm J. Oberlin's ulnar nerve transfer to the biceps motor nerve in obstetric

brachial plexus palsy: indications, and good and bad results. Microsurgery 2004;24:182–7.

83. Shigematsu K, Yajima H, Kobata Y, et al. Oberlin partial ulnar nerve transfer for restoration in obstetric brachial plexus palsy of a newborn: case report. J Brachial Plex Peripher Nerve Inj 2006;1:3.

84. Siqueira MG, Socolovsky M, Heise CO, et al. Efficacy and safety of Oberlin's procedure in the treatment of brachial plexus birth palsy. Neurosurgery 2012;71(6):1156–61.

85. Al-Qattan MM, Al-Kharfy TM. Median nerve to biceps nerve transfer to restore elbow flexion in obstetric brachial plexus palsy. Biomed Res Int 2014; 2014(4):1–4.

86. Little KJ, Zlotolow DA, Soldado F, et al. Early functional recovery of elbow flexion and supination following median and/or ulnar nerve fascicle transfer in upper neonatal brachial plexus palsy. J Bone Joint Surg Am 2014;96:215–21.

87. Estrella EP, Mella PM. Double nerve transfer for elbow flexion in obstetric brachial plexus injury: a case report. J Plast Reconstr Aesthet Surg 2013; 66(3):423–6.

88. McRae MC, Borschel GH. Transfer of triceps motor branches of the radial nerve to the axillary nerve with or without other nerve transfers provides antigravity shoulder abduction in pediatric brachial plexus injury. Hand 2012;7(2):186–90.

89. Blaauw G, Slooff ACJ. Transfer of pectoral nerves to the musculocutaneous nerve in obstetric upper brachial plexus palsy. Neurosurgery 2003;53(2): 338–42.

90. Wellons JC III, Tubbs RS, Pugh JA, et al. Medial pectoral nerve to musculocutaneous nerve neurotization for the treatment of persistent birth-related brachial plexus palsy: an 11-year institutional experience. J Neurosurg Pediatr 2009;3(5): 348–53.

Nerve Transfers for the Restoration of Wrist, Finger, and Thumb Extension After High Radial Nerve Injury

Mitchell A. Pet, MD[a], Angelo B. Lipira, MD[a], Jason H. Ko, MD[b],*

KEYWORDS

• Nerve transfer • Radial nerve injury • Wrist extension • Finger extension • Thumb extension

KEY POINTS

- High radial nerve injuries have traditionally been reconstructed using techniques of nerve repair, nerve grafting, and/or tendon transfer.
- Nerve transfer has emerged as an alternative reconstructive strategy that is supported by the literature and offers several advantages.
- For classic high radial nerve injury, nerve transfer is a reliable option to restore wrist, finger, and thumb extension.
- Nerve transfer is also applicable to radial nerve dysfunction of other etiologies, including brachial plexopathy, cervical spinal cord injury, and stroke.

 Video content accompanies this article at http://www.hand.theclinics.com

INTRODUCTION

High radial nerve palsy can occur after a variety of traumatic, compressive, and iatrogenic insults to the upper extremity. It presents most commonly in association with humeral shaft fractures, complicating approximately 11.8% of these injuries.[1] The radial nerve can be injured by bony fragments during the original trauma or reduction, iatrogenic injury during open reduction and internal fixation, and by entrapment within bony callus and scar surrounding the healing fracture.

The classic high radial nerve palsy reflects injury at the level of the humeral shaft and presents with the inability to actively extend the wrist, fingers, and thumb. Unchecked by the extensors, the intact wrist and finger flexors produce a resting position characterized by a flexed wrist ("wrist drop") and partially closed palm. This leaves the patient unable to fully open the hand for the purpose of initiating grasp, rendering tasks requiring manual dexterity quite difficult.[2] Furthermore, because of the inability to stabilize the wrist during activation of the wrist and finger flexors, power grip is also diminished significantly. Without consistent splinting, passive motion can be lost and fixed flexion at the wrist and finger joints may be observed.

There is a considerable body of literature surrounding the optimal management of high radial nerve palsy, especially in the setting of humeral shaft fracture.[2] Although most authors agree that open injuries should be explored acutely, differing opinions exist regarding the timing and type of reconstruction offered when a radial nerve discontinuity is identified. The management of

a Division of Plastic and Reconstructive Surgery, Harborview Medical Center, University of Washington School of Medicine, 325 9th Avenue, Mailstop #359796, Seattle, WA 98104, USA; b Division of Plastic Surgery, Northwestern University Feinberg School of Medicine, 675 N. St. Clair Street, Suite 19-250, Chicago, IL 60611, USA
* Corresponding author.
E-mail address: Jason.ko@nm.org

Hand Clin 32 (2016) 191–207
http://dx.doi.org/10.1016/j.hcl.2015.12.007
0749-0712/16/$ – see front matter © 2016 Elsevier Inc. All rights reserved.

closed injuries is even more controversial, with some authors advocating early exploration and others preferring a period of observation to allow a chance for spontaneous recovery. Recent publications, including a rigorous decision analysis[3] and metaanalysis,[1] seem to demonstrate that there is no evidence of inferior outcomes when a waiting period of several months is allowed, and waiting has become a popular strategy.

Although areas of controversy persist, most published algorithms[1,4,5] for the management of high radial nerve palsy have several key features in common:

- Early exploration of open or very high-energy injuries and acute or subacute reconstruction by primary repair or nerve grafting, based on the zone of injury;
- Observation of closed injuries for a period of 3 to 6 months, followed by nerve exploration and reconstruction in patients who demonstrate no evidence of clinical or electromyographic recovery; and
- Tendon transfers for wrist, finger, and thumb extension for patients with a failed nerve reconstruction or delayed presentation.

Despite their increasing acceptance as a viable alternative to tendon transfer for the restoration of wrist, finger, and thumb extension, nerve transfers are notably absent from this outline. As such, this article aims to summarize the development of nerve transfers applicable to this clinical scenario, review the supporting literature, and provide illustrative case examples. Classic high radial nerve palsy will be examined first, followed by a discussion of nerve transfers for radial nerve dysfunction of other etiologies.

ANATOMY

The course of the radial nerve in the upper arm, and how this relates to its propensity for traumatic injury, have been extensively studied and carefully documented.[2] More pertinent to this article is a review of the branching pattern of the radial nerve in the forearm and the key anatomic relationships that guide safe and reliable dissection during nerve transfer surgery. Familiarity with the median nerve and its branches is equally important, because it is the principal donor in these nerve transfers. Branch sizes and axon counts are not discussed but are well-described in multiple anatomic studies.[6–8]

Radial Nerve

After piercing the lateral intermuscular septum in the upper arm, the radial nerve courses between the brachialis and brachioradialis muscles. Within this interval, the radial nerve branches first to the brachioradialis muscle. At or just above the interepicondylar line, the extensor carpi radialis longus (ECRL) branch arises and runs for a short distance between the brachioradialis and ECRL. The radial nerve then enters the forearm by passing anterior to the lateral epicondyle before splitting into a superficial radial sensory nerve (RSN) (which travels beneath the brachioradialis) and a deep motor branch. The deep motor component gives a branch to the extensor carpi radialis brevis (ECRB) approximately 2 to 3 cm distal to the interepicondylar line. Just proximal to the leading edge of the supinator (arcade of Frohse), 1 or 2 branches to the supinator arise from the deep surface of the motor branch. After coursing beneath the tendinous leading edge of the supinator and traversing the supinator muscle, the deep motor branch becomes the posterior interosseous nerve (PIN). During exposure, the PIN is found to be the most radial branch, the RSN is the most ulnar, and the smaller ECRB branch lies in between.

Median Nerve

The first branch from the median nerve as it travels medial to the brachial artery in the antecubital fossa is to the pronator teres (PT). This branch originates from the superficial surface of the nerve near the interepicondylar line and may be duplicate or of a single origin with rapid bifurcation before entering the PT. The median nerve then travels underneath the tendinous arch of the flexor digitorum superficialis (FDS), which must be divided to expose the underlying branches. Further distal, branches to the flexor carpi radialis (FCR) and palmaris longus (if present) originate from the deep ulnar aspect of the nerve individually, or as a single trunk with rapid bifurcation. Two or 3 FDS branches then arise from the ulnar side of the nerve, and the larger anterior interosseous nerve (AIN) arises from the radial side. The main trunk of the median nerve goes on to give rise to the palmar cutaneous branch in the distal forearm before entering the carpal tunnel.

SURGICAL TREATMENT OF HIGH RADIAL NERVE INJURY
Primary Repair and Nerve Grafting

In cases of high radial nerve injury without a nerve gap, an expedient and tension-free primary repair is a time-tested reconstructive strategy[2] that is applicable most commonly in cases of sharp laceration from penetrating trauma or iatrogenic injury during open treatment of a humerus fracture. It is only in these cases of sharp nerve transection that the cut nerve ends are likely to be in suitable condition for tension-free primary repair.

In blunt, blast, or traction mechanisms, the extended zone of injury usually necessitates considerable nerve resection to obtain healthy proximal and distal stumps. When exploring open injuries in the acute setting, the zone of injury is not obvious. As such, intraoperative histologic examination of nerve sections or nerve tagging followed by delayed reconstruction may be indicated. Once the zone of injury has been resected and the gap defined, nerve grafting with 1 or multiple cables can be undertaken. Owing to the proximal innervation of muscle targets, the outcomes for nerve graft reconstruction of the proximal radial nerve are better than for other major upper extremity nerves.[9] However, even in large volume centers, recovery is hardly reliable. In a series of 220 radial nerve gaps repaired with sural nerve grafting, Shergill and colleagues[10] documented an overall failure rate of 42%. Results were worst in cases of "untidy" wounds, long gaps, and extended delay before surgical repair.

When considering primary repair or nerve grafting of a high radial nerve injury, we recommend attention to the following pearls:

- Any tension on a nerve coaptation will lead to an inferior result. When performing a primary repair, neurolyse both proximally and distally to allow a tension-free coaptation throughout the entire range of motion. If this cannot be accomplished, consider an alternative method of reconstruction.
- At the time of nerve reconstruction, identify and release all anatomic points of distal nerve compression.
- While awaiting reinnervation, maintain supple joints and avoid flexion contracture at the wrist and fingers with judicious splinting and therapy.
- Follow these patients closely. Failure to observe an advancing Tinel's and/or motor recovery in the 6 to 9 months after primary repair or nerve grafting should prompt electrodiagnostic evaluation and consideration of nerve transfer before motor endplate degeneration occurs.

Tendon Transfer and Nerve Transfer

Most hand and upper extremity surgeons are comfortable and facile with their preferred set of tendon transfers to restore wrist, finger, and thumb extension. Indeed, several tendon transfer combinations have been shown to provide consistent and satisfactory outcomes for this indication.[11–13]

However, despite their reliability, tendon transfers have several disadvantages that have invited improvement and innovation in the area of nerve transfer surgery. The advantages and limitations of tendon and nerve transfers for the indication of high radial nerve injury are summarized and compared in **Table 1**. Given its favorable profile, nerve transfer has become an accepted, and often preferred, treatment for reconstructing wrist, finger, and thumb extension after high radial nerve injury and radial nerve dysfunction of other etiologies.

Nerve Transfer for High Radial Nerve Injury: Review of the Literature

Nerve transfer was first proposed as a treatment for radial nerve gaps associated with humeral fracture by A. S. Lurje in 1948.[14] Lurje had developed a technique of anterior transposition of the radial nerve into the interval between the biceps and brachialis muscles, which allowed him to perform primary repair of nerve gaps of up to 6 cm. However, in performing this transposition procedure on longer nerve gaps, the author noted considerable difficulty in stretching the ends of the radial nerve, and admitted some "doubt whether the central end of the nerve would be able to neurotize its peripheral end due to considerable tension."

Having routinely observed the branches of the musculocutaneous nerve to the biceps and brachialis coursing in the same intermuscular interval used for transposition, Lurje changed his approach and performed nerve transfer of the uninjured musculocutaneous nerve to the distal radial nerve stump in 2 patients with particularly long nerve gaps. To preserve critical elbow flexion, the donor was taken proximal to the expendable brachialis branches but distal to the biceps branches. Both patients treated with this procedure recovered some wrist extension between 13 to 15 months postoperatively, but experienced no recovery of finger or thumb extension.

The techniques described by Lurje were remarkable for their creativity, but in retrospect, it is clear that the proposed musculocutaneous to radial nerve transfer technique fails to follow several fundamental principles of nerve transfer, which had yet to be elucidated. Specifically, this technique uses a nonsynergistic donor–recipient pair and foregoes the opportunity to convert the proximal injury into a more distal one.

In 2001, Ustün and colleagues[6] published a cadaver-based anatomic study establishing the feasibility of transferring median nerve branches to the PIN. By moving the surgical repair to the level of the forearm, this strategy offered an

Table 1
Comparison of the advantages and limitations of tendon and nerve transfer for high radial nerve injury

Tendon Transfer	Nerve Transfer
Can be done at any time	Must be done before motor endplate degeneration (<10 mo)
Shorter surgical time	Longer surgical time
Extensive muscle dissection required	Muscle is not dissected
Muscle biomechanics significantly altered.	Muscle remains in situ without alteration of biomechanics
Donors should have at least MRC 4/5 strength	Donors should have at least MRC 4/5 strength
Donor deficit related to complete sacrifice of donor muscle/tendon function has been documented (PT, FDS, PL)	Donor should be expendable, but deficit often limited by choosing redundant nerve branches for transfer
Single transfer can restore a single function Separate finger and thumb extension transfers are necessary, and independent finger extension is not provided	One nerve transfer can restore multiple functions. A single nerve transfer can provide thumb and independent finger extension.
Prolonged postoperative immobilization is necessary, leading to decreased passive range of motion	No postoperative immobilization is required
High frequency, short duration hand therapy	Low frequency, long duration hand therapy for motor reeducation
Rapid return of function	Delayed return of function (10–12 mo)
Tendon repair at risk for rupture or adhesion	Complications of tendon repair are not applicable

Abbreviations: FDS, flexor digitorum superficialis; MRC, medical research council; PL, palmaris longus; PT, pronator teres.
   Adapted from Davidge KM, Yee A, Kahn LC, et al. Median to radial nerve transfers for restoration of wrist, finger, and thumb extension. J Hand Surg Am 2013;38(9):1826; with permission.

opportunity to deliver regenerating donor axons to the radial nerve branches very close to the extensor musculature, facilitating prompt reinnervation before motor endplate degeneration. Furthermore, given the reliable radial nerve branching pattern and wealth of expendable median nerve branches in the forearm, this marriage has offered surgeons extensive flexibility in selecting donor–recipient branch pairs that facilitate easy motor reeducation and promote good outcomes.

Transfer of median nerve branches for the reconstruction of high radial nerve palsy was first described in a clinical setting by Susan Mackinnon's group in 2002.[15] In their initial 2 cases, wrist extension was restored using a branch to the FDS transferred to the ECRB. Finger extension was restored with transfer of the palmaris longus branch, with or without an additional FDS fascicle to the PIN. Recovery of 40° to 45° of wrist extension with MRC grade 4 strength was seen in both patients. Finger extension recovered fully in 1 patient and partially in the other.

Although FDS to ECRB has remained their preferred transfer for wrist extension, Mackinnon's group has refined their technique for finger/thumb extension and now considers the FCR a better donor for transfer to the PIN than the palmaris longus/FDS branches. This modified set of transfers pairs donor and recipient nerve functions that are complementary based on the tenodesis effect.[16] This is advantageous during rehabilitation, allowing the patient to activate a substituted motor function that was already cortically linked to the function being replaced. In cases where antagonistic donors were used, this group has observed a more difficult (and in 1 case, completely unsuccessful) course of postoperative motor reeducation, despite successful muscle reinnervation.[17] Donor deficits in median nerve function are mild and transient, owing to redundant donor muscle innervation, as well as compensation by the flexor carpi ulnaris for the FCR and the flexor digitorum profundus for the FDS.[18]

In a subsequent publication, Mackinnon's group went on to describe adjuvant PT to ECRB end-to-side tendon transfer performed at the time of nerve transfer to offer some early recovery of wrist extension. This serves as a functional bridge during the 9 to 12 months spent awaiting reinnervation after nerve transfer, and may act to preserve passive range of motion in the wrist, which might otherwise be lost during this time.[19] They recommend this adjuvant tendon transfer in all cases where the patient is a suitable candidate. Potential exclusion criteria include wrist joint stiffness or complex regional pain syndrome that might be exacerbated by prolonged immobilization, or cases where the PT nerve or muscle/tendon is nonfunctional, nonexpendable, or is required for another transfer.

García-López and colleagues[20,21] have published an alternative set of nerve transfers for high radial nerve palsy. Although this group also recommends FCR to PIN transfer for finger extension, they advocate pairing this with transfer of a PT nerve branch to the ECRL to reconstruct wrist extension. They found that 2 branches of the median nerve innervate the PT and that transfer of 1 branch to the ECRL resulted in restoration of M4 wrist extension in 6 patients, while preserving at least M4 pronation strength.

García-López and colleagues advocate targeting of the ECRL rather than the ECRB because they find the ECRB branch to be more variable in its origin, and the ECRL to be quite easily identified. Because the ECRL tendon inserts more radially than the ECRB, they have observed some radial deviation with wrist extension during early recovery. This resolved shortly thereafter as the ECU became reinnervated via the PIN. The stated impetus for choosing a donor for wrist extension other than the FDS comes from this group's experience in patients with C5 to C8 root avulsion that underwent isolated FDS to ECRB transfer. Although some wrist extension was restored, these patients were unable to maintain the wrist in neutral position without flexing the fingers.[22] This is problematic, because this motion precludes the act of reaching forward with an extended wrist and open hand, as one would to grasp an object placed in front of them. Although this concern is certainly valid in the population studied, it is not necessarily applicable to patients with high radial nerve palsy who undergo concomitant FCR to PIN transfer for finger extension. When these transfers are performed as a pair, it is likely that the restoration of active finger extension mitigates the unwanted finger flexion observed with wrist extension when FDS to ECRB transfer alone was performed. This concern aside, the outcomes documented for FCR to PIN and PT to ECRL nerve transfer are encouraging, and this seems to be a viable strategy for addressing high radial nerve palsy.

A summary of published outcomes for all of the various median-to-radial nerve transfers described in the literature is provided in **Table 2**.

Evaluation and Management of the Patient with High Radial Nerve Injury: A Clinical Algorithm

In **Fig. 1** we present our clinical algorithm for evaluation and surgical management of acute, traumatic isolated high radial nerve palsy. This encompasses the majority of patients we treat, but special consideration must be given to several groups. Delayed presentations necessarily alter this course, because nerve transfers should ideally be performed at a maximum of 10 months after injury. In patients presenting more than 10 months after injury, nerve transfers are usually inadvisable, and we recommend tendon transfer, which can be done at any time. Furthermore, although nerve transfer is our method of choice, patients who prioritize expedient functional recovery (ie, manual laborers who need to return to work) may benefit more from tendon transfer. Similarly, patients who are unwilling to commit to a prolonged course of motor reeducation may fare better with tendon transfers rather than nerve transfers. Whereas nerve grafting is not routinely part of our algorithm for motor recovery, it may play a role in children (where the distance to target is decreased), in cases of oncologic nerve resection where the zone of injury is well-defined, and in patients with limited nerve and/or tendon donors.

BEYOND HIGH RADIAL NERVE INJURY: MOTOR NERVE TRANSFERS FOR RADIAL NERVE DYSFUNCTION OF OTHER ETIOLOGIES

Because most radial nerve transections occur along the spiral groove of the humerus, nerve transfer techniques were first developed to address the resultant high radial nerve palsy. Given the encouraging results seen with this initial application, several groups have investigated nerve transfer as a method of reconstructing radial nerve dysfunction of other etiologies. This has included the application of previously described median-to-radial transfers to new problems, in addition to the introduction of transfers that are altogether novel. This body of work is organized by indication and summarized elsewhere in this paper.

Upper Cervical Root Injury

Extended upper brachial plexus injuries affecting the fifth, sixth, and seventh cervical roots cause radial nerve dysfunction, and affected patients often have severely compromised extensor function at the wrist and fingers (in addition to the elbow, which is beyond the scope of this review). To address the wrist extension deficit, Ukrit and

Table 2
Summary of all nerve transfers in the literature targeting wrist and/or finger/thumb extension

Author, Year	Nerve Transfer	Indication	n	Mean Follow-Up	Outcomes	Donor Deficit	Notes
Lurje,[14] 1948	MCN to RN	High radial nerve palsy	2	14 mo	Some wrist extension No finger or thumb extension restored	No serious impairment of elbow flexion	MCN taken distal to biceps branch
Ray and Mackinnon,[17] 2011	FDS to ECRB, FCR to PIN (7) FDS to PIN, FCR to ECRB (2) FDS to PIN, PL to ECRB (3) FDS to PIN (2) FDS to ECRB and PIN (3) FCR to ECRB and PIN (1) FDS to ECRB, FPL to PIN (1)	High radial nerve palsy	19	20 mo	Wrist extension: M5 in 1, M4 in 15, M0 in 1 Finger extension: M5 in 1, M4 in 10, M3 in 2, Minimal or M0 in 6	NR	Supplemental PT to ECRB tendon transfer performed in 9 patients Isolated FDS to PIN transfer performed in 2 patients with preserved wrist extension
García-López et al,[20] 2014	PT to ECRL FCR to PIN	High radial nerve palsy (4) Posterior cord lesion (2)	6	20 mo	Wrist extension: M4 in all Finger extension: M4 in 4, M3 in 2 Thumb extension/abduction: M4 in all	Pronation downgraded from M5 to M4 in 3 patients Wrist flexion downgraded from M5 to M4 in 2 patients	Independent motor control was achieved
Ukrit et al,[7] 2009	FDS to ECRB	C5-7 root avulsion	2	24 mo	Wrist extension: M4 in both AROM: 0°–30° in 1, 0°–70° in 1	No deficit of finger flexion	—
Bertelli and Ghizoni,[22] 2012	FDS to ECRB (all) PL to PIN (1)	C5-8 root avulsion	3	32 mo	Wrist extension: M3- in 2, M3 in 1 Finger extension: M0 in 1	No deficit of finger flexion	Wrist extension independent of finger flexion was not achieved Wrist extension beyond neutral not achieved

Study	Transfer	Diagnosis	No.	Follow-up	Motor result	Deficit	Comments
Bertelli et al,[23] 2012	PQ to ECRB	C5-8 root avulsion	4	12 mo	Wrist extension: M4 in all, full AROM	Transient deficit of pronation recovered completely by 12 mo	Wrist extension independent of forearm pronation was achieved. PQ reinnervated by concomitant transfer of redundant thenar or FDS motor branch
Bertelli et al,[36] 2012	Supinator to PIN	C6 tetraplegia	1	6 mo	Finger extension: M4 Full AROM at MCPJ, slight deficit at PIPJ Thumb extension: 8 cm from thumb pulp to index finger during maximal extension	No deficit of supination	Bilateral procedure, symmetric result. Finger and thumb extension independent of supination was achieved
Bertelli and Ghizoni,[25] 2010	Supinator to PIN	C7-T1 root avulsion	4	12 mo	Finger and thumb extension: M3 in all	No deficit of supination	Finger and thumb extension independent of supination was achieved
Xu et al,[26] 2015	Supinator to PIN	C7-T1 root avulsion	10	43 mo	Finger extension: M4 in 6, M3 in 3, M2 in 1 Thumb extension: M3 in 7, M2 in 2, M1 in 1	No deficit of supination	ECU neurotization resolved radial deviation during wrist extension in 7 of 10 patients
Fox et al,[27] 2014	Supinator to PIN (1) Supinator to ECU (1)	C5 or C6 tetraplegia	2	N/A	N/A	No deficit of supination	Too early in postoperative course to expect recovery
Fridén and Gohritz,[31] 2012	Brachialis to ECRL	C5 tetraplegia	1	5 mo	Wrist extension: M3	No deficit of elbow flexion	Early result, further improvement expected

(continued on next page)

Table 2
(continued)

Author, Year	Nerve Transfer	Indication	n	Mean Follow-Up	Outcomes	Donor Deficit	Notes
Palazzi et al,[32] 2006	Brachialis to PIN (with nerve graft)	C7-T1 root avulsion	1	26 mo	Finger extension: M3 Thumb extension: M1 Wrist extension (ECU): M3+	NR	—
Plate et al,[37] 2013	PT to PIN	Posterior cord lesion	1	36 mo	Finger extension: M4, full AROM Wrist extension: M4+, AROM to 40° of extension	NR	Concomitant posterior cord grafting may have contributed to wrist extension recovery via radial wrist extensors
Brown, 2011[33]	Anterior and middle deltoid fascicles of axillary nerve to wrist and finger extensor fascicles of radial nerve	C5 tetraplegia	1	N/A	N/A	No deficit of deltoid function	Too early in postoperative course to expect recovery Very proximal transfer, performed at shoulder level

Abbreviations: AROM, active range of motion; ECRB, extensor carpi radialis brevis; ECRL, extensor carpi radialis longus; ECU, extensor carpi ulnaris; FCR, flexor carpi radialis; FDS, flexor digitorum sublimis; FPL, flexor pollicus longus; MCN, musculocutaneous nerve; MCPJ, metacarpophalangeal joint; N/A, not applicable; PIN, posterior interosseous nerve; PIPJ, proximal interphalangeal joint; PL, palmaris longus; PQ, pronator quadratus; PT, pronator teres; RN, radial nerve.
Data from Refs.[7,14,17,20,22,23,25–27,31–33,36,37]

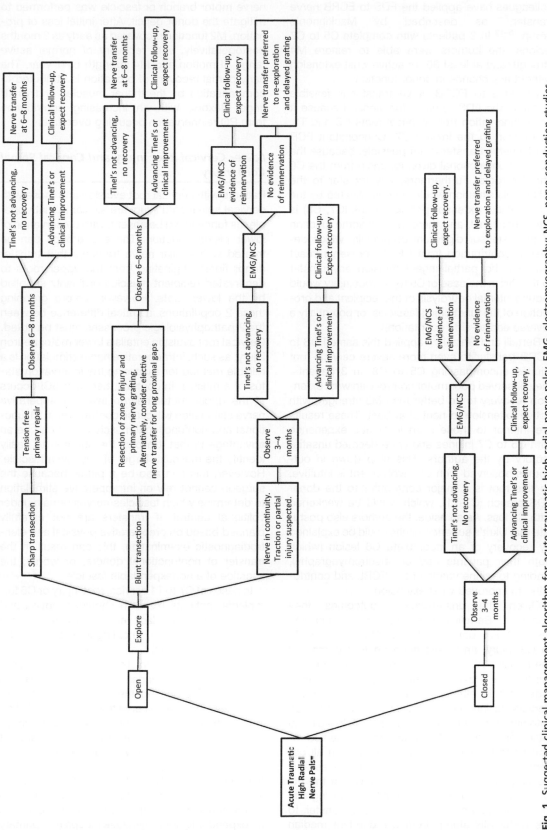

Fig. 1. Suggested clinical management algorithm for acute traumatic high radial nerve palsy. EMG, electromyography; NCS, nerve conduction studies.

colleagues have applied the FDS to ECRB nerve transfer,[7] as described by Mackinnon's group.[15–19] In 2 patients with complete C5 to C7 lesions, the authors were able to restore M4 strength and at least 30° of active wrist extension without any change in donor function.

The FDS to ECRB nerve transfer is feasible because the FDS remains functional, because it gains innervation from cervical roots C8 and T1, in addition to the injured C7. Concomitant FCR to PIN nerve transfer is not possible, because the FCR is nonfunctional given its origin from the C6 and C7 roots. Furthermore, any transfer to the PIN in this situation would be complicated by the fact that the extensor pollicis longus (C7, C8) is often functional, and there may be some function of the extensor digitorum communis, which derives a contribution from C8. To preserve intact thumb and/or partial finger extension, any transfer to the PIN in the case of C5 to C7 root injury would require internal neurolysis of the recipient and protection of the functioning fascicles, or potentially a reverse end-to-side coaptation.

Bertelli and Ghizoni[22] applied this same FDS to ECRB transfer to even more severe cervical root injuries encompassing C5 to C8. In 3 patients, they observed poor motor control with wrist extension recovery to no better than M3 strength, with active extension to neutral at best. These results are inferior to those seen in Ukrit's experience with C5 to C7 injuries and were deemed unsatisfactory by the authors. This step down in outcomes observed with C8 involvement is intuitive, as this root is a major contributor to the donor FDS branch (C7-T1), which would be weakened with C8 loss. As an aside, the authors also postulate that Ukrit's superior results could be explained by recovery of an incomplete C8 lesion (which both their patients had on electromyography), leading to reinnervation of the ECRL and contributing to improved wrist extension.

Given the unsatisfactory outcomes they observed, Bertelli and colleagues[23] abandoned the FDS as a donor to the ECRB in cases of C5 to C8 injury, and have gone on to recommend the terminal AIN innervating the pronator quadratus (PQ) as a better donor. The theoretic advantage of this alternative donor is that the PQ derives its innervation mainly from the T1 root, with only a minor contribution from C8. In 4 clinical cases of PQ to ECRB transfer, they observed recovery of M4 wrist extension strength in all patients. Of note, because the PT is necessarily denervated in these patients, sacrifice of the PQ was expected to result in a nontrivial downgrade in pronation. As such, concomitant transfer to the distal AIN stump from a redundant median

nerve motor branch or fascicle was performed to mitigate the donor deficit. After initial loss of pronation, M2 function recovered as early as 2 months postoperatively, with recovery of normal active range of motion and M4 strength by 1 year. The early partial recovery of pronation is attributed to compensation by the thenar muscles and wrist/finger flexors, with an increasing contribution from PQ reinnervation occurring over time.

Lower Cervical Root Injury and Cervical Spinal Cord Injury

Patients with cervical root avulsion and those with cervical spinal cord injury are similar in that upper plexus function will be absent, with preservation of lower plexus function. These 2 groups can be treated with similar nerve transfers that transfer donor fibers originating from the upper roots to denervated recipient muscles ordinarily supplied by the lower roots. However, before grouping these 2 populations, a critical difference between the 2 pathophysiologic processes must be noted. Cervical root avulsion entails a lower motor neuron injury; as such, intraoperative nerve stimulation is a reliable method for assessing the innervation status of a muscle. In contrast, because SCI occurs at the upper motor neuron level, intraoperative nerve stimulation will cause contraction of all functional and nonfunctional muscles. This can be an advantage in that it allows the surgeon to easily identify the muscular target of any given fascicle. However, this can also be a pitfall, because the surgeon cannot rely on intraoperative stimulation to determine which fascicles/nerves remain under volitional control. If transfers are not carefully planned based on preoperative physical and electrodiagnostic examination, this can result in the transfer of nonfunctional donors, or worse, the sacrifice of a nonexpendable fascicle.

In cases of C7 to T1 cervical root injury or C6 tetraplegia, patients maintain shoulder motion and elbow flexion, but lack elbow extension, wrist flexion, finger flexion, and finger extension. The radial wrist extensors are often functional, but are of variable strength. To address the dysfunction of thumb and finger extension, Bertelli and colleagues[24] proposed the transfer of supinator branches of the radial nerve to the PIN.[25–27] At first glance, this transfer is counterintuitive, because both the donor and recipient are components of the deep branch of the radial nerve. However, in C7 to T1 root avulsion and C6 tetraplegia, the C7 to C8 innervated PIN is not under volitional control, whereas the C5 to C6 innervated supinator remains functional. Furthermore, the supinator is an expendable donor because biceps (the primary supinator of the forearm) function remains intact. In patients who have intact active wrist extensors, the restoration of finger and thumb extension maximizes the functionality of tenodesis grip. When tenodesis grip is not possible or is insufficient, supinator to PIN transfer can be performed with concomitant brachialis to AIN transfer,[28–30] thus restoring both active opening and closure of the hand. In addition to performing these nerve transfers to improve function for tetraplegia, we have used this supinator to PIN transfer in a patient with weak wrist extension after stroke (case 3).

In C5 tetraplegia or C6 to T1 root injury, there is preservation of elbow flexion, but minimal to no function below the elbow. In this case, one of the few available donors is the brachialis branch of the musculocutaneous nerve, which is expendable owing to preservation of the biceps. Fridén and Gohritz have transferred this branch to the ECRL to restore wrist extension,[31] thus providing a tenodesis grip and a platform for passive procedures that may allow a key or pincer grip. This reconstructed functionality, in the setting of preserved elbow flexion, may allow a patient to grasp a utensil and feed himself or herself independently. Transfers of the brachialis branch to the PIN[32] (with nerve graft) and from anterior deltoid branches of the axillary nerve to the wrist/finger extensor fascicles of the radial nerve[33] have also been described.

SENSORY NERVE TRANSFER

Sensory branches of the radial nerve include the posterior brachial cutaneous nerve, the inferior lateral brachial cutaneous nerve, the posterior antebrachial cutaneous nerve, and the RSN. Because the former 3 branches originate high in the arm or axilla, they are less infrequently injured in the common pattern of high radial nerve injury in association with mid or distal humerus fracture. Even when injured, sensory loss in the distribution of these cutaneous nerves over the dorsal arm and forearm causes little functional deficit.

Because it arises distal to the elbow, the RSN is routinely denervated in cases of high radial nerve injury. This leads to numbness on the radial dorsum of the distal forearm and hand. Although not profoundly disabling, a lack of protective sensation in this area can lead to accidental injury. End-to-end lateral antebrachial cutaneous nerve to RSN transfer has been performed to restore sensation in this area, and can be completed through the same exposure as the median-to-radial motor transfers described elsewhere in this paper (**Fig. 2**). Although a donor deficit of lateral forearm numbness is expected, this is outweighed by recovery in the higher priority distribution of the RSN.[16,18] Additionally, transfer of the first branch of the dorsal ulnar cutaneous nerve to the RSN has been proposed based on anatomic study,[34] although clinical implementation of this technique has yet to be documented.

Leechavengvongs and colleagues[35] published a series of 8 patients with severe pain in the RSN distribution owing to deafferentation from C5 to C6 root avulsion injuries. Each was treated with end-to-side transfer of the RSN into the median nerve based on the hypothesis that sensory reinnervation could mitigate their intractable pain. Significant pain relief and sensory recovery to the S2 or S3 level was observed in all patients, representing the effective provision of at least protective sensation in the RSN distribution. Although the implications of this study for pain relief are quite complex, it clearly demonstrates that this end-to-side nerve

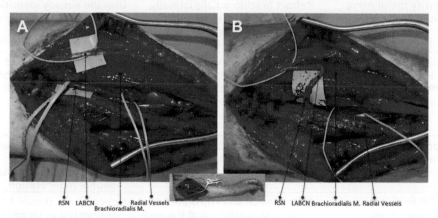

RSN LABCN Radial Vessels
Brachioradialis M.

RSN LABCN Brachioradialis M. Radial Vessels

Fig. 2. (*A*) Exposure of the lateral antebrachial cutaneous and radial sensory nerves (RSN) superficial and deep to the brachioradialis muscle, respectively. This sensory transfer was performed as an adjunct to the motor transfer described in our preferred technique. (*B*) Donor and recipient nerve prepared for tensionless end-to-end coaptation (lateral antebrachial cutaneous nerve [LABCN] to RSN).

Table 3
Authors' preferred technique for treatment of high radial nerve palsy

	Step	Technique	Rationale
1	Positioning and tourniquet.	Patient is positioned supine with the arm extended on a hand table. Tourniquet can be used if donor exposure and identification can be accomplished within 30–40 min.	After 30–40 min, tourniquet neurapraxia may preclude the use of nerve stimulation.
2	Incision.	Straight incision from lateral antecubital fossa along medial aspect of brachioradialis to midpoint of the forearm.	Allows exposure of median and radial nerves. Extend distally and radially if PT-ECRB tendon transfer planned.
3	Subcutaneous dissection.	Identify and protect LABCN that runs with cephalic vein.	LABCN may be transferred to RSN for sensation.
4	Identify and retract brachioradialis.	Retract laterally and identify RSN and radial vessels beneath.	Provides visualization of PT tendon, which runs between RSN and vessels.
5a	Identify and step-lengthen PT tendon (if PT-ECRB tendon transfer not planned).	Step-cut through tendon, leaving adequate tendon on both sides to perform repair.	Allows superficial head of PT to be reflected medially, exposing deep head of PT.
5b	PT tendon division (if PT-ECRB tendon transfer planned).	Elevate PT tendon as distal as possible on radius including slip of periosteum.	Maximum length of PT tendon for transfer to ECRB. Exposes deep head of PT.
6	Release deep head of PT.	Release with cautery until median nerve is well-exposed.	Exposes and decompresses median nerve in proximal forearm.
7	Release tendinous edge of FDS.	Divide using cautery until underlying median nerve is decompressed.	Decompresses median nerve and allows more distal visualization of branches.
8	Identify median nerve and dissect distally to isolate its branches.	Use nerve stimulator to confirm branches from proximal to distal: PT, multiple to PL and FCR, FDS, AIN. Mark donor nerves with vessel loops (Video 1).	Confidently identify all regional branches of median nerve. Preservation of the PT and AIN branches is critical.
9	Identify radial nerve main trunk.	Retract brachioradialis laterally, follow RSN proximally until radial nerve is identified. Divide leash of Henry.	Uses the already identified RSN as a guide to locate the radial nerve proper.
10	Dissect the radial nerve distally and identify PIN and ECRB branches.	ECRB branch is small and directly radial to RSN. PIN is larger, further radial, and dives deep to the supinator. Mark recipient nerves with vessel loops.	The easily recognizable RSN is used as a reference point for recipient nerve identification.
11	Expose/decompress radial nerve branches.	Release tendinous leading edge of ECRB and supinator (arcade of Frohse).	Allows maximal mobilization of recipient nerves. Decompression facilitates axonal regeneration.
12	Mobilize and transect donor nerves.	Mobilize FCR and FDS branches as distal as possible, and transect distally.	Donor nerves should be transected as far distal as possible to allow tensionless coaptation.

(continued on next page)

Table 3
(continued)

	Step	Technique	Rationale
13	Mobilize and transect recipient nerves.	Mobilize PIN and ECRB branches as proximal as possible and transect proximally.	Recipient nerves should be transected as far proximal as possible to allow tensionless coaptation.
14	Nerve coaptation.	FCR coapted to PIN and FDS to ECRB. Performed under operating microscope using 9-0 nylon, 2-3 epineurial sutures per nerve followed by fibrin glue.	Minimal suturing to minimize trauma and foreign body reaction. Ensure tension free throughout wrist and elbow range of motion.
15	LABC to RSN (optional).	Transfer LABC (donor) to RSN (recipient).	Restore sensation to dorsoradial hand.
16a	Repair PT tendon	If step-lengthening was performed, repair with 3–0 braided nonabsorbable sutures.	PT function preservation; step-lengthening prevents compression of nerves.
16b	PT to ECRB tendon transfer.	Set appropriate tension, Pulvertaft weave using 3-0 braided nonabsorbable suture.	Tendon transfer provides early wrist extension and can help maintain passive motion until nerve function returns.
17	Hemostasis and closure.	Release tourniquet (if used), ensure hemostasis, deep dermal and subcuticular sutures.	Meticulous hemostasis recommended as hematoma leads to increased scarring that can hinder nerve regeneration.
18	Splint.	Elbow 90°, forearm pronated, wrist neutral, fingers free. Remove in 3–5 d and removable wrist cock-up splint. If tendon transfer performed, splint with wrist in extension and thumb spica for 4 wk.	Important to maintain passive motion. Patient removes splint frequently and performs early gentle motion (unless protecting tendon transfer).
19	Hand therapy	Initiate 2 wk postoperatively with early motor reeducation, edema and gentle range of motion. At 1 mo begin light strengthening.	Important to begin motor reeducation before reinnervation.

Transfer of the FCR and FDS nerves to the PIN and ECRB respectively is described. PT to ECRB tendon transfer and LABCN to RSN sensory nerve transfer are included as optional adjunct procedures.

Abbreviations: AIN, anterior interosseous nerve; ECRB, extensor carpi radialis brevis; FCR, flexor carpi radialis; FDS, flexor digitorum superficialis; LABCN, lateral antebrachial cutaneous nerve; PIN, posterior interosseous nerve; PL, palmaris longus; PT, pronator teres; RSN, radial sensory nerve.

Adapted from Davidge KM, Yee A, Kahn LC, et al. Median to radial nerve transfers for restoration of wrist, finger, and thumb extension. J Hand Surg Am 2013;38(9):1814; with permission.

transfer is a reasonable option for reinnervation of the RSN distribution. Although it was demonstrated in a brachial plexus injury population, this transfer should be considered applicable to patients with classical high radial nerve injury.

AUTHORS' PREFERRED TECHNIQUE

When nerve transfer is indicated for the restoration of wrist, finger, and thumb extension after high radial nerve injury, we prefer FDS to ECRB and FCR to PIN transfer with concomitant PT to ECRB transfer. Our technique, based on Mackinnon's description,[15–18] is outlined in **Table 3** and Video 1. In cases of incomplete high radial nerve palsy, we have modified this technique to include reverse end-to-side nerve transfer, or performed only one of the component nerve transfers in cases of isolated wrist or finger/thumb extensor paralysis.

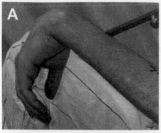

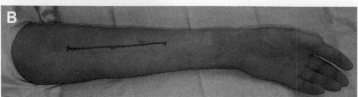

Fig. 3. Illustrative case 1. Complete high radial nerve palsy after gunshot wound. (*A*) Preoperative examination, attempting wrist, finger, and thumb extension. (*B*) Planned incision over the volar forearm.

ILLUSTRATIVE CASES

Case 1: Complete High Radial Nerve Palsy After Gunshot Wound

A 36-year-old right-hand dominant man presented with a gunshot wound to the left arm and complete inability to extend the wrist, fingers, or thumb indicating a high radial nerve palsy. Three months after this injury, no recovery had been observed, and electrodiagnostic testing showed no evidence of reinnervation.

Given the complete lack of function of this patient's radial nerve branches to ECRB and the PIN with normal median nerve function, we planned nerve transfers from FCR to PIN and FDS to ECRB, as well as tendon transfer from PT to ECRB. This procedure was performed 15 weeks after his nerve injury, and was conducted using the

technique described in **Table 3**. Intraoperative photographs are shown in **Figs. 3** and **4**. Eight months after the procedure, he has strong active wrist extension, presumably from the tendon transfer. Finger and thumb extension have yet to recover, but this is not expected until 10 to 12 months postoperatively.

Case 2: Partial Recovery from High Radial Nerve Injury with Weak Finger and Thumb Extension

A 55-year-old right-hand dominant man fell 20 feet from a rooftop sustaining multiple injuries including a left elbow dislocation. At initial presentation, weak wrist, finger, and thumb extension were noted. Over the ensuing 6 months, he had good recovery of wrist extensor function, but

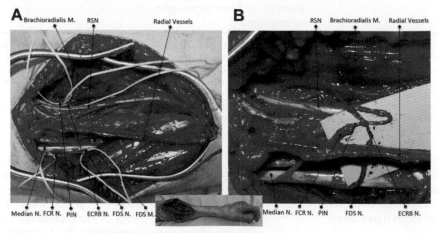

Fig. 4. Illustrative case 1. Complete high radial nerve palsy after gunshot wound. (*A*) Exposure of the median and radial nerves with isolation of the donor (flexor carpi radialis [FCR] and flexor digitorum superficialis [FDS]) and recipient (posterior interosseous nerve [PIN] and extensor carpi radialis brevis [ECRB]) nerves. (*B*) Zoom view of donor and recipient nerve prepared for tensionless end-to-end coaptation (FCR to PIN, FDS to ECRB). RSN, radial sensory nerve.

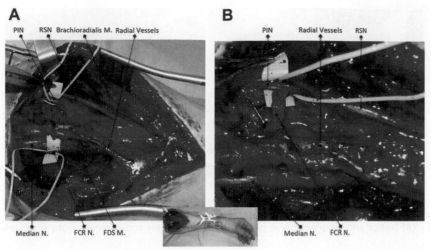

Fig. 5. Illustrative case 2. Partial recovery from high radial nerve injury with weak finger and thumb extension. (A) Exposure of the median and radial nerves with isolation of the donor (flexor carpi radialis [FCR]) and recipient (posterior interosseous nerve [PIN]) nerves. The positioning and incision are similar to **Fig. 2**. (B) Zoom view of donor and recipient nerve prepared for tensionless reverse end-to-side coaptation (FCR to PIN). FDS, flexor digitorum superficialis; RSN, radial sensory nerve.

finger and thumb extension plateaued at MRC 2 (Video 2). Electrodiagnostic testing demonstrated partial denervation of the PIN innervated musculature with poor chance of recovery. Given the persistent deficit of PIN function, we discussed options for nerve reconstruction. In an effort to augment his recovery without sacrificing existing PIN function, we planned a reverse end-to-side transfer of the FCR branch to PIN. Exposure was performed according to the procedure described in **Table 3**. Reverse end-to-side coaptation was carried out by creating an epineurial window in the PIN, to which the cut end of the FCR branch was coapted using 9-0 nylon suture and fibrin glue. Intraoperative photographs are shown in **Fig. 5**. Six months after this operation, the patient has recovered 5/5 strength of finger and thumb extension with full active range of motion (Video 3).

Case 3: Finger and Thumb Extension Deficit After Stroke

A 40-year-old right-hand dominant man suffered an ischemic left basal ganglia stroke 5 years before presentation, leaving him with a partial right hemiplegia. His chief complaint upon presentation to our upper extremity clinic was that he could not open his hand to grasp or release objects. Physical examination revealed no active finger or thumb extension, weak but functional wrist flexion and extension, and normal finger flexion, supination, and elbow/shoulder function. Electrodiagnostic studies confirmed sparse voluntary motor recruitment in the finger and thumb extensors, weak recruitment in the wrist flexors, and normal recruitment of the supinator and finger flexors.

Given the patient's chief complaint, nerve transfer to the PIN was planned. The supinator nerve was chosen as our preferred donor given the weakness of the FCR and antagonistic nature of finger flexor to extensor transfers. Both branches to the supinator were transferred to the PIN in and end-to-end fashion according to the technique of Bertelli and colleagues.[24,25] Intraoperative photographs can be found in **Figs. 6** and **7**. Sufficient time to expect reinnervation has not yet elapsed.

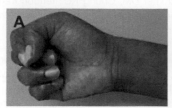
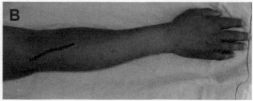

Fig. 6. Illustrative case 3. Finger and thumb extension deficit after stroke. (A) Preoperative examination, attempting finger and thumb extension. (B) Planned incision over the dorsal forearm.

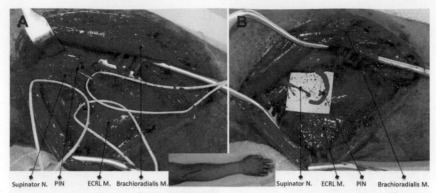

Fig. 7. Illustrative case 3. Finger and thumb extension deficit after stroke. (*A*) Exposure of the posterior interosseous (PIN) and supinator nerves within the interval between the brachioradialis and the extensor carpi radialis longus (ECRL). (*B*) Donor and recipient nerve prepared for tensionless end-to-end coaptation (supinator to PIN).

SUMMARY

Since the original description of median-to-radial nerve transfer 13 years ago,[15] considerable data have accumulated supporting this as an effective option for the reconstruction of high radial nerve injuries. For the indication of classical high radial nerve palsy, transfer of the FCR to the PIN, and FDS to the ECRB with or without PT to ECRB tendon transfer, has proven to be a reliable and synergistic reconstruction capable of restoring strong, independent extension of the wrist, fingers, and thumb. Based on this success, additional donor–recipient pairings have been used to reconstruct radial nerve deficits resulting from brachial plexus injury, stroke, and spinal cord injury. Given this advancement in the field of radial nerve reconstruction, an updated clinical management algorithm for acute traumatic high radial nerve palsy has been offered.

SUPPLEMENTARY DATA

Supplementary data related to this article can be found at http://dx.doi.org/10.1016/j.hcl.2015.12.007.

REFERENCES

1. Shao YC, Harwood P, Grotz MR, et al. Radial nerve palsy associated with fractures of the shaft of the humerus: a systematic review. J Bone Joint Surg Br 2005;87(12):1647–52.
2. Ljunquist KL, Martineau P, Allan C. Radial nerve injuries. J Hand Surg Am 2015;40(1):166–72.
3. Bishop J, Ring D. Management of radial nerve palsy associated with humeral shaft fracture: a decision analysis model. J Hand Surg Am 2009;34(6):991–6.e1.
4. Mohler LR, Hanel DP. Closed fractures complicated by peripheral nerve injury. J Am Acad Orthop Surg 2006;14(1):32–7.
5. Li Y, Ning G, Wu Q, et al. Review of literature of radial nerve injuries associated with humeral fractures: an integrated management strategy. PLoS One 2013; 8(11):e78576.
6. Ustün ME, Ogün TC, Büyükmumcu M. Neurotization as an alternative for restoring finger and wrist extension. J Neurosurg 2001;94(5):795–8.
7. Ukrit A, Leechavengvongs S, Malungpaishrope K, et al. Nerve transfer for wrist extension using nerve to flexor digitorum superficialis in cervical 5, 6, and 7 root avulsions: anatomic study and report of two cases. J Hand Surg Am 2009;34(9):1659–66.
8. Bertelli JA, Kechele PR, Santos MA, et al. Anatomical feasibility of transferring supinator motor branches to the posterior interosseous nerve in C7–T1 brachial plexus palsies. J Neurosurg 2009; 111(2):326–31.
9. Roganovic Z, Pavlicevic G. Difference in recovery potential of peripheral nerves after graft repairs. Neurosurgery 2006;59(3):621–33.
10. Shergill G, Bonney G, Munshi P, et al. The radial and posterior interosseous nerves. Results of 260 repairs. J Bone Joint Surg Br 2001;83(5):646–9.
11. Jones NF, Machado GR. Tendon transfers for radial, median, and ulnar nerve injuries: current surgical techniques. Clin Plast Surg 2011;38(4):621–42.
12. Sammer DM, Chung KC. Tendon transfers: part I. Principles of transfer and transfers for radial nerve palsy. Plast Reconstr Surg 2009;123(5): 169e–77e.
13. Seiler JG, Desai MJ, Payne SH. Tendon transfers for radial, median, and ulnar nerve palsy. J Am Acad Orthop Surg 2013;21(11):675–84.
14. Lurje A. On the use of n. musculocutaneous for neurotization on n. radialis in cases of very large defects of the latter. Ann Surg 1948;128(1):110–5.

15. Lowe JB, Tung TR, Mackinnon SE. New surgical option for radial nerve paralysis. Plast Reconstr Surg 2002;110(3):836–43.

16. Mackinnon SE, Roque B, Tung TH. Median to radial nerve transfer for treatment of radial nerve palsy. J Neurosurg 2007;107(3):666–71.

17. Ray WZ, Mackinnon SE. Clinical outcomes following median to radial nerve transfers. J Hand Surg Am 2011;36(2):201–8.

18. Davidge KM, Yee A, Kahn LC, et al. Median to radial nerve transfers for restoration of wrist, finger, and thumb extension. J Hand Surg Am 2013;38(9):1812–27.

19. Brown JM, Tung TH, Mackinnon SE. Median to radial nerve transfer to restore wrist and finger extension. Neurosurgery 2010;66:75–83.

20. García-López A, Navarro R, Martinez F, et al. Nerve transfers from branches to the flexor carpi radialis and pronator teres to reconstruct the radial nerve. J Hand Surg Am 2014;39(1):50–6.

21. García-López A, Perea D. Transfer of median and ulnar nerve fascicles for lesions of the posterior cord in infraclavicular brachial plexus injury: report of 2 cases. J Hand Surg Am 2012;37(10):1986–9.

22. Bertelli JA, Ghizoni MF. Transfer of a flexor digitorum superficialis motor branch for wrist extension reconstruction in C5-C8 root injuries of the brachial plexus: a case series. Microsurgery 2012;33(1):39–42.

23. Bertelli JA, Tacca CP, Winkelmann Duarte EC, et al. Transfer of the pronator quadratus motor branch for wrist extension reconstruction in brachial plexus palsy. Plast Reconstr Surg 2012;130(6):1269–78.

24. Bertelli JA, Tacca CP, Ghizoni MF, et al. Transfer of supinator motor branches to the posterior interosseous nerve to reconstruct thumb and finger extension in tetraplegia: case report. J Hand Surg Am 2010;35(10):1647–51.

25. Bertelli JA, Ghizoni MF. Transfer of supinator motor branches to the posterior interosseous nerve in C7–T1 brachial plexus palsy. J Neurosurg 2010; 113(1):129–32.

26. Xu B, Dong Z, Zhang C-G, et al. Clinical outcome following transfer of the supinator motor branch to the posterior interosseous nerve in patients with C7–T1 brachial plexus palsy. J Reconstr Microsurg 2015;31(02):102–6.

27. Fox IK, Davidge KM, Novak CB, et al. Use of peripheral nerve transfers in tetraplegia: evaluation of feasibility and morbidity. Hand (N Y) 2015;10(1): 60–7.

28. Hawasli A, Chang J, Reynolds M, et al. Transfer of the brachialis to the anterior interosseous nerve as a treatment strategy for cervical spinal cord injury: technical note. Global Spine J 2015; 05(02):110–7.

29. Gu Y, Wang H, Zhang L, et al. Transfer of brachialis branch of musculocutaneous nerve for finger flexion: anatomic study and case report. Microsurgery 2004; 24(5):358–62.

30. Zhang C-G, Dong Z, Gu Y-D. Restoration of hand function in C7–T1 brachial plexus palsies using a staged approach with nerve and tendon transfer. J Neurosurg 2014;121(5):1264–70.

31. Fridén J, Gohritz A. Brachialis-to-extensor carpi radialis longus selective nerve transfer to restore wrist extension in tetraplegia: case report. J Hand Surg Am 2012;37(8):1606–8.

32. Palazzi S, Palazzi J-L, Caceres J-P. Neurotization with the brachialis muscle motor nerve. Microsurgery 2006;26(4):330–3.

33. Brown J. Nerve transfers in tetraplegia I: background and technique. Surg Neurol Int 2011;2(1):121.

34. Suppaphol S, Watcharananan I, Tawonsawatruk T, et al. The sensory restoration in radial nerve injury using the first branch of dorsal ulnar cutaneous nerve–a cadaveric study for the feasibility of procedure and case demonstration. J Med Assoc Thai 2014;97(3):328–32.

35. Leechavengvongs S, Ngamlamiat K, Malungpaishrope K, et al. End-to-side radial sensory to median nerve transfer to restore sensation and relieve pain in C5 and C6 nerve root avulsion. J Hand Surg Am 2011;36(2):209–15.

36. Bertelli JA, Tacca CP, Ghizoni MF, et al. Transfer of supinator motor branches to the posterior interosseous nerve to reconstruct thumb and finger extension in tetraplegia: case report. J Hand Surg Am 2010;35(10):1647–51.

37. Plate JF, Ely LK, Pulley BR, et al. Combined proximal nerve graft and distal nerve transfer for a posterior cord brachial plexus injury. J Neurosurg 2013; 118(1):155–9.

High Median Nerve Injury
Motor and Sensory Nerve Transfers to Restore Function

Francisco Soldado, MD, PhD[a], Jayme A. Bertelli, MD, PhD[b,c,*],
Marcos F. Ghizoni, MD, PhD[c]

KEYWORDS

- Median nerve • Nerve injury • Motor and sensory deficits • Motor nerve transfers
- Sensory nerve transfers

KEY POINTS

- Clinically significant deficits following high median nerve injuries (HMNIs) are: (1) absent thumb and index finger flexion; (2) thumb-index-middle finger pulp anesthesia; and (3) grasp and pinch weakness.
- Absent thumb and index finger flexion and thumb-index-middle finger pulp anesthesia are the most problematic deficits these patients experience.
- HMNIs and their distal targets (pulp sensation, thenar weakness) experience no benefit from nerve grafting but are amenable to nerve transfers.
- The authors prefer supinator to flexor digitorum superficialis, extensor carpi radialis brevis to anterior interosseous nerve, thumb-index dorsal digital nerve to palmar digital nerve; and abductor digiti minimi to median thenar branch nerve transfers.
- Median nerve repair is mandatory in patients with concomitant pain.

INTRODUCTION

High median nerve injuries (HMNIs) or above-the-elbow median nerve lesions occur proximal to the origin of the anterior interosseous nerve (AIN).[1] Collectively, these injuries are uncommon, accounting for only 0.1% of the injuries involving upper extremity nerves, which makes it difficult to draw definitive conclusions regarding the ideal reconstructive strategy.[2]

There is considerable discrepancy between the motor and sensory deficits observed in clinical practice and those described in the classic literature, the latter generally based on what is known about the anatomic distribution of the median nerve.[2] Redundant innervation and compensatory muscle function could explain this discrepancy.[2,3]

The first half of this article describes the real motor and sensory deficits that occur post-HMNI that necessitate surgical treatment. The second addresses the indications for, limitations of, and outcomes achieved after surgical reconstruction using nerve transfers. The authors reinforce the view that combining nerve transfers with nerve grafting is of interest, particularly with respect to managing pain related to nerve injury.

The authors have no conflicts of interest to disclose.

[a] Pediatric Hand Surgery and Microsurgery Unit, Hospital Sant Joan de Deu, Universitat de Barcelona, Passeig de Sant Joan de Déu, 2, 08950 Esplugues de Llobregat, Barcelona, Spain; [b] Department of Orthopedic Surgery, Governador Celso Ramos Hospital, Rua Irmã Benwarda, 297, 88025-301-Florianópolis - SC, Brazil; [c] Department of Neurosurgery, Center of Biological and Health Sciences, University of the South of Santa Catarina (Unisul), Avenida José Acácio Moreira, 787, Bairro Dehon, 88704-900 - Tubarão-SC, Brazil
* Corresponding author. Rua Newton Ramos 70, Apto 901, Florianópolis, Santa Catarina 88015395, Brazil.
E-mail address: drbertelli@gmail.com

Hand Clin 32 (2016) 209–217
http://dx.doi.org/10.1016/j.hcl.2015.12.008
0749-0712/16/$ – see front matter © 2016 Elsevier Inc. All rights reserved.

hand.theclinics.com

MOTOR AND SENSORY DEFICITS FOLLOWING HIGH MEDIAN NERVE INJURIES

Classic anatomy describes the median nerve as innervating both pronators, the flexor carpi radialis (FCR), palmaris longus, flexor digitorum superficialis (FDS), flexor pollicis longus (FPL), flexor digitorum profundus of the index and middle fingers, and some of the thenar muscles.[4,5] In terms of sensory innervation, the median nerve's distribution includes the radial aspect of the palm, as well as the thumb and the index, middle and half of the ring finger.[6]

In accordance with this, at the beginning of the last century, Tinel[5] stated that after an HMNI, pronation is impossible, wrist flexion is feeble, flexion of the thumb, index, and middle finger is absent, thumb opposition is compromised to some extent, and sensation over the radial aspect of the hand and the radial-side fingers is abolished.[7] Although still accepted today, these proposed clinical deficits are highly discrepant with the authors' findings and those reported by Boswick and Stromberg[2] in 1967. Median nerve motor and sensory distribution and significant clinical problems are summarized in **Table 1**.

Motor Deficits

Motor deficits observed after an isolated HMNI in a cohort of patients from the lead author's department (Bertelli[3]) are very similar to those reported by Boswick and Stromberg.[2]

The clinical findings, occurring in all patients, were

- Pronation largely preserved, to more than 50° with M4 strength, as measured using the British Medical Research Council (BMRC) scale

---

Table 1
Median nerve motor and sensory distribution and significant clinical problems

Median Nerve Innervation	Hypothetical Functional Loss	Clinical Deficits	Nerve Transfer
Motor			
Pronator teres Pronator quadratus	Pronation	No loss of complete range of pronation 50° range of pronation still possible	Exceptional Possible improvement if the median nerve is grafted
FCR Palmaris longus	Wrist flexion	None	None
FDS Flexor digitorum profundus (index and middle)	Index and middle finger flexion, grasping strength	Grasping weakness[a] No index flexion Middle finger flexion present	Supinator branch to FDS plus nerve grafting ECRB to AIN None
FPL	Thumb IP flexion Pinch strength	No thumb IP flexion Pinch weakness[b]	ECRB to AIN
Thenar muscles (partial)	Opposition Pinch strength	Loss of opposition in 15%–30% of patients Pinch weakness[b]	ADM to median nerve thenar branch[c]
Sensory			
Radial palm of the hand	Anesthesia	No loss of protective sensation	None
Thumb Index Middle Radial ring	Anesthesia	Loss of protective sensation predominantly in thumb, index, and middle finger pulps No loss of protective sensation in ring finger	Dorsal radial sensory nerves to thumb and index finger palmar nerves None

According to classic literature.
Abbreviations: ADM, abductor digiti minimi; ECRB, extensor carpi radialis brevis; IP, interphalangeal.
[a] 40% of the contralateral side.
[b] 35% of the contralateral side.
[c] In all cases, to improve pinch strength.

- Wrist flexion scoring M5, performed without any lateral deviation
- Complete middle finger flexion, scoring M4[8]
- Thumb opposition largely preserved, scoring 5 or greater on the Kapandji scale, which ranges from 1 to 10.[9]

However, all the patients also exhibited

- Absent interphalangeal (IP) flexion in the thumb and index finger distal phalanx
- Severely decreased grasp and pinch strength, averaging just 40% and 35% of the normal, contralateral side, respectively.

Consequently, motor deficits warranting reconstruction relate to thumb and index IP flexion, and pinch and grasp strength.[3] Loss of thumb opposition has been described to occur in between 14% and 30% of patients with a median nerve injury, and the need for pronation reconstruction has been rarely reported post-HMNI.[10–12]

Sensory Deficits

Classic literature and even current perceptions suggest that there is anesthesia over the radial aspect of the palm with median nerve lesions.[7,13] However, in our and other investigators' experiences, sensation of the palm is largely preserved.[3,5,14–16]

In fact, patients with HMNI exhibit altered sensation that is clinically significant (ie, the lack of protective sensation) predominantly over the palmar distal phalanx of the thumb and the middle and distal phalanges of the index and middle fingers[3,5,14–16] (**Fig. 1**). Hence, strategies for sensory reconstruction for HMNI should preferentially address the fingertips.[17]

The authors also found that sensory function in the ring finger was largely preserved because the ulnar nerve supplied the median palmar nerve, thereby requiring no reconstruction. This is because reinnervation of a single palmar nerve can restore sensation to the entire pulp.[17–19]

NERVE TRANSFERS FOR RECONSTRUCTION OF HIGH MEDIAN NERVE INJURIES

Indications for nerve transfers in HMNI vary according to the duration of time since the initial nerve injury and the remoteness of the target.

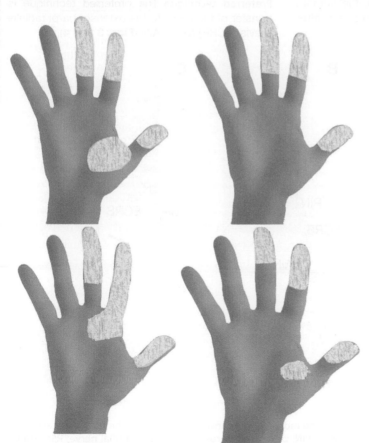

Fig. 1. Zones of absent protective sensation (*gray*) after a proximal injury to the median nerve. Sensorial deficits are more predominant in the fingertips than on the palm of the hand.

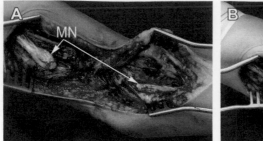
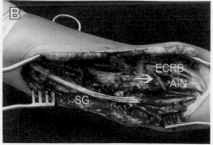

Fig. 2. Combined nerve grafting and nerve transfer (nerve to the extensor carpi radialis brevis [ECRB] to the AIN) in a 32-year-old man operated on 5 months post-HMNI. The patient complained of neurogenic pain, which resolved after median nerve grafting. (*A*) *Arrows* indicate the proximal and distal median nerve stumps (MN). (*B*) The MN is repaired with 3 cables of the sural nerve grafts (SG). *Arrow* indicates the site o coaptation of the ECRB with the AIN.

Proximal nerve injuries (proximal arm) and distal targets (thenar muscles and sensory pulp restoration) are amenable to nerve transfers. Depending on these 2 factors, combining nerve transfers and median nerve repair might be necessary. In addition, the presence of pain warrants median nerve repair (**Fig. 2**). Nerve transfers should be performed preferentially within 6 months of the injury, with 12 months the limit postinjury for motor transfers. The time window for sensory nerve transfers is controversial and, considering the low morbidity of these procedures, the authors find that these can be performed even 3 years after the injury.

Motor deficits treated later than 12 months after the injury should be addressed through tendon transfers. The authors' preferred techniques, by clinical deficit, are listed in **Table 1**.

Restoring Index Finger and Thumb Flexion, and Grasp and Pinch Strength

Restoring index and thumb flexion
Indication Median nerve lesion above the elbow preferentially within 6 months of injury.

Preferred technique The preferred technique is transfer of the nerve to the extensor carpi radialis brevis (ECRB) to the AIN (**Figs. 3 and 4**).[20]

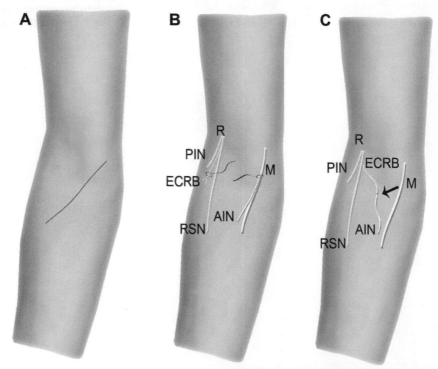

Fig. 3. (*A–C*) Surgical technique used to transfer the radial nerve branch to the ECRB to the AIN. In (*C*) *arrow* indicates the site of nerve repair. M, median nerve; PIN, posterior interosseous nerve; R, radial nerve; RSN, superficial branch of the radial nerve.

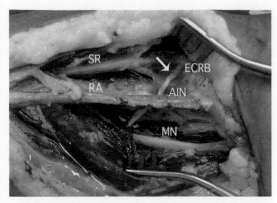

Fig. 4. Surgical field view showing the nerve to the ECRB coapted to the AIN (*arrow*). MN, median nerve; RA, radial artery; SR, superficial branch of the radial nerve.

Transferring the nerve to the ECRB to the AIN results in full finger flexion, with averages for grasp and pinch strength of 5 kg and 2 kg, respectively.[20] Recovery begins in the FPL, whereas active finger flexion returns during the third and fourth postoperative months.

Alternative nerve transfers to the anterior interosseous nerve Three case reports describe reconstruction of the AIN. One uses the branch to the supinator, the second uses the branch to the brachioradialis muscle, and the third uses the branch to the brachialis muscle.[11,21,22] Results seem mediocre relative to those obtained when the nerve to the ECRB is transferred.

Restoration of grasp weakness
Indication The indication is median nerve lesion at the level of the middle or lower arm, preferentially within 6 months of the injury.

Preferred technique The preferred technique is transfer of the nerves to the supinator muscle to the nerve to the FDS.[3,20]

Transferring the nerves to the supinator muscle to a motor branch of the FDS improves grasp strength.[20]

Restoration of pinch strength
Indication The indication is an above elbow lesion of the median nerve preferentially within 6 months of the injury.

Preferred technique The preferred technique is transferring the nerve to the abductor digiti minimi (ADM) to the thenar median nerve branch (**Fig. 5**).[3]

Pinch weakness, as well as grasp weakness, can result from paralysis of both extrinsic and intrinsic muscles of the hand.[23] Thus, pinch weakness results from paralysis of both the FPL and thenar muscles. In fact, even when FPL innervation is preserved, as in median nerve lesions in the wrist, pinch strength is diminished by an average of 60%.[23] Restoring thumb flexion through a nerve transfer to the AIN improves pinch strength. However, to achieve further gains in pinch strength, the nerve to the abductor digiti minimi can be transferred to the median thenar branch, even if some opposition is present (see later discussion). **Box 1** depicts the authors' strategy to restore index and thumb flexion, and reverse grasp and pinch weakness.

Restoration of Thumb Opposition

Indication
The indication is an above elbow lesion of the median nerve preferentially within 6 months of the injury.

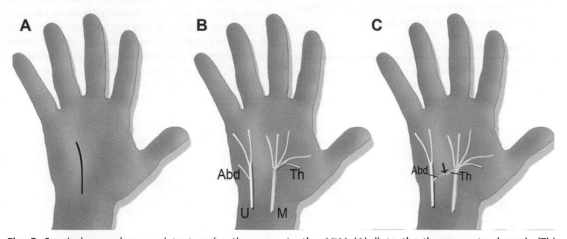

Fig. 5. Surgical procedure used to transfer the nerve to the ADM (Abd) to the thenar motor branch (Th). (*A*) Surgical approach through a longitudinal palmar incision over Guyon canal. (*B*) Ulnar (U) and median (M) terminal branches in the palmar region. (*C*) After nerve transfer. Surgical field view showing the nerve to the ECRB coapted to the AIN (*arrow*).

Box 1
Strategy to restore of index and thumb flexion, and grasp and pinch weakness

- Nerve to the ECRB to AIN
- Nerves to the supinator to the nerve to the FDS
- Nerve to the ADM to the thenar branch of median nerve

Preferred technique

The preferred technique is transferring the nerve to the ADM to the median nerve thenar branch (see **Fig. 5**).

Even when an HMNI was repaired urgently by end-to-end suture, reinnervation of thenar muscles did not occur in one series of 54 adult subjects.[2] Thus, achieving thenar muscle reinnervation requires a distal nerve transfer.[24]

The authors preference is to use the motor branch to the ADM for neurotization of the thenar branch of the median nerve.[3] This transfer is performed in all patients because the aim is not only to restore thumb opposition but also to increase pinch strength.

Alternative nerve transfers to the thenar motor branch

Other theoretically possible donors for transfer to the thenar motor branch are the nerves to the flexor digiti minimi brevis and opponens digiti minimi. However, sacrificing these motor branches compromises elevation of the hypothenar region during thumb opposition.[25] Also described is transfer of the ulnar nerve branch to the third lumbrical to the thenar branch of the median nerve.[26] In the authors' experiences, this branch is very thin, its anatomy is unpredictable, and it frequently originates together with the motor branch to the interosseous muscles of the fourth space.

Pronation Palsy

Most patients do not require pronation reconstruction.[2,3] None of the subjects in the Bertelli[3] series exhibited significantly weak pronation. Two nerve transfers have been described for this purpose that could be used for those exceptional cases with absent pronation. Hsiao and colleagues[11] successfully transferred the ECRB motor branch to the pronator teres (PT) motor branch. Meanwhile, Vasconcellos[27] proposed transferring the brachialis motor branch to the epitrochlear branch of the median nerve, which innervates the PT. Transferring the brachialis motor branch seems an interesting option in cases of deficient pronation because, in the authors' reconstruction strategy, the ECRB motor branch is transferred to the AIN.

Sensory Reconstruction

Indication

The indication is an above elbow lesion of the median nerve preferentially within 6 months of the injury.

Preferred technique

The preferred technique is transfer of the ulnar thumb and radial index dorsal digital nerve to the corresponding palmar digital nerve (**Figs. 6 and 7**).[17]

The authors consider only areas with no protective sensation (no perception of a 2.0 g Semmes-Weinstein filament) to be significantly impaired and warranting reconstruction.[17] The rationale is that after sensory nerve reconstruction improved sensation beyond 2.0 g monofilaments rarely, if ever, occurs and is considered a good result.[28] Hence, our criterion is linked to our capacity for surgical reconstruction.

As opposed to median nerve injuries in the wrist for which protective sensation in the fingertips can be restored predictably by direct suture or nerve grafting, sensory recovery tends to be poor in proximal injuries of the median nerve because of the long distance between the site of nerve injury or repair and the target cutaneous receptors.[17,29,30] Thus, to achieve sensory reinnervation after an HMNI, a nerve transfer is necessary,

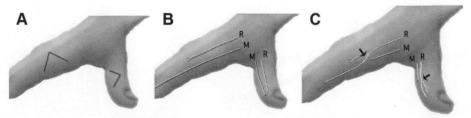

Fig. 6. Surgical procedure for transferring dorsal sensory branches of the radial nerve (ie, dorsal digital nerves) to palmar digital nerves in the index finger and thumb. (*A*) Surgical approach through V-shaped incisions. (*B*) Identification and transfer of the dorsal digital nerve (R) to the radial index finger and ulnar thumb to the ipsilateral palmar digital nerve (M). (*C*) Nerve stumps are coapted without tension (*arrows*).

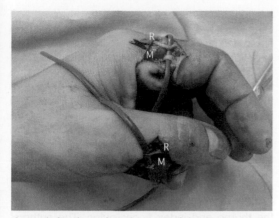

Fig. 7. (M) palmar digital nerves of the median nerve, (R) dorsal digital nerves of the radial nerve. In general, the ulnar side of the thumb is the target for sensory reconstruction. In this patient, surgery was performed on the radial side of the thumb because of a concomitant cutaneous lesion on the medial side of the pulp of the thumb with potenticial damage to the palmar ulnar digital nerve.

aiming to approximate the site of nerve repair to sensory end organs.

The authors' preference is to perform a very distal sensory nerve transfer under the hypothesis of decreasing the risk of faulty location and neuropathic pain relative to more proximal sensory nerve transfers.[17] Dorsal branches of the radial nerve (eg, dorsal digital nerves) harvested at the level of the proximal phalanx of the radial side of the index and ulnar side of the thumb are transferred to the ipsilateral palmar digital nerve. With this technique, restoration of protective sensation or better to the fingertips occurred in all our patients, with better results observed in the thumb. Locognosia was acquired in all thumbs and 50% of index fingers. No patient developed neuropathic pain.[17]

Because patients do not complain of the loss of protective sensation in the middle finger, the authors do not believe it necessary to perform sensory transfers at this level. We propose nerve transfer to a single palmar digital nerve because repairing one of the palmar nerves ensures sensory recovery to the entire pulp.[17–19]

Timing limitations for this sensory nerve transfer are unknown. Bertelli and Ghizoni[17] reported good results even in patients who had undergone surgery later than 6 months postinjury. Bedeschi and colleagues,[31] and Matloubi,[32] reported good outcomes with reconstructions performed up to 3 years after the injury.

Alternative sensory nerve transfers
Several sensory transfers using the dorsal sensory radial nerve or either the palmar or dorsal sensory

ulnar nerve for transfer to the median nerve branches at the level of the wrist, palm or dorsum of the hand have resulted in positive outcomes.[31–39] However, sensory nerve transfers at this level commonly result in mislocognosia.[17,35]

SURGICAL TECHNIQUES FOR THE RECOMMENDED NERVE TRANSFERS

The surgical techniques for recommended nerve transfers consist of the following.

Transfer of the Radial Nerve Branch to the Extensor Carpi Radialis Brevis to the Anterior Interosseous Nerve, and of Supinator Branches to the Flexor Digitorum Superficialis Branch

- Oblique incision over the anterior aspect of the elbow alongside the PT (see **Fig. 2**)
- Division of the lacertus fibrosus to identify the median nerve and the AIN and FDS branch
- Identification of the superficial radial nerve deep to the brachioradialis margin
- Identification of the branch of the radial nerve to the ECRB, deep and parallel to the superficial radial nerve
- Identification of the supinator branches alongside the posterior interosseous nerve and proximal to the arcade of Frohse
- Dissection of the AIN and FDS branches proximal within the median nerve to ensure tension-free coaptation
- Donor and recipient nerve suspension on a vessel loop, with electrical stimulation to confirm preservation of the donor and paralysis of the recipient nerve
- Distal division of the radial nerve branch to the ECRB and the supinator and proximal divisions of recipient nerves
- Nerve coaptation under the microscope using 9-0 nylon sutures.

Transfer of the Motor Branch Nerve to the Abductor Digiti Minimi to the Median Thenar Branch

- Longitudinal palmar incision lateral to the hypothenar mass, reaching proximally to Guyon canal and the distal forearm (see **Fig. 5**)
- Division of the flexor retinaculum (the motor thenar branch is identified and dissected intraneurally roughly 3 cm in a proximal direction)
- Division of Guyon canal retinaculum to identify the ulnar motor branch and the nerve to the ADM
- Dissection of both nerves proximally within the median and ulnar nerves, respectively, to ensure tension-free coaptation

- Donor and recipient nerve suspension on a vessel loop, with electrical stimulation to confirm preservation of the donor and paralysis of the recipient nerve
- Distal division of the nerve to the ADM and proximal division of recipient nerve
- Coaptation under the microscope using 9-0 nylon sutures.

Transfer of the Ulnar Thumb and Radial Index Dorsal Digital Nerve to the Ipsilateral Palmar Digital Nerve

- A volar V incision is created at the base of the thumb on the ulnar side and the index finger on its radial side (see **Figs. 6** and **7**)
- Identification and sectioning of the dorsal digital nerve (for the index finger and thumb, sectioning is planned at least 1 cm proximal to the distal boundaries of preserved sensation on the dorsal aspect, as determined during the preoperative evaluation)
- Sectioning of the palmar digital nerve is performed more proximally to allow for redundancy of the nerve stumps and tension-free nerve repair
- Nerve coaptation using 9-0 nylon sutures.

Nerve Grafting

Whenever possible, the authors recommend grafting the median nerve combined with a distal nerve transfer. If performed within 6 months of the injury, viable axons can be redirected to reinnervate forearm muscles. Although pronation is not totally paralyzed, it can be ameliorated by grafting due to the proximal origin of PT motor branches. Additionally, some axons may reach the FCR. The FDS superficialis has multiple motor branches.[40] Following supinator nerve transfer, only one FDS branch is reinnervated. Hence, additional FDS branches remain available to be reinnervated by axons stemming from the proximal stump of the median nerve. Theoretically, because we perform distal sensory nerve transfers to a single palmar nerve, the remaining nerves and those to the middle finger remain available to recipient axons via nerve grafting.

All patients with pain complaints must undergo median nerve repair. In all of the authors' patients, nerve grafting eliminated pain immediately after surgery. Failure to address the median nerve proximal stump may contribute to persistent pain, even if a distal nerve transfer is performed concomitantly.[20,29,41]

SUMMARY

Following a HMNI, wrist flexion and third finger flexion do not warrant reconstruction. In a small minority of cases, pronation is compromised and needs restoration. Thumb and index flexion and grasp and pinch weakness require surgical reconstruction because most patients consider these deficits the most debilitating after an HMNI, along with thumb and finger pulp anesthesia. Transfer of the ECRB branch to the AIN improves thumb and index finger flexion. Transfer of the nerve to the supinator to the FDS improves grip strength. Though a low percentage of patients experience compromised opposition, the authors always transfer the nerve to the ADM to the thenar branch of the median nerve to improve pinch strength. Clinically significant sensory deficits are only found over the thumb and index finger pulps. The authors' preferred technique to restore sensation at this level is a very distal radial sensory nerve transfer to the palmar digital nerves. All patients presenting with pain should have their injured median nerve repaired.

REFERENCES

1. Ko JW, Mirarchi AJ. Late reconstruction of median nerve palsy. Orthop Clin North Am 2012;43(4): 449–57.
2. Boswick JA, Stromberg WB. Isolated injury to the median nerve above the elbow. A review of thirteen cases. J Bone Joint Surg Am 1967;49(4):653–8.
3. Bertelli JA, Soldado F, Lehn VL, et al. Reappraisal of clinical deficits following high median nerve injuries. J Hand Surg Am 2016;41(1):13–9.
4. Cooney WP, Linscheid RL, An KN. Opposition of the thumb: An anatomic and biomechanical study of tendon transfers. J Hand Surg Am 1984;9(6): 777–86.
5. Tinel J. Nerve wounds. New York: William Wood & Company; 1917. p. 175–8.
6. Mazurek MT, Shin AY. Upper extremity peripheral nerve anatomy: current concepts and applications. Clin Orthop Relat Res 2001;383:7–20.
7. Greene WB. Netter's orthopaedics. New York: Saunders; 2006. p. 1.
8. Soldado F, Ghizoni MF, Bertelli JA. The ulnar nerve consistently drives flexion of the middle finger. J Hand Surg Eur Vol 2014;9(2):211–2.
9. Kapandji A. Clinical test of apposition and counter-apposition of the thumb. Ann Chir Main 1986;5(1): 67–73.
10. Boatright JR, Kiebzak GM. The effects of low median nerve block on thumb abduction strength. J Hand Surg Am 1997;22(5):849–52.
11. Hsiao EC, Fox IK, Tung TH, et al. Motor nerve transfers to restore extrinsic median nerve function: Case report. Hand (N Y) 2009;4(1):92–7.
12. Jensen EG. Restoration of opposition of the thumb. Hand 1978;10(2):161–7.

13. Stopford JS. The variation in distribution of the cutaneous nerves of the hand and digits. J Anat 1918; 53(Pt 1):14–25.

14. Letiévant JJE. Traité des sections nerveuses. Paris (France): J.B. Bailliere et Fils; 1873. p.66.

15. Sherren J. Injuries of nerves and their treatment. New York: William Wood and Company; 1908. p. 263–7.

16. Stiles HJ, Forrester-Brown MF. Treatment of injuries of the peripheral spinal nerves. London: Oxford Medical Publications; 1922. p. 16.

17. Bertelli JA, Ghizoni MF. Very distal sensory nerve transfers in high median nerve lesions. J Hand Surg Am 2011;36(3):387–93.

18. Tadjalli HE, McIntyre FH, Dolynchuk KN, et al. Importance of crossover innervation in digital nerve repair demonstrated by nerve isolation technique. Ann Plast Surg 1995;35(1):32–5.

19. Weinzweig N. Crossover innervation after digital nerve injury: myth or reality? Ann Plast Surg 2000; 45(5):509–14.

20. Bertelli JA. Transfer of the radial nerve branch to the extensor carpi radialis brevis to the anterior interosseous nerve to reconstruct thumb and finger flexion. J Hand Surg Am 2015;40(2):323–8.e2.

21. García-López A, Sebastian P, Martinez F, et al. Transfer of the nerve to the brachioradialis muscle to the anterior interosseous nerve for treatment for lower brachial plexus lesions: Case report. J Hand Surg Am 2011;36(3):394–7.

22. Ray WZ, Yarbrough CK, Yee A, et al. Clinical outcomes following brachialis to anterior interosseous nerve transfers. J Neurosurg 2012;117(3):604–9.

23. Kozin SH, Porter S, Clark P, et al. The contribution of the intrinsic muscles to grip and pinch strength. J Hand Surg Am 1999;24(1):64–72.

24. Ustün ME, Oğün TC, Karabulut AK, et al. An alternative method for restoring opposition after median nerve injury: an anatomical feasibility study for the use of neurotisation. J Anat 2001;198(5): 635–8.

25. Sunderland S. Voluntary movement and the deceptive action of muscles in peripheral nerve lesions. Aust N Z J Surg 1944;13(3):160–83.

26. Schultz RJ, Aiache A. An operation to restore opposition of the thumb by nerve transfer. Arch Surg 1972;105(5):777–9.

27. Accioli de Vasconcellos ZA. Contribution à l'étude des neurotisations intra- et extra-plexuelles du plexus brachial et de ses branches terminals. Étude chez le Rat et chez l'Homme [dissertation]. Paris (France): René Descartes University; 1999.

28. Bertelli JA. Distal sensory nerve transfers in lower-type injuries of the brachial plexus. J Hand Surg Am 2012;37(6):1194–9.

29. Roganovic Z, Petkovic S. Missile severances of the radial nerve. Results of 131 repairs. Acta Neurochir (Wien) 2004;146(11):1185–92.

30. Ruijs AC, Jaquet JB, Kalmijn S, et al. Median and ulnar nerve injuries: A meta-analysis of predictors of motor and sensory recovery after modern microsurgical nerve repair. Plast Reconstr Surg 2005;116(2): 484–94 [discussion: 495–6].

31. Bedeschi P, Celli L, Balli A. Transfer of sensory nerves in hand surgery. J Hand Surg Br 1984;9(1):46–9.

32. Matloubi R. Transfer of sensory branches of radial nerve in hand surgery. J Hand Surg Br 1988;13(1):92–5.

33. Brunelli GA. Sensory nerves transfers. J Hand Surg Br 2004;29(6):557–62.

34. Ducic I, Dellon AL, Bogue DP. Radial sensory neurotization of the thumb and index finger for prehension after proximal median and ulnar nerve injuries. J Reconstr Microsurg 2006;22(2):73–8.

35. Harris RI. The treatment of irreparable nerve injuries. Can Med Assoc J 1921;11(11):833–41.

36. Ozkan T, Ozer K, Gülgönen A. Restoration of sensibility in irreparable ulnar and median nerve lesions with use of sensory nerve transfer: Long-term follow-up of 20 cases. J Hand Surg Am 2001;26(1):44–51.

37. Rapp E, Lallemand S, Ehrler S, et al. Restoration of sensation over the contact surfaces of the thumb-index pinch grip using the terminal branches of the superficial branch of the radial nerve. Chir Main 1999;18:179–83.

38. Tung TH, Mackinnon SE. Nerve transfers: Indications, techniques, and outcomes. J Hand Surg Am 2010;35(2):332–41.

39. Turnbull F. Restoration of digital sensation after transference of nerves. J Neurosurg 1963;20:238.

40. Ye F, Lee H, An C, et al. Anatomic localization of motor entry points and accurate regions for botulinum toxin injection in the flexor digitorum superficialis. Surg Radiol Anat 2011;33(7):601–7.

41. Murphy RK, Ray WZ, Mackinnon SE. Repair of a median nerve transection injury using multiple nerve transfers, with long-term functional recovery. J Neurosurg 2012;117(5):886–9.

High Ulnar Nerve Injuries
Nerve Transfers to Restore Function

Jennifer Megan M. Patterson, MD

KEYWORDS

- Nerve transfer • Ulnar nerve injury • Intrinsic ulnar neuropathy • End-to-side

KEY POINTS

- Adults with high ulnar nerve injuries show very poor intrinsic recovery after traditional reconstructive techniques (nerve repair and nerve grafting).
- Distal motor nerve transfer of the anterior interosseous nerve to the ulnar motor nerve results in improved ulnar intrinsic recovery after a high ulnar nerve injury.
- Distal sensory nerve transfers from the median to the ulnar nerve allow for restoration of protective sensation along the ulnar border of the hand and in the ulnar digits.
- End-to-side transfers should be considered in proximal ulnar nerve injuries, where less than complete recovery is expected.

INTRODUCTION

Peripheral nerve injuries occur frequently and are challenging problems to treat. Ulnar nerve injuries are the most common upper extremity peripheral nerve injury and result in distal numbness and weakness in the hand.[1] High ulnar nerve injuries pose an additional challenge given the long distance from the site of injury to the distal motor endplates. Adult patients with ulnar nerve lacerations in the proximal forearm and cubital tunnel show very poor intrinsic recovery after nerve repair or grafting compared with more distal injuries.[2–4] Nerve transfers provide the advantage of being close to the targeted muscle, which minimizes the time to reinnervation and maximizes potential recovery. Nerve transfers for ulnar nerve injuries were first described in 1997 and have been refined over the years, resulting in improved patient outcomes after high ulnar nerve injuries.[5–15]

INDICATIONS

Distal motor and sensory nerve transfers are indicated in proximal fourth-, fifth-, and sixth-degree ulnar nerve injuries, where distal recovery after nerve repair or grafting is likely to be poor[16] (Table 1). Motor transfers can be performed end to end (ETE) or reverse end to side (also referred to as supercharged end to side, SETS). ETE transfers are appropriate in proximal fourth- and fifth-degree injuries when no recovery is expected through the native nerve. The indications for SETS transfers have not been fully defined. They may be indicated in patients with proximal fourth- and fifth-degree injuries where some recovery may be expected after primary repair (young children or adults with a Martin-Gruber anastomosis) or in second- and third-degree ulnar nerve injuries, where there is concern about the ability to obtain complete recovery.

When considering nerve transfers, several important principles must be taken into account.[16,17] There must be a donor nerve that is expendable and close to the target motor endplates. A "pure" motor donor should be used to reconstruct motor deficits, and a "pure" sensory nerve should be used to reconstruct sensory deficits. The donor and recipient should be of similar cross-sectional size. Finally, the function of the donor nerve should be synergistic with that of the recipient.

Department of Orthopaedic Surgery, University of North Carolina, Chapel Hill, 3135 Bioinformatics Building, Campus Box 7055, Chapel Hill, NC 27599, USA
E-mail address: megan_patterson@med.unc.edu

Hand Clin 32 (2016) 219–226
http://dx.doi.org/10.1016/j.hcl.2015.12.009
0749-0712/16/$ – see front matter © 2016 Elsevier Inc. All rights reserved.

hand.theclinics.com

Table 1
Indications for supercharged end to side nerve transfer

	Degree	FIBS	MUPS	Transfer Type
Acute injury				
High ulnar	II/III	+	Collateral sprouting, nascent	SETS
	VI/V	+	—	ETE
	VI/V (Martin-Gruber)	+	Normal	SETS
Mid ulnar	II/III	+	Collateral sprouting, nascent	SETS
	VI/V	+	—	SETS
Cubital tunnel				
Acute/chronic injury	II/III	+	+/−	SETS

Abbreviations: FIBS, fibrillations; MUPS, motor unit potentials.
Courtesy of S.E. Mackinnon, MD, St Louis, MO; with permission.

Tendon transfers remain an option in treating high ulnar nerve lesions, and many different tendon transfers have proven to be successful.[18] Tendon transfers require a supple extremity preoperatively and will allow for a quicker return of function, often within 2 to 3 months. The results of nerve transfers take longer to occur but have the benefit of maintaining the original origin, insertion, and line of pull of the denervated muscle, which may ultimately allow for an improved outcome. Nerve transfers for ulnar nerve injury do not preclude subsequent additional tendon transfers.

CONTRAINDICATIONS

Nerve transfers are contraindicated in the following patients[16]:

- Those patients wherein a different treatment method will result in a better or equivalent outcome with less morbidity.
- Patients with distal nerve injuries close to the site of motor and sensory innervation. These injuries should be repaired primarily or with a nerve graft.
- Patients with neurapraxic (I) or axonotmetic (II, III) injuries. These injuries should be treated with observation without surgical intervention as recovery is to be expected.
- Patients who have already experienced irreversible muscle atrophy and fibrosis due to the time that has passed from their injury. Tendon transfers are more appropriate in these patients.

PREOPERATIVE CONSIDERATIONS

As with any reconstructive procedure, the patient must be optimized before surgery. The soft tissues should be healed and stable without infection. The joints powered by the transfer should have full passive motion.[16] Electrodiagnostic studies are helpful for preoperative planning. They provide information on the extent of injury as well as the status of available donor nerves.

SURGICAL OPTIONS

The easiest way to restore distal ulnar motor function is with a transfer of the median innervated anterior interosseous nerve (AIN) branch to the pronator quadratus (PQ), either ETE or SETS. In patients with both median and ulnar nerve injuries where the AIN is not available, branches of the posterior interosseous nerve (PIN) may be transferred through the interosseous membrane to the ulnar nerve, although the results of these transfers have not been as satisfying as those using AIN.[9,10] Ulnar sensory deficits maybe be reconstructed using median nerve branches to the third web space, median sensory fascicles in the distal forearm (end to side), palmar cutaneous branch of the median nerve, or the terminal branches of the lateral antebrachial cutaneous nerve.[6,19]

SURGICAL TECHNIQUE

- The patient should be positioned supine with the upper extremity extended on a hand table.
- A nonsterile pneumatic tourniquet is placed high on the upper arm.
- The operating microscope should be available throughout the procedure.

Nerve Transfers to Restore Ulnar Motor Function: Anterior Interosseous Nerve to Ulnar Motor

Decompression of Guyon canal

- A curved incision is made just ulnar to the thenar crease in the palm and taken across the wrist in a zigzag fashion, extending up the forearm between the palmaris longus and the flexor carpi ulnaris (FCU) for approximately 12 to 14 cm (**Fig. 1**).
- Identify the ulnar neurovascular bundle (UNVB) proximally in the distal forearm and follow it distally.
- Release the tight fascial bands volar to the UNVB just proximal to the wrist.
- Divide palmaris brevis if present and open Guyon canal (**Fig. 2**).
- Retract the UNVB ulnarly and palpate the hook of the hamate.
- Release the hypothenar fascia just ulnar to the hook of the hamate to reveal the underlying ulnar motor branch (**Fig. 3**).
- Decompress the ulnar motor branch around the hook of the hamate to the level of the small finger flexor tendons.
- Stimulate the ulnar motor branch to confirm absent function.

Identification of ulnar nerve topography and isolation of the ulnar motor branch

- The ulnar nerve has predictable fascicular topography in the distal forearm. The motor fascicular group lies between the 2 sensory fascicular groups.
- After identification of the ulnar motor branch distally, it is "visually" neurolysed proximally

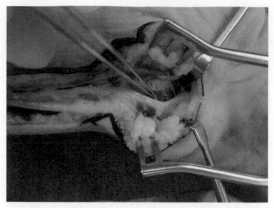

Fig. 2. Decompression of Guyon canal. Forceps are pointing to the hook of the hamate and leading edge of hypothenar fascia.

into the distal forearm. It is useful to place a small vessel loop around the motor branch distally so it can be quickly identified. The motor and sensory branches remain distinct, and they can easily be followed proximally by visual neurolysis and do not need to be formally separated along their entire length. A longitudinally running vessel is often seen between the sensory and motor fascicles that can aid in their visual neurolysis.

- The motor branch is separated from the adjacent sensory branches at about 8 to 9 cm proximal to the wrist crease and marked with a second vessel loop (**Fig. 4**).

Identify the anterior interosseous nerve

- Sweep the volar flexor tendons (except for the FCU) radially to expose the PQ.

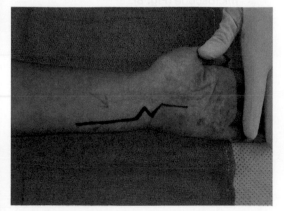

Fig. 1. Incision for anterior interosseous to ulnar motor nerve transfer and distal median to ulnar sensory transfers. The incision is extended proximally up the forearm as needed to allow adequate exposure of the anterior interosseous and dorsal ulnar sensory nerves.

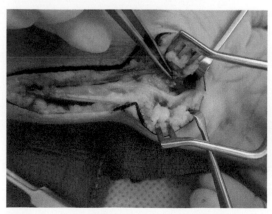

Fig. 3. Exposure of the deep motor branch of the median nerve after release of the hypothenar fascia.

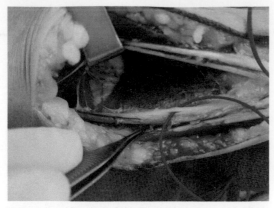

Fig. 4. Identification of the motor fascicle proximally in the forearm. The motor fascicle is found ulnar to the sensory branch and has been marked with a vessel loop.

- Identify the AIN and its adjacent vessels proximally entering the midline of the PQ (**Fig. 5**).
- Separate the AIN from the adjacent vessels and follow it distally to its branching point in the midportion of the PQ, dividing the overlying PQ muscle fibers.
- Mobilize the AIN proximally to increase mobility.
- Transect the AIN at its branching point.
- Pass the AIN toward the ulnar nerve obliquely and divide any vessels or muscle attachments that would otherwise impair a straight pass.

Coaptation

- End to end:
  - Drape the AIN over the ulnar motor branch to determine the exact location to divide the motor branch. The motor branch is divided proximally to allow for a tension-free transfer (**Fig. 6**).

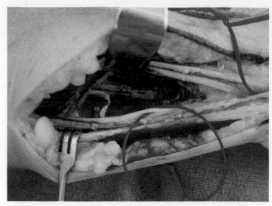

Fig. 6. The AIN has been divided distally at its branching point and draped over the ulnar motor fascicle. For an ETE transfer, the ulnar motor fascicle is divided proximal to allow for a tension-free transfer. For an SETS transfer, an epineural window is made in the ulnar motor fascicle to allow a tension-free transfer.

  - Suture the 2 ends together using a 9-0 nylon suture and the operating microscope. The repair may be further augmented with fibrin glue (**Fig. 7**).
- Supercharged end to side:
  - Drape the AIN over the motor branch of the ulnar nerve and create a large epineural window in the motor fascicle at this level (usually 8–9 cm proximal to volar wrist crease). A wide epineural window is important to allow the maximal number of regenerating neurons to sprout from the AIN to the ulnar nerve (see **Fig. 6**).
  - Suture the AIN into the epineural window with a 9-0 nylon suture and the operating microscope (**Fig. 8**).

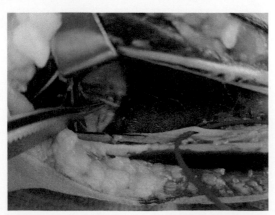

Fig. 5. Identification of the AIN entering the proximal aspect of the PQ in its midline.

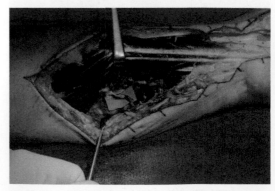

Fig. 7. The AIN has been sutured to the ulnar motor fascicle (*marked blue with surgical ink*) after dividing the motor fascicle proximally. Note the lack of tension on the transfer. (*Courtesy of* S.E. Mackinnon, MD, St Louis, MO; with permission.)

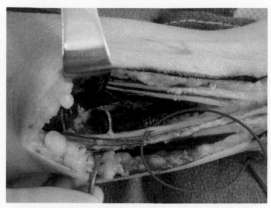

Fig. 8. The AIN has been sutured to the ulnar motor fascicle through a large epineural window. Note the lack of tension on the transfer.

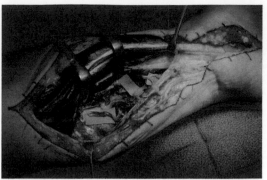

Fig. 9. Sensory transfers to restore ulnar nerve sensation. From left to right, the transfers are as follows: AIN motor to ulnar motor; third web space median to ulnar sensory; palmar cutaneous branch of median nerve to dorsal ulnar sensory nerve; distal end of third web space branch transferred end to side to main median sensory nerve. Note that these transfers are placed deep to the forearm flexors and proximal to the wrist crease. (*Courtesy of* S.E. Mackinnon, MD, St Louis, MO; with permission.)

- Regardless of technique (ETE vs SETS), assess tension on the transfer after placing one suture by bringing the hand and wrist through full range of motion. After a tension-free transfer is confirmed throughout, arc-of-motion additional sutures are placed.

In patients with combined proximal median and ulnar nerve injuries, transfer of the terminal branches of the PIN to the ulnar motor nerve has been described. Nerve branches extensor indicis proprius (EIP), abductor pollicis longus (APL), and extensor pollicis brevis (EPB) may be transferred through a window in the interosseous membrane ETE to the ulnar motor fascicle. Transferring branches to extensor digiti minimi (EDM) and extensor carpi ulnaris (ECU) has also been described, although this transfer requires the use of a nerve graft. Although this technique remains a reconstructive option in this challenging patient population, its utility has yet to be shown in large patient populations.[9,10]

Nerve Transfers to Restore Ulnar Sensory Function

Third web space median to ulnar sensory transfer

- Identify the median nerve in the distal forearm (**Fig. 9**)
- Identify the third web space fascicle of the median nerve:
  - In distal forearm: A natural cleavage plane exists between this fascicle and the remainder of the median nerve in the distal forearm. After identification of the fascicle in the distal forearm, stimulate it to confirm the absence of motor function.
  - Distally in the palm: If the third web space fascicle cannot be easily identified in the distal forearm, the carpal tunnel should be released so it can be found distally in the palm and followed proximally.
  - Small plexus located proximal to radial styloid can be divided if they are small.
- Divide the third web space fascicle distally at the proximal edge of or within the carpal tunnel.
- Divide ulnar sensory fascicle proximally.
- Coaptation:
  - Suture the 2 ends together using a 9-0 nylon suture and the operating microscope.
  - Perform transfer deep to the flexor tendons.
  - Plan coaptation to lie 5 to 6 cm proximal to volar wrist crease to avoid placement at the wrist joint.
  - Distal aspect of the third web space branch is placed end to side into the remainder of the sensory component of the main body of the median nerve to allow recovery of rudimentary protective sensation to the third web.

End-to-side reinnervation of the dorsal ulnar cutaneous nerve

- Divide dorsal ulnar cutaneous nerve proximally.
- Drape the end of the dorsal ulnar cutaneous nerve over the median nerve along its ulnar border in a relaxed position.
- Create an epineural window in the median nerve at this level.
- Coapt the dorsal ulnar cutaneous nerve to the epineural window in the median nerve.

Other sensory nerve transfers have been described to restore ulnar sensation. The palmar cutaneous branch of the median nerve may be used to restore sensation to the ulnar border of the hand and ulnar digits.[8] Use of this transfer is an option if the third web space branch is not available. The lateral antebrachial cutaneous nerve, extended with a sural nerve graft, may be used to restore sensation to the dorsal ulnar sensory branch.[6]

ADJUNCT PROCEDURES

Several adjunct procedures have been described to augment the nerve transfers described above.

- Extensor digiti quinti to extensor digiti communis tendon transfer to correct Wartenberg position.[7]
- Flexor tenodesis of the ulnar innervated flexor digiti profundus (FDP) tendons to the median innervated FDP tendons to restore extrinsic function.[7]
- Metacarpophalangeal joint capsulodesis and pulley advancement, to serve as an "internal splint" during recovery.[20]

POSTOPERATIVE MANAGEMENT

The patient is immobilized in a long arm splint with the wrist in neutral and the elbow at 90° of flexion for 2 to 3 days. After the postoperative dressing is removed, the patient wears a sling for comfort, and gentle range-of-motion exercises are begun. For distal AIN transfers, the patient is kept in a volar wrist splint in neutral for 2 weeks, removing it multiple times a day for gentle range-of-motion exercises. At 4 weeks postoperatively, the patient is advanced to strengthening and motor re-education, focusing on exercises that recruit the donor nerve. For AIN to ulnar motor transfers, the focus is placed on recruiting pronation, and for radial to ulnar nerve transfers, the focus is placed on recruiting wrist and finger extension.

OUTCOMES

Reports of recovery of intrinsic ulnar nerve function after repair or grafting of high ulnar nerve injuries in adults have been uniformly poor.[2–4] Published results after AIN to ulnar motor nerve transfer have been promising, with many investigators reporting recovery of intrinsic ulnar nerve function. Novak and Mackinnon[11] reported on the results after AIN to ulnar motor nerve transfer in 8 patients. All patients showed reinnervation of the ulnar intrinsics with an approximate 6-fold increase in lateral pinch strength and grip strength.

A secondary tendon transfer was required in only one patient, and there were no reports of functional deficits related to pronation strength. Battiston and Lanzetta[8] reported similar results in 7 patients with high ulnar nerve injuries who were treated with distal motor and sensory transfers from the median nerve. At an average of 2.5 years after surgery, 5 of these patients had good results; one 11-year-old patient had an excellent result, and only one patient was reported to have a poor result. None of these patients reported weakness in pronation. Haase and Chung[12] reported on the results after AIN to ulnar motor nerve transfer in 2 patients with high ulnar nerve injuries. Both patients showed evidence of ulnar intrinsic recovery, which was confirmed by electrodiagnostic studies. Flores[21] published the first study comparing patients with high ulnar nerve lesions treated with nerve grafting to those treated with distal motor and sensory nerve transfers. He retrospectively reviewed the charts of 20 patients treated with proximal ulnar nerve grafts and 15 patients treated with both AIN and third web space sensory transfers. He found that the nerve transfer group showed better strength recovery (higher recovery of M3/M4 strength and higher hand grip measurements), but that both groups showed similar sensory recovery. The patients treated with nerve transfer also had better disabilities of the arm, shoulder, and hand (DASH) scores, indicating better functional recovery.

Although the indications for ETE AIN to ulnar motor transfer are quite clear, those for SETS transfers are still being defined.[14,22,23] Kale and colleagues[22] compared SETS and ETE nerve transfers in a rat model and demonstrated that similar axonal regeneration and muscle mass preservation occurred between these 2 experimental groups. They suggested that SETS nerve transfers might be used to augment recovery in situations where incomplete recovery is expected. The same group[23] sought to clarify this hypothesis in a rat study in 2013. They evaluated recovery in 3 nerve injury groups—an incomplete recovery model (IRM), an SETS-only model, and an IRM augmented with an SETS transfer. They found increased myelinated axon counts, motor neuron counts, and muscle force in the IRM augmented with SETS transfer, again concluding that SETS transfer enhances recovery in the setting of incomplete injuries and recommended its use in proximal second- and third-degree injuries. Davidge and colleagues[15] retrospectively reviewed their clinical experience with SETS nerve transfers in the setting of in-continuity proximal ulnar neuropathy in 55 adult patients. Their indications for SETS transfer was proximal in-continuity ulnar neuropathy (most commonly chronic compressive neuropathy and traction injuries). All patients had preoperative ulnar intrinsic weakness and FDI denervation demonstrated by clinical examination and electrodiagnostic studies. The investigators found that all patients showed improvement postoperatively in their FDI strength, grip and pinch strength, and DASH scores, although they were unable to determine what degree of intrinsic recovery was attributable to the SETS transfer versus native ulnar nerve recovery. Although this is something that can be measured in animal models, it is much more difficult to prove in the clinical situation and is the focus of future research. Current literature supports the use of the SETS AIN to ulnar motor nerve transfer in the setting of proximal incontinuity ulnar neuropathy with evidence of acute and chronic intrinsic denervation and in situations where incomplete recovery is expected after proximal ulnar nerve injury.

Combined proximal median and ulnar nerve injuries represent a unique challenge. Transfer of expendable branches of the radial nerve to the distal ulnar motor fascicle allow for the potential recovery of ulnar intrinsic strength. Phillips and colleagues[9] presented a case report on this technique in a 17-year-old boy with a proximal ulnar and median nerve laceration. They repaired the nerves proximally to allow for recovery of extrinsic function. For intrinsic ulnar recovery, they performed a transfer of the radial nerve branches to APL, EPB, and EIP. The patient had transient loss of index finger extension, which returned after a few months. There was no reported functional loss to the thumb. One year after nerve transfer, the patient was noted to have recovered extrinsic function and early evidence of ulnar intrinsic function (ability to place and hold in the intrinsic plus position and volitional twitching of the first dorsal interosseous). Tung and colleagues[10] performed an anatomic study detailing the transfer of branches of the PIN to EDM and ECU to the ulnar motor fascicle and included in their report a single case example. They noted that a nerve graft was always required to allow for coaptation of the EDM and ECU branches to the ulnar motor fascicle. This need for nerve graft makes this transfer less desirable to restore ulnar intrinsic function than the other described techniques that do not require grafting, although it does leave EIP innervated and available for tendon transfer, which in cases of combined median and ulnar nerve injury is often needed. The patient described in this study was a 22-year-old woman with a high combined median and ulnar nerve laceration after a motor vehicle accident. At 4 years after cable grafting of her proximal nerve injuries and

EDM/ECU transfer to the ulnar motor fascicle with sural nerve grafting, she was noted to have good but incomplete recovery of her ulnar intrinsic muscles. She had 4/5 strength of the first dorsal interossei, recovery of lumbrical function. She had reduced thumb and finger abduction and adduction but reported overall good hand dexterity and graded her overall function of the upper extremity at approximately 70%. The investigators acknowledge that these PIN transfers require a longer reinnervation distance than the AIN transfer, but still provide a shorter distance when compared with primary repair or grafting of lacerations at the level of the antecubital fossa.

SUMMARY

Peripheral nerve injuries are challenging problems. Nerve transfers are one of many options available to surgeons caring for these patients, although they do not replace tendon transfers, nerve graft, or primary repair in all patients. Distal nerve transfers for the treatment of high ulnar nerve injuries allow for a shorter reinnervation period and improved ulnar intrinsic recovery, which is critical to function of the hand.

REFERENCES

1. Lad SP, Nathan JK, Schubert RD, et al. Trends in median, ulnar, radial, and brachioplexus nerve injuries in the United States. Neurosurgery 2010; 66(5):953–60.
2. Gaul JS. Intrinsic motor recovery – a long-term study of ulnar nerve repair. J Hand Surg Am 1982;7(5):502–8.
3. Sakellarides H. A follow-up study of 172 peripheral nerve injuries in the upper extremity in civilians. J Bone Joint Surg Am 1962;44(1):140–8.
4. Roganovic Z. Missile-caused ulnar nerve injuries: outcomes of 128 repairs. Neurosurgery 2004;59: 621–33.
5. Wang Y, Shengxiu Z. Transfer of a branch of the anterior interosseous nerve to the motor branch of the median nerve and ulnar nerve. Chin Med J 1997;110(3):216–9.
6. Oberlin C, Teboul F, Severin S, et al. Transfer of the lateral cutaneous nerve of the forearm to the dorsal branch of the ulnar nerve, for providing sensation on the ulnar aspect of the hand. Plast Reconstr Surg 2003;112(5):1498–500.
7. Brown JM, Yee A, Macinnon SE. Distal median to ulnar nerve transfers to restore ulnar motor and sensory function within the hand: technical nuances. Neurosurgery 2009;65(5):966–78.
8. Battiston B, Lanzetta M. Reconstruction of high ulnar nerve lesions by distal double median to ulnar nerve transfer. J Hand Surg Am 1999;24(6):1185–91.

9. Phillips BZ, Franco MJ, Yee A, et al. Direct radial to ulnar nerve transfer to restore intrinsic muscle function in combined proximal median and ulnar nerve injury: case report and surgical technique. J Hand Surg Am 2014;39(7):1358–62.

10. Tung TH, Barbour JR, Gontre G, et al. Transfer of the extensor digiti minimi and extensor carpi ulnaris branches of the posterior interosseous nerve to restore intrinsic hand function: case report and anatomic study. J Hand Surg Am 2013;38:98–103.

11. Novak CB, Mackinnon SE. Distal anterior interosseous nerve transfer to the deep motor branch of the ulnar nerve for reconstruction of high ulnar nerve injuries. J Reconstr Microsurg 2002;18:459–64.

12. Haase SC, Chung KC. Anterior interosseous nerve transfer to the motor branch of the ulnar nerve for high ulnar nerve injuries. Ann Plast Surg 2002; 49(3):285–90.

13. Ustun ME, Ogun TC, Buyukmumcu M, et al. Selective restoration of motor function in the ulnar nerve by transfer of the anterior interosseous nerve. J Bone Joint Surg Am 2001;83-A(4):549–52.

14. Barbour J, Yee A, Kahn LC, et al. Supercharged end-to-side anterior interosseous to ulnar motor nerve transfer for intrinsic musculature reinnervation. J Hand Surg Am 2012;37:2150–9.

15. Davidge KM, Yee A, Moore AM, et al. The supercharge end-to-side anterior interosseous-to-ulnar motor nerve transfer for restoring intrinsic function: clinical experience. Plast Reconstr Surg 2015; 136(3):344–52.

16. Mackinnon SE, Colbert SH. Nerve transfers in the hand and upper extremity surgery. Tech Hand Up Extrem Surg 2008;12(1):20–33.

17. Mackinnon SE, Novak CB. Nerve transfers – new options for reconstruction following nerve injury. Hand Clin 1999;15(4):643–66.

18. Richards RR. Tendon transfers for failed nerve reconstruction. Clin Plast Surg 2003;30:223–45.

19. Tung TH, Mackinnon SE. Nerve transfers: indications, technique, and outcomes. J Hand Surg Am 2010;35:332–41.

20. Atiyya AN, Nassar WA. Ulnar nerve repair with simultaneous metacarpophalangeal joint capsulorraphy and pulley advancement. J Hand Surg Am 2015; 40(9):1818–23.

21. Flores LP. Comparative study of nerve grafting versus distal nerve transfer for treatment of proximal injuries of the ulnar nerve. J Reconstr Microsurg 2015;31(9):647–53.

22. Kale SS, Glaus SW, Yee A, et al. Reverse end-to-side nerve transfer: from animal model to clinical use. J Hand Surg Am 2011;36:1631–9.

23. Farber SJ, Glaus SW, Moore AM, et al. Supercharge nerve transfer to enhance motor recovery: a laboratory study. J Hand Surg Am 2013;38:466–77.

Nerve Transfers in Tetraplegia

Ida K. Fox, MD

KEYWORDS

- Nerve transfer • Tetraplegia • Spinal cord injury

KEY POINTS

- Nerve transfer techniques can be applied to restore hand and upper extremity function in the setting of cervical spinal cord injury (tetraplegia).
- Late transfers restore volitional control by bypassing the irreparable central nervous system zone of injury.
- Early transfers can be used to restore volitional control *and* innervate motor units within the zone of injury.
- Utmost care to avoid downgrading function, burning bridges, or collateral damage is imperative in this particular patient population, which has such high-demand use of the upper extremities.

INTRODUCTION: NATURE OF THE PROBLEM

Restoring upper extremity function in the setting of cervical spinal cord injury (SCI) harnesses the unique knowledge and skill set of the upper extremity surgeon. By the use of peripheral nerve transfer techniques, volitional control of previously absent motion (such as elbow extension and finger flexion and/or extension) provides improved function and quality of life.

In SCI, upper extremity loss of function occurs in a descending segmental fashion. People with upper cervical injury may have shoulder motion only. In midcervical injury patterns, people have heterogeneous patterns of elbow extension, wrist extension and flexion, forearm pronosupination, and hand motion; elbow flexion is present. Those with lower cervical level injury may only be missing intrinsic hand muscle function (**Table 1**).

Traditional surgeries in SCI include combinations of tendon transfers, tenodesis, and fusion procedures. Significant previous work with tendon transfers,[1-8] functional neuro-prostheses,[9,10] and

continued advances[11-13] are encouraging. However, eligible patients, particularly in the United States, have failed to benefit for a variety of complex surgical and societal reasons.[14-16]

More recent novel application of nerve transfer techniques to this unique population demands an understanding of the following:

- Pathophysiology of peripheral and central nervous system injury
- Unique use patterns, adaptations, and compensations
- Social, psychological, and financial constraints.

The patterns of trauma that lead to the SCI vary and simultaneous superimposed brachial plexus or peripheral nerve injury, subsequent compression neuropathy, and overuse and instability issues (with shoulder dysfunction and pain), as well as spasticity, can further complicate the clinical scenario.

The bottom line is to figure out what function is present, what of this is redundant and expendable,

Disclosure: Grant funding from the Craig H. Neilsen Foundation for Spinal Cord Injury Research on the Translational Spectrum: Nerve Transfers to Restore Hand Function in Cervical Spinal Cord Injury.
Division of Plastic Surgery, Washington University School of Medicine, 660 South Euclid Avenue, Box 8238, Saint Louis, MO 63110, USA
E-mail address: foxi@wudosis.wustl.edu

Hand Clin 32 (2016) 227–242
http://dx.doi.org/10.1016/j.hcl.2015.12.013
0749-0712/16/$ – see front matter © 2016 Elsevier Inc. All rights reserved.

Table 1		
The International Classification for Surgery of the Hand in Tetraplegia		
Group	Muscle Function	Description
0	No muscles below elbow for transfer	Elbow flexion and forearm supination
1	BR	Expendable elbow flexor
2	ECRL	Extension of wrist
3	ECRB	Expendable wrist extensor
4	PT	Pronation of forearm
5	FCR	Flexion of wrist
6	Finger extensors	Extrinsic finger extension (can be partial)
7	Thumb extensor	Thumb extension at IPJ
8	Digital flexors	Thumb and finger flexion (often partial)
9	Intrinsic minus	Full finger flexion; lacks only intrinsic muscle function
10	Exceptions	Mixed patterns

Sensibility at the thumb is assessed; O-Occulo indicates that two-point discrimination is >10 mm; Cu-cutaneous indicates that two-point discrimination is <10 mm.

Abbreviations: BR, brachioradialis; ECRB, extensor carpi radialis brevis; ECRL, extensor carpi radialis longus; FCR, flexor carpi radialis; PT, pronator teres.

Modified from McDowell CL, Moberg E, House JH. The second international conference on upper limb rehabilitation of the upper limb in tetraplegia. J Hand Surg Am 1986;11:607; with permission.

and what is missing. If the pattern of injury is established and no further spontaneous recovery of function is expected, nerve transfer surgery may be a reasonable treatment option. There are 2 basic time schedules for intervention: time-independent and time-dependent (the rescue transfer).

In clear-cut, isolated, cases of SCI with a narrow zone of anterior horn cell damage, a transfer done in the periphery can reconnect the brain to the motor unit and restore muscle movement. In this scenario, unlike that of peripheral nerve injury, the transfer can be done at any time post-SCI.[17,18] The transfer necessarily creates an iatrogenic peripheral nerve injury to swap motor control from the redundant and expendable donor to the critical and absent recipient muscle group (**Fig. 1**).

In time-dependent rescue transfers, the zone of injury is more extensive and/or involves the brachial plexus and peripheral nerves. In this challenging situation, there may be reasonable expendable donors to use in a twofold fashion: (1) restore volitional control and (2) reinnervate muscle that would otherwise become nonreinnervatable as seen in peripheral nerve or brachial plexus injury patterns See **Fig. 1**.

Although, the surgical technique may be relatively straightforward to the trained peripheral nerve and hand surgeon, the perioperative and intraoperative decision-making, management and counseling is not. Therefore, a comprehensive team approach with input from the person with SCI; the caretakers; SCI or physical and rehabilitation medicine specialists; and physical, occupational, and hand therapists, among others, is critical for optimal management.

SURGICAL TECHNIQUE
Preoperative Planning

Preoperative planning is critical to success. Several overarching principles are described in the following discussion.

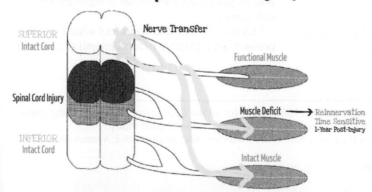

Level of Spinal Cord Injury

Fig. 1. The 2 types of nerve transfers that may be performed in terms of the extent of SCI. The bottom arrow depicts a time-independent nerve transfer, which is performed to restore volitional control of motor function or bypass the zone of SCI. This may be done at any time post-SCI. The top arrow depicts a time-dependent rescue transfer, which is performed to restore volitional control and reinnervate nonfunctioning muscles. (*Courtesy of* nervesurgery.wustl.edu, 2015.)

Patient history

Patient history includes

- Delineating the nature of the underlying injury, including any recent improvement or decline in function:
  - Continued gradual gain in new function should be left alone before surgical intervention (recovery of function can occur months to even years post-SCI)[19,20] and spontaneous gains should not be interrupted.
  - Loss of function is concerning for an underlying structural problem (eg, a posttraumatic syrinx) or medical issue (eg, underlying infection) and must be assessed before proceeding with surgery.
- Ruling out major biologic, psychologic, and social contraindications for surgery is imperative:
  - Skin, urinary, and respiratory health must be discussed and monitored; the presence of pressure sores, untreated urinary and respiratory infections, and/or other medical comorbidities may preclude surgical intervention.
  - Patients (and caregivers) must demonstrate psychological readiness for any semielective surgical procedure.
    - There are some perioperative restrictions on activity.
    - There is a risk of down-grading function.
    - There are other risks entailed with general anesthetic and a surgical procedure (damage to neighboring structures such as sensory nerves, infection, bleeding, wound healing problems, anesthetic, and other complications).
    - Results will take a long time to become apparent and gain of function is slow, gradual, and not to preinjury levels.
  - Social support, including transport to and from therapy and other postoperative follow-up visits, assistance with non–weight bearing transfers, and perioperative use of a motorized wheel chair, ensure proper perioperative care and improved outcomes.
- Defining patient goals and needs is critical:
  - Patients, caregivers, family members, and treating health care providers must have realistic expectations about the expected time-course and extent of recovery.
  - Some patients may benefit from alternative treatments such as tendon transfer (see later discussion on diagnostic testing), adaptive strategies, or other treatments.

Patient examination

Table 2 outlines a detailed description of the physical examination by area of the upper extremity. Examination entails:

- Comprehensive examination of both upper extremities is crucial to understanding overall use patterns, differences in function, and specific factors that may influence surgical decision making.
  - Time of day, temperature, coexisting infection, or other issues can lead to changes in motor function.
  - Providing truncal support by an assistant or supportive belts allows for a focused examination of upper extremity muscle function.
- Careful evaluation of potential redundant donors and putative recipients is critical.
  - Be careful of adaptive strategies, such as use of gravity (for elbow extension, pronation, and wrist motion) and the tenodesis-effect finger motion (volitional wrist flexion and extension with reflexive finger extension and flexion).
  - Carefully delineate muscle motion that is due to volitional control and differentiate from spasticity (the patient is often aware of what is what).
- Ensure joint suppleness:
  - Elbow flexion contractures will preclude optimal restoration of volitional elbow extension.
  - Posturing in profound forearm supination and wrist extension puts wrist and finger flexors in a disadvantaged position for reinnervation and successful motor recovery.
  - Finger flexion contractures may initially seem useful for augmenting tenodesis-driven hand function but can make hand opening more challenging.

Diagnostic testing

There is no gold standard diagnostic test that will provide all of the information necessary to determine eligibility and appropriateness of nerve transfer surgery in this patient population. The following diagnostic tests may be useful and should be ordered on a case by case basis:

- Confirm spinal stability and the absence of a syrinx by appropriate imaging as needed.
- Although not completely refined, preoperative electrodiagnostic testing is often helpful (particularly in late time-independent transfers) to confirm the integrity of the motor unit below the level of the SCI.
- Nerve conduction studies that show intact compound motor action potentials for

Table 2
Physical examination

Area to Examine	Description
Shoulder	
General Tips	Assess for scapular winging, rotator cuff issues
Movement	Check overall patterns of external and internal rotation, abduction and adduction, extension and flexion
Muscle function	Individually palpate and resist anterior, middle, or posterior deltoid
Elbow	
General Tips	Assess for elbow flexion contracture
Movement	Check overall patterns of flexion and extension
Muscle function	Individually palpate and resist • Triceps function (against gravity, with gravity eliminated) • Biceps (with forearm in supinated position) • Brachialis (with forearm in pronated position, palpate on either side of biceps tendon) • Brachioradialis (displaceable, not displaceable)
Forearm	
General Tips	Assess natural resting posture of forearm and position as patient uses hands: pronated or supinated position
Movement	Check passive and active pronosupination
Muscle function	Individually palpate and resist • Supinator function: palpate muscle belly at dorsoradial forearm along border of radius with resisted supination (remember biceps also supinates the forearm so direct palpation is important) • Resist pronation and palpate pronator teres to confirm active function
Wrist	
General Tips	Assess all of the wrist flexor and extensors individually
Movement	Check passive and active wrist flexion; flexor muscle spasticity may limit wrist extension; try and differentiate between loss of passive motion due to spasticity (treatable with nerve transfer) vs joint level contracture (may require serial splinting or surgical release)

Muscle function	Individually palpate and resist
	• ECRL: if only working wrist extensor is ECRL, wrist will have extreme radial deviation with extension
	• ECRB: If ECRL and ECRB are functioning, wrist will have moderate radial deviation with extension; can palpate ECRL or ECRB tendons and visualize proximal forearm bean sign or sulcus between the 2 muscle bellies if both are functional
	• ECU: if all 3 wrist extensors are working, wrist will have central wrist extension; ECU will contribute to ulnar deviation of the wrist; palpate tendon to ensure volitional true function and not effect of gravity
	• Resist wrist flexion and palpate FCR and FCU tendons; ensure volitional function and not effect of gravity or spasticity

Hand

General Tips	Assess resting posture of the hand, atrophy, contractures, skin lesions
Movement	Careful evaluation of passive and active motion, presence or absence of contractures, and joint laxity will permit individual tailoring of the treatment plan:
	• Contractures and/or stiffness: assess for extrinsic tightness and/or spasticity vs true joint contractures; assess the MPJ and IPJ separately; note that some degree of IPJ flexion contracture can augment tenodesis-driven grip and preoperative stretching to improve PROM should be balanced with current functional patterns
	• Laxity: in particular, a floppy thumb may be problematic for functional fusion is an option but postoperative immobilization and modification of transfer techniques (bed to wheelchair, etc.) will be required
	• Assess degree of clawing
Muscle function	Individually palpate tendons and resist to test the following:
	• Extrinsic flexors and extensors of the thumb and fingers including FPL, FDP, FDS, EDC, EIP, EDQ, EPL
	• Intrinsic function

A detailed physical examination is complicated and takes a significant amount of time; repeated examinations are often necessary to confirm findings; discussion of use patterns and collaboration with hand, physical, and occupational therapists, as well as the patient and caretaker, helps complete this careful examination.

Abbreviations: ECU, extensor carpi ulnaris; EDC, extensor digitorum communis; EDQ, extensor digitorum quinti minimi (to small finger); EIP, extensor indicis proprius (to index finger); EPL, extensor pollicis longus; FCU, flexor carpi ulnaris; FDP, flexor digitorum profundus; FDS, flexor digitorum superficialis; FPL, flexor pollicis longus; IPJ, interphalangeal joint; MPJ, metacarpophalangeal joint.

Courtesy of r.nervesurgery.wustl.edu, 2015.

recipient nerve roots of interest suggest a receptive recipient.

- Electromyography can be used to assess both donors and recipients:
  - Donor muscles should be essentially normal and without evidence of denervation.
  - For delayed transfer, even years after injury, recipient muscles should not have any evidence of denervation (ie, no fibrillations) nor should there be any evidence of volitional control (ie, no motor unit potentials).
  - For early rescue transfer, in which the goal is restoration of volitional function and reinnervation of the motor unit at the level of the SCI, there may be evidence of denervation but there should not be any evidence of volitional control.
- The role of functional electrical stimulation and other diagnostic testing modalities is yet undefined in this field.

Preparation and Patient Positioning

Perioperative care of SCI patients undergoing nerve transfer surgery is a little different from that of peripheral nerve or brachial plexus patients. Systemic complications should be avoided by careful attention to skin integrity, respiratory and urinary system health, maintaining normothermia, and recognizing and treating autonomic dysreflexia.

Preoperative care tips
Preoperative care includes the following:

- Patients should transfer directly from their home wheelchair to a specialty low-air-loss or other pressure distributing bed (not a stretcher).
- A warming blanket or warm room helps avoid preoperative hypothermia.
- Skin integrity should be assessed.
- Any evidence of respiratory, urinary, or other infection should lead to delay in surgery.

Intraoperative positioning and care
Intraoperative positioning and care include the following:

- The operating room should be warmed before patient arrival.
- Nonparalytic general anesthesia (or a very short acting paralytic) is necessary to allow for intraoperative neuromuscular stimulation.
- Insertion of a Foley catheter (for longer multi-transfer surgeries) should be done once the patient is completely anesthetized.

- Padding of pressure points, especially for prone positioning, should be undertaken carefully (eg, avoid over-stretching of pectoral muscles from use of too large shoulder rolls).
- The entire upper extremity should be prepped into the field so that intraoperative stimulation of the appropriate muscle groups can be confirmed by direct visualization and palpation.

Surgical Approach

The main nerve transfers used in this population are aimed at restoring the following major functions: elbow extension, wrist extension, and finger flexion and extension (**Fig. 2**). Other more unusual transfers have been also been described.[21,22]

As with all nerve transfers, detailed knowledge of the internal topography of the peripheral nerve permits intraneural dissection and identification of the appropriate donor and recipient fascicles. In contrast to peripheral nerve and brachial plexus injury, in SCI, stimulation of recipient nerve fascicles outside of the zone of SCI will often result in a muscle contracture. In SCI, the goal is primarily to restore volitional control; reinnervation is a secondary goal in cases of early, time-dependent rescue nerve transfers.

Therefore, in SCI, the surgeon must have a very clear idea of what muscles are under volitional control and which are not:

- This ability to stimulate the recipient nerve can make the internal neurolysis somewhat easier from a technical standpoint (eg, median nerve motor fascicles can more easily be separated from the sensory fascicles).
- Over-aggressive dissection and inadvertent transection of a nerve that is under volitional control (such as pronator teres nerve) must be avoided.

Surgical Procedures

General tips
Surgical procedures include the following:

- Remember to prepare the entire extremity.
- In prone position cases, the arm is positioned in adduction and supported on 1 or 2 arm boards.
- In supine position cases, the arm is positioned in abduction and a standard hand table is used to support it.
- For most of these procedures, an arm tourniquet is not used because it would be in the operative field.
- A tourniquet can be used for short periods with caution to avoid a potential tourniquet

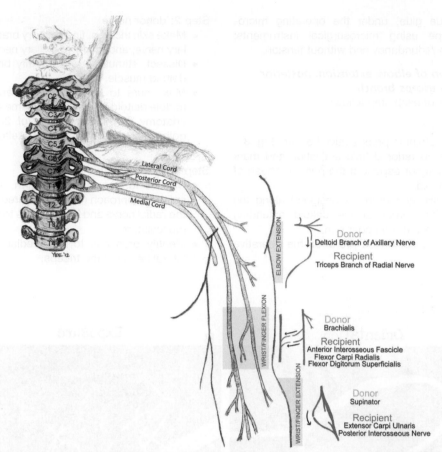

C2
C3
C4
C5
C6
C7
T1
T2
T3
T4

YEE '12

Lateral Cord
Posterior Cord
Medial Cord

ELBOW EXTENSION

Donor
Deltoid Branch of Axillary Nerve

Recipient
Triceps Branch of Radial Nerve

WRIST/FINGER FLEXION

Donor
Brachialis

Recipient
Anterior Interosseous Fascicle
Flexor Carpi Radialis
Flexor Digitorum Superficialis

WRIST/FINGER EXTENSION

Donor
Supinator

Recipient
Extensor Carpi Ulnaris
Posterior Interosseous Nerve

Fig. 2. The most commonly described nerve transfers that have been used in the setting of cervical SCI. Transfer of branches of the axillary nerve (usual donor includes branches to teres minor or posterior deltoid) to the triceps branches of the radial nerve restore elbow extension. Transfer of branches of the musculocutaneous nerve to brachialis muscle may be used to restore wrist extension or finger flexion. Transfer of the supinator branch of the radial nerve may be used to restore finger and thumb extension and abduction (by reinnervation of the posterior interosseous nerve branch) or wrist extension (by reinnervation of the nerve to extensor carpi ulnaris). (*Courtesy of* nervesurgery.wustl.edu, 2015.)

palsy and the inability to perform intraoperative nerve stimulation.

- A diluted epinephrine solution (1:1 million) can be injected along incision lines to help control dermal oozing.
- Use vessel loops to encircle identified donor and recipient nerve branches before transection.
- Stimulate both donor and recipient nerves before transection and coaptation.
- Confirm the donor activation is sufficient and powerful enough.
- Confirm that recipient nerve is properly identified:
  - Anatomic identification is required in rescue time-dependent transfers, in which the

goals are to restore volitional function and reinnervate motor units whose anterior horn cells (motor neuron cell body) is within the zone of the direct SCI.
  - Identification through intraoperative stimulation is possible in cases in which motor units are preserved and the goal is restoration of volitional function.
- Use fastidious technique throughout with the following goals:
  - Minimize collateral damage (to adjoining nerves, soft tissue, and musculature) by use of bipolar cautery and gentle tissue handling.
  - Optimize regeneration by precise coaptation of nerve ends with 9-0 nylon and fibrin

tissue glue, under the operating microscope using microsurgical instruments; with redundancy and without tension.

Restoration of elbow extension: posterior deltoid to triceps branch

The details of each step follow:

Step 1: incision
- Mark patient in preoperative holding (**Fig. 3**).
- Resist posterior deltoid activation and mark the posterior aspect of the posterior head of the deltoid.
- A curvilinear incision is designed along the posterior border of the deltoid extending distally along the upper arm.
- Patient is positioned prone on the operative table.

Step 2: donor nerve
- Make skin incision, find sensory branch of axillary nerve, and follow to axillary nerve proper.
- Dissect, stimulate, and identify branches to deltoid muscle.
- Make sure to leave adequate anterior and middle deltoid function. Sometimes fascicular anatomy permits use of 1 (of 2) branches going to middle and posterior deltoid.

Step 3: recipient nerve
- Dissect further distally in arm. A muscle-splitting approach may be required to expose the radial nerve and its branches to the triceps musculature.
- Identify branches to the medial, long, and lateral heads of the triceps.

A   Orientation
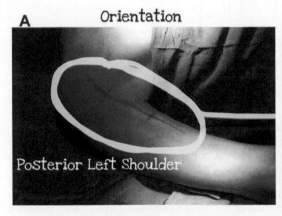
Posterior Left Shoulder

B   Exposure
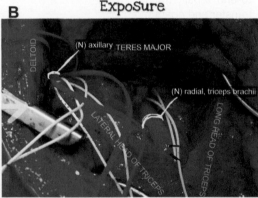

DONOR Posterior Deltoid Branch

Posterior Deltoid to Medial Triceps Nerve Transfer
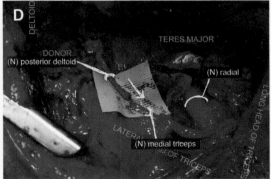

Fig. 3. For restoration of elbow extension, a posterior approach is used to transfer the posterior deltoid branch of the axillary nerve to nonfunctioning triceps muscle branches of the radial nerve. An anterior approach using the teres minor branch as the donor is also described. (*A*) The patient is positioned prone and a curvilinear incision is made over the posterior shoulder and arm. (*B*) The axillary and radial nerves are identified and stimulated. (*C*) An intraneural dissection is performed to separate the posterior deltoid branch donor from the anterior and middle deltoid branches, which are left in continuity to provide continued shoulder abduction function. (*D*) The coaptation is performed in an end-to-end, tension-free fashion. (*Courtesy of* nervesurgery. wustl.edu, 2015.)

- Review preoperative electromyography to help decide which recipient to chose:
  - Recipient muscle with denervation and no motor unit potentials is appropriate for rescue restoration of volitional control and reinnervation.
  - Nerve branches to triceps muscle that had evidence of denervation but motor unit potentials is under volitional control and may contribute to elbow extension function. These branches should not be used a recipients because this may ultimately lead to downgraded function.

Step 4: coaptation and closure
- Once putative recipients and donors are identified and confirmed, dissect proximally along the donor nerve and distally along the recipient.
- Ensure adequate redundancy for direct end-to-end repair, transect nerves, and perform transfer and coaptation.
- Irrigate, achieve hemostasis, and consider drain placement.
- Reapproximation of the longitudinally split triceps may be completed. Otherwise, subcutaneous tissues are reapproximated and skin is closed with deep dermal and running subcuticular stiches. Additional reinforcing nylon mattress sutures may be used in very active or patients with less robust dermis.

Restoration of wrist extension: brachialis to extensor carpi radialis longus
The details of each step follow:

Step 1: incision
- Mark patient in preoperative holding.
- Resist elbow flexion with the forearm in neutral pronosupination and identify and mark the brachioradialis muscle belly.
- A longitudinal incision for exposure of the brachialis donor is made at the medial aspect of the arm at the intermuscular groove between the biceps and triceps muscles.
- A second longitudinal is designed at the lateral aspect of the elbow between the brachioradialis laterally and the biceps medially. This permits identification and isolation of the recipient extensor radialis longus branch of the radial nerve.
- The patient is in the supine position with the surgeon seated at the axilla and facing the medial aspect of the arm.

Step 2: donor nerve
- Make the medial arm skin incision and identify and protect branches of the medial antebrachial cutaneous nerves.
- Identify the biceps muscle and retract it superolaterally away from the triceps. Identify the lateral antebrachial cutaneous nerve and, more proximally, the branches to the brachialis muscle.
- Continued proximal dissection to identify the biceps branches is usually unnecessary if biceps function is entirely normal on preoperative examination and electrodiagnostic testing.
- Dissect, stimulate, and identify branches to brachialis muscle.

Step 3: recipient nerve
- Pronate the forearm, make the lateral arm incision, and dissect between the biceps muscle medially and the brachioradialis and extensor carpi radialis longus muscles laterally.
- The surgeon may need to move to the end of the hand table or above the shoulder to perform the proximal internal neurolysis required to gain adequate length of the recipient nerve branch.
- The brachioradialis branch comes off proximally and should be preserved.
- The next branch of the radial nerve is to extensor carpi radialis longus. This will require extensive proximal neurolysis to separate it from the radial nerve proper and achieve adequate length of the recipient nerve.

Step 4: coaptation and closure
- Once putative recipients and donors are identified and confirmed, dissect proximally along the donor nerve and distally along the recipient.
- Ensure adequate redundancy for direct end-to-end repair and transect the nerves.
- The extensor carpi radialis recipient branch is tunneled under the biceps and delivered into the medial arm incision.
- A tension-free coaptation is performed.
- For this particular transfer; careful evaluation of the length of recipient and donor nerve fascicles is critical to making sure the nerve transfer is free of tension. This may require significant proximal neurolysis of the recipient nerve branch.
- Irrigate and achieve hemostasis.
- For this procedure, if dissection is limited, no drain is necessary and a layered skin closure with dissolvable stiches is completed.

Restoration of digit extension: supinator to posterior interosseous nerves

The details of each step follow:

Step 1: incision
- Mark patient in preoperative holding (**Fig. 4**).
- Resist elbow flexion with the forearm in neutral pronosupination and identify and mark the brachioradialis muscle belly.
- A longitudinal incision is marked just posterior (or lateral) to the brachioradialis muscle belly for exposure of the supinator and posterior interosseous nerves.
- The patient can be in either the supine (or prone position), depending on what other surgery is being done.
- Dissection is carried through the subcutaneous tissue down the muscle fascia: the interval between the brachioradialis and extensor carpi radialis longus muscles (the posterior cutaneous nerve marks this interval).
- The fascia is divided and the 2 muscles are separated to expose the radial sensory nerve, posterior interosseous nerve, and extensor carpi radialis brevis branch.

Step 2: donor nerve
- Supinator branches are identified and transected as distally as possible once

intraoperative stimulation of donor and recipient branches is completed.

Step 3: recipient nerve
- The posterior interosseous nerve is identified diving under the leading edge of the supinator muscle proximal edge.
- The supinator muscle is partially divided to aid exposure and facilitate subsequent regeneration.
- The posterior interosseous nerve is dissected and transected proximally to allow for a tension-free coaptation to the supinator branches once intraoperative stimulation is completed and adequate redundancy is confirmed.

Step 4: coaptation and closure
- Once putative recipients and donors are identified and confirmed as previously discussed, dissect proximally along the donor nerve and distally along the recipient.
- Ensure adequate redundancy for direct end-to-end repair and transect the nerves.
- A tension-free coaptation is performed.
- Irrigate and achieve hemostasis.
- If dissection is limited, no drain is necessary and a layered skin closure with dissolvable stiches is completed.

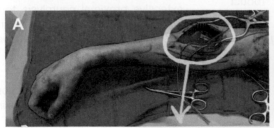
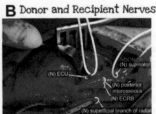

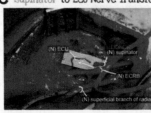

Fig. 4. For restoration of finger and thumb extension (and/or augmentation of wrist extension) a supinator to posterior interosseous nerve (PIN) transfer can be performed. Although these images depict an isolated supinator to extensor carpi ulnaris (ECU) branch of PIN transfer, the approach is the same for the supinator to PIN transfer. (*A*) An incision is made and dissection is carried between the brachioradialis and extensor carpi radialis longus muscles. (*B*) The supinator and PIN branches of the radial nerves are identified and stimulated. The radial sensory nerve and branch to the extensor carpi radialis brevis are protected. (*C*) Although here the supinator branch was coapted to the ECU only, more commonly, the supinator should be coapted to the entire PIN (which includes branches to the thumb extensors and abductor, extrinsic finger extensors and ECU). (*Courtesy of* nervesurgery. wustl.edu, 2015.)

Restoration of digit flexion: brachialis to median nerve-innervated flexors

The details of each step follow:

Step 1: incision
- A longitudinal incision is made at the medial aspect of the arm at the intermuscular groove between the biceps and triceps muscles (**Fig. 5**).
- For cases of rescue restoration of volitional control and reinnervation transfer, a more extensile approach with distal continuation in a zig-zag fashion across the antecubital fossa permits exposure and identification of the anterior interosseous nerve and other relevant recipients.
- The patient is positioned in the supine position.

Step 2: donor nerve
- Make the skin incision and identify and protect any branches of the medial antebrachial cutaneous nerves
- Identify the biceps muscle and retract it superolaterally away from the triceps. Identify the lateral antebrachial cutaneous nerve and, more proximally, the branches to the brachialis muscle.
- Continued proximal dissection to identify the biceps branches is usually unnecessary if biceps function is entirely normal on preoperative examination and electrodiagnostic testing.
- Dissect, stimulate, and confirm the branches to brachialis muscle.

Step 3: recipient nerve
- Using same incision, proceed back slightly more proximally and superficially to identify the median nerve proper.
- The anterior interosseous nerve and flexor digitorum superficialis branches of the median nerve are identified and separated from other branches of the median nerve.
- Deliberate exclusion of the following median nerve branches is important and can be done based on internal topography and/or intraoperative nerve stimulation:
  - Exclude working fascicles under volitional control such as those to flexor carpi radialis and pronator teres.

A

BRACHIALIS TO AIN/FDS
NERVE TRANSFER

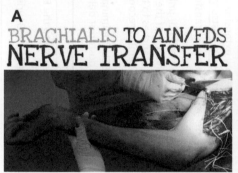

B DONOR Brachialis Nerve

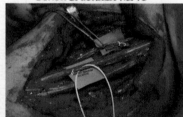

RECIPIENT AIN/FDS Fascicle

C Brachialis to AIN/FDS Nerve Transfer

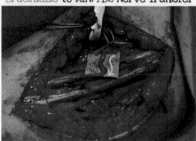

Fig. 5. For restoration of finger flexion, the brachialis branch of the musculocutaneous nerve can be transferred to branches of the median nerve. (*A*) A medial arm incision is made and the donor and recipient nerves are identified. (*B*) The donor brachialis nerve branches are identified. The median nerve has been turned to expose the deep side of the nerve where the anterior interosseous nerve (AIN) and flexor digitorum superficialis (FDS) fascicles can be identified using a hand held nerve stimulator. This more limited dissection is possible in cases of time-independent nerve transfers in SCI in which the recipient fascicles can be stimulated and the transfer is completed to restore volitional control. (*C*) The brachialis branches were dissected distally and transected at the neuromuscular junction and the recipient median branches were dissected proximally to gain adequate length for a tension free closure. (*Courtesy of* nervesurgery.wustl.edu, 2015.)

Table 3
Clinical results

Description	Results
Historical	
MC to median nerve transfer	Variable likely due to more limited knowledge about internal topography of relevant nerves available at that time. These limitations, as well as the more limited use of surgical magnification, precluded intraneural dissection to avoid downgrading functioning median nerve innervated muscles.[33,34]
For elbow extension	
Teres minor to triceps	The teres minor branch of the axillary nerve is transferred to a triceps branch of the radial nerve through an axillary incision[31] • Bilateral transfer at 9 mo post-SCI; M4 elbow extension achieved; no loss of shoulder external rotation at 14 mo postsurgery.[31] • Unilateral transfer at 6 mo post-SCI; M4 elbow extension achieved no loss of shoulder external rotation; ability to extend elbow holding 2-kg weights × 10 repetitions at 19 mo postsurgery.[26]
Posterior deltoid to triceps	The posterior deltoid branch of the axillary nerve is transferred to triceps branches of the radial nerve through a posterior shoulder/arm incision: • Case series included in 7 subjects at <24 mo post-SCI; unilateral or bilateral transfers to restore elbow extension were completed. Donors included the posterior division of the axillary nerve (9 limbs), middle or posterior deltoid branches (2 limbs) and the anterior deltoid (2 limbs). Recipient branches to the long and upper medial triceps were reinnervated. Results included elbow extension of M4 (11 limbs) and M3 (2 limbs) recorded an average of 19 mo postsurgery. There were no reported donor site deficits.[25] • 2 subjects underwent transfer at <1 y post-SCI. Preliminary data suggests variable results: 1 with antigravity elbow extension restored, 1 without gain in function. Partial posterior deltoid function was preserved as only 1 of the 2 branches to middle and posterior deltoid was taken.[24]
For wrist extension	
Brachialis to ECRL	The brachialis branch of the MC nerve is transferred to the ECRL through a medial arm incision that extends across the antecubital fossa to the proximal forearm: • 1 subjects underwent transfer at 12 mo post-SCI; M3 wrist extension at 5 mo postsurgery and improved hand use through the tenodesis effect.[29]
Supinator to ECU	The supinator branch of the radial nerve is transferred to the ECU through a posterior arm incision: • 1 subject underwent transfer at 20 mo post-SCI; increased wrist stability was noted but antigravity wrist extension was not achieved; (the authors recommend supinator to entire PIN transfer instead of this particular transfer)[24]

For finger extension	
Supinator to PIN	The supinator branch is transferred to the PIN (including nerves to EDC, EPL, APL, and EPB) through a posterior forearm incision: • Bilateral transfer at 7 mo post-SCI; M4 finger MPJ extension at 6 mo postsurgery and improved thumb abduction or extension; no loss of forearm supination (biceps muscle function preserved).[32] • Bilateral staged transfer at 6 and 8 mo post-SCI; M4 finger extension and M3 independent thumb extension at 17/19 mo post-transfer; no loss of forearm supination.[26] • Case series included in 7 subjects at <24 mo post-SCI; bilateral transfers to restore digit extension were completed. Most subjects achieved M4 thumb and finger extension. Results were recorded an average of 19 mo postsurgery. There were no reported donor site deficits.[25]

For finger flexion	
Brachialis to AIN	The brachialis branch of the MC nerve is transferred to the AIN through a medial arm incision: • Bilateral staged transfer at 23 mo post-SCI; M3 thumb and finger extension at 8 (left)/10 (right) months post-transfer; pre-existing joint stiffness limits motion in this 71 yo but self-reported functional and quality of life gains were significant; no downgrading of elbow flexion noted.[28] • Bilateral staged transfer at 6 and 8 mo post-SCI; M4 finger flexion at 17/19 mo post-transfer; achieved measurable pinch and grip using a pinch gauge and dynamometer; temporary loss of wrist flexion on 1 side recovered by 9 mo postsurgery.[26]
Brachialis to AIN/FDS	The brachialis branch of the MC nerve is transferred to the AIN and, sometimes, to FDS nerve branches through a medial arm incision: • Case series includes 13 surgeries in 9 patients 4.8 (range 0.6–12) y post-SCI; in this heterogeneous population results varied. Follow-up ranged from 1 mo to 3 y postsurgery; M1-2 flexion (with wrist and MPJ blocking) was measured; patients reported increase in tenodesis-effect grasp and improved function (ability to self-catheterize, lift light objects using prehension); subtle temporary decreases in elbow flexion subjects and new onset paresthesias were the main complications.[23,24]

Information from the literature on nerve transfer surgery in the setting of cervical SCI. There are several case reports and series describing the clinical results; however, this approach is relatively new and final clinical outcomes take several years to be fully realized. Ongoing outcomes assessment and critical appraisal of the indications, specific surgical approaches, and role of these techniques is essential.

Abbreviations: AIN, anterior interosseous nerve; APL, abductor pollicis longus; EPB, extensor pollicis brevis; M, British Medical Research Council motor function; MC, musculocutaneous; PIN, posterior interosseous nerve; yo, year old.

Courtesy of nervesurgery.wustl.edu, 2015; *and Data from* Refs.[23–26,28,29,31–34]

- ○ Avoid sensory branches so as not to disrupt working sensation and waste valuable motor donors.
- ○ Exclude distal thenar and pronator quadratus nerve fibers that are too far away from the nerve coaptation site to achieve meaningful recovery.

Step 4: coaptation and closure

- Once putative recipients and donors are identified and confirmed, dissect proximally along the donor nerve and distally along the recipient.
- Ensure adequate redundancy for direct end-to-end repair, transect nerves, and perform transfer and coaptation.
- If there are enough donor brachialis branches, direct repair of these branches to separate anterior interosseous and flexor digitorum superficialis branches may be possible. Otherwise, a grouped fascicular repair can be completed.
- It seems that brachialis nerve alone permits some reinnervation to all of these muscles. Flexor pollicis longus function is often the least impressive; however, any degree of function will likely lead to improved tenodesis-effect grasp and some strength and holding power.
- For this procedure, if dissection is limited, no drain is necessary, and a layered skin closure with dissolvable stiches is completed.

Immediate Postoperative Care

Continued attention to normothermia, skin integrity, and resumption of normal bowel and bladder routines is important. Monitoring for autonomic dysreflexia by early recognition of any unusual painful stimulus (eg, too tight sequential stocking or blocked Foley catheter tubing) will avoid this life-threatening complication. Of note, most people with SCI have lower baseline blood pressure, so routine call house officer orders may require notification to permit early detection of subtle rises in pressure over preoperative norms.

Placement of indwelling pain pump catheters at the surgical site can help with management of perioperative pain but this, as well as the nerve manipulation during intraoperative neurolysis, can result in a temporary neurapraxia. Patients and caregivers should be warned of this effect.

Immediate resumption of light use of the effected extremity for activities of daily living, such as eating, self-catheterizing, and grooming, are permitted because all transfers are completed in a tension-free fashion. Most incisions are closed with dissolvable sutures and a simple airstrip dressing. The dressing is removed at 48 hours and routine bathing is resumed. Drains (used primarily for the shoulder area surgeries) are removed when drain output is less than 30 mL per day.

Full weight-bearing activity, such as use of extremity for transfers or manual wheelchair propulsion, is allowed at 2 to 4 weeks postsurgery. This varies according to surgery and patient healing and can be started when all drains are out, edema has resolved, and skin incisions appear well-healed. Sports and strengthening exercises are permitted at 4 weeks postsurgery barring complications.

REHABILITATION AND RECOVERY

The rehabilitation and recovery after nerve transfers for SCI takes time. Function improves gradually over months to years postsurgery.

At 2 to 4 weeks postsurgery, a therapy visit is made to provide the following:

- Education about the nerve transfer with review of nerve injury and recovery time course and what to expect.
- Teaching of cocontraction exercises, which include activating or firing the donor and passive recipient, and range of motions exercises.
- Scar, edema, stiffness, and other general management principles are instituted.

Monthly or bimonthly visits continue for 1 to 2 years after transfer for

- Upper extremity strengthening
- Cocontraction exercises
- Motor re-education
- Early identification of reinnervation, which proceeds very slowly from a flicker of motion (with donor cocontraction) to function with gravity eliminated
- Depending on the transfer, antigravity or even greater strength may be achieved in the recipient muscles
- Continued motor re-education and integration into functional activities and the daily routine maximizes independent recipient muscle function and optimizes patient outcomes.

CLINICAL RESULTS IN THE LITERATURE

The literature on nerve transfers to restore upper extremity function in the setting of cervical SCI is limited due the relatively novel application of these techniques to this patient population and the time required for regeneration and restoration of function. Most of the published case reports and case series reported to date show excellent return of function with limited donor deficits[18,21–34] (Table 3).

SUMMARY

There is a role for nerve transfers in the armamentarium of the hand and upper extremity and peripheral nerve surgeon who take care of patients with cervical SCI. Although the exact role for nerve transfers in this patient population deserves further evaluation, they may be combined with tendon transfers or used as a stand-alone procedure. For this critically underserved patient population, any opportunity to restore function, as challenging and time-consuming as this may be, deserves careful and meticulous attention.

REFERENCES

1. Lamb DW, Landry R. The hand in quadriplegia. Hand 1971;3(1):31–7.
2. Moberg E. Surgical treatment for absent single-hand grip and elbow extension in quadriplegia. Principles and preliminary experience. J Bone Joint Surg Am 1975;57(2):196–206.
3. Zancolli E. Surgery for the quadriplegic hand with active, strong wrist extension preserved. A study of 97 cases. Clin Orthop Relat Res 1975;(112):101–13.
4. House JH, Gwathmey FW, Lundsgaard DK. Restoration of strong grasp and lateral pinch in tetraplegia due to cervical spinal cord injury. J Hand Surg Am 1976;1(2):152–9.
5. Hentz VR, Brown M, Keoshian LA. Upper limb reconstruction in quadriplegia: functional assessment and proposed treatment modifications. J Hand Surg Am 1983;8(2):119–31.
6. Lamb DW, Chan KM. Surgical reconstruction of the upper limb in traumatic tetraplegia. A review of 41 patients. J Bone Joint Surg Br 1983;65(3):291–8.
7. Zancolli EA, Zancolli ER. Surgical reconstruction of the upper limb in middle level tetraplegia. In: Tubiana R, editor. The Hand. Vol. IV, Chapter 36. Philadelphia: WB Saunders; 1993. p. 548–63.
8. Hentz VR, Ladd AL. In: Piemer CA, editor. Functional reconstruction of the upper extremity in tetraplegia. New York: McGraw Hill; 1996.
9. Keith MW, Kilgore KL, Peckham PH, et al. Tendon transfers and functional electrical stimulation for restoration of hand function in spinal cord injury. J Hand Surg Am 1996;21(1):89–99.
10. Taylor P, Esnouf J, Hobby J. The functional impact of the Freehand System on tetraplegic hand

11. Kozin SH. Biceps-to-triceps transfer for restoration of elbow extension in tetraplegia. Tech Hand Up Extrem Surg 2003;7(2):43–51.
12. Friden J, Reinholdt C. Current concepts in reconstruction of hand function in tetraplegia. Scand J Surg 2008;97(4):341–6.
13. Friden J, Reinholdt C, Turcsanyii I, et al. A single-stage operation for reconstruction of hand flexion, extension, and intrinsic function in tetraplegia: the alphabet procedure. Tech Hand Up Extrem Surg 2011;15(4):230–5.
14. Curtin CM, Gater DR, Chung KC. Upper extremity reconstruction in the tetraplegic population, a national epidemiologic study. J Hand Surg Am 2005; 30(1):94–9.
15. Curtin CM, Hayward RA, Kim HM, et al. Physician perceptions of upper extremity reconstruction for the person with tetraplegia. J Hand Surg Am 2005; 30(1):87–93.
16. Squitieri L, Chung KC. Current utilization of reconstructive upper limb surgery in tetraplegia. Hand Clin 2008;24(2):169–73, v.
17. Coulet B, Allieu Y, Chammas M. Injured metamere and functional surgery of the tetraplegic upper limb. Hand Clin 2002;18(3):399–412, vi.
18. Oppenheim JS, Spitzer DE, Winfree CJ. Spinal cord bypass surgery using peripheral nerve transfers: review of translational studies and a case report on its use following complete spinal cord injury in a human. Experimental article. Neurosurg Focus 2009; 26(2):E6.
19. Ditunno JF Jr, Cohen ME, Hauck WW, et al. Recovery of upper-extremity strength in complete and incomplete tetraplegia: a multicenter study. Arch Phys Med Rehabil 2000;81(4):389–93.
20. Steeves JD, Kramer JK, Fawcett JW, et al. Extent of spontaneous motor recovery after traumatic cervical sensorimotor complete spinal cord injury. Spinal Cord 2011;49(2):257–65.
21. Bertelli JA, Ghizoni MF. Transfer of nerve branch to the brachialis to reconstruct elbow extension in incomplete tetraplegia: case report. J Hand Surg Am 2012;37(10):1990–3.
22. Bertelli JA, Mendes Lehm VL, Tacca CP, et al. Transfer of the distal terminal motor branch of the extensor carpi radialis brevis to the nerve of the flexor pollicis longus: an anatomic study and clinical application in a tetraplegic patient. Neurosurgery 2012;70(4): 1011–6 [discussion: 6].
23. Fox IK, Davidge KM, Novak CB, et al. Use of peripheral nerve transfers in tetraplegia: evaluation of feasibility and morbidity. Hand (N Y) 2015;10(1): 60–7.
24. Fox IK, Davidge KM, Novak CB, et al. Nerve transfers to restore upper extremity function in cervical

spinal cord injury: update and preliminary outcomes. Plast Reconstr Surg 2015;136(4):780–92.

25. Bertelli JA, Ghizoni MF. Nerve transfers for elbow and finger extension reconstruction in midcervical spinal cord injuries. J Neurosurg 2015;122(1):121–7.

26. van Zyl N, Hahn JB, Cooper CA, et al. Upper limb reinnervation in C6 tetraplegia using a triple nerve transfer: case report. J Hand Surg Am 2014;39(9):1779–83.

27. Bertelli JA, Ghizoni MF. Single-stage surgery combining nerve and tendon transfers for bilateral upper limb reconstruction in a tetraplegic patient: case report. J Hand Surg Am 2013;38(7):1366–9.

28. Mackinnon SE, Yee A, Ray WZ. Nerve transfers for the restoration of hand function after spinal cord injury. J Neurosurg 2012;117(1):176–85.

29. Friden J, Gohritz A. Brachialis-to-extensor carpi radialis longus selective nerve transfer to restore wrist extension in tetraplegia: case report. J Hand Surg Am 2012;37(8):1606–8.

30. Bertelli JA, Tacca CP, Winkelmann Duarte EC, et al. Transfer of axillary nerve branches to reconstruct elbow extension in tetraplegics: a laboratory investigation of surgical feasibility. Microsurgery 2011;31(5):376–81.

31. Bertelli JA, Ghizoni MF, Tacca CP. Transfer of the teres minor motor branch for triceps reinnervation in tetraplegia. J Neurosurg 2011;114(5):1457–60.

32. Bertelli JA, Tacca CP, Ghizoni MF, et al. Transfer of supinator motor branches to the posterior interosseous nerve to reconstruct thumb and finger extension in tetraplegia: case report. J Hand Surg Am 2010;35(10):1647–51.

33. Kiwerski J. Recovery of simple hand function in tetraplegia patients following transfer of the musculocutaneous nerve into the median nerve. Paraplegia 1982;20(4):242–7.

34. Benassy J. Transposition of the musculo-cutaneous nerve upon the median nerve. Case report. Med Serv J Can 1966;22(7):695–7.

Free Functional Muscle Transfers to Restore Upper Extremity Function

Emily M. Krauss, MSc, MD, Thomas H. Tung, MD*,
Amy M. Moore, MD

KEYWORDS

- Muscle transfer • Microsurgery • Free tissue transfer • Brachial plexus • Nerve regeneration
- Nerve transfer • Nerve graft • Intercostal nerves

KEY POINTS

- Free functional muscle transfer provides an option for functional restoration once target muscle re-innervation is no longer feasible.
- Critical requirements include a functioning donor motor nerve, proper tension insetting, and physical therapy for motor re-education and strengthening.
- Adequate time should be provided for nerve regeneration if performed in 2 stages, with a long nerve graft.

INTRODUCTION

Free functional muscle transfer (FFMT) provides a reconstructive option for functional improvement in the setting of severe upper extremity nerve and brachial plexus injuries. With the advent of microsurgery, followed by the development of free muscle and musculocutaneous flaps for wound coverage,[1] an FFMT expands the use of free tissue transfer for dynamic reconstruction. Paired with nerve transfer, it provides an opportunity to restore volitional control of the upper extremity after nerve injury.

FFMT has numerous requirements for success. First, there must be an expendable donor muscle that is available for transfer. Second, an expendable donor motor nerve outside of the zone of injury must be available in proximity to the recipient site to power the transferred muscle. Next, proper insetting of the muscle is required to maintain an ideal muscle length-tension ratio.[2] Last, cooperation of the patient with the surgical team

and a dedicated hand therapist postoperatively is essential for proper splinting and motor re-education to maximize function.

This review outlines the indications for FFMT, focusing on the reconstructive goals for FFMT in brachial plexus palsy, and reviews commonly used donor muscles and nerves. The authors' preferred approach to these complicated nerve injuries is also discussed.

INDICATIONS

FFMT is a reconstructive option after 3 broad groups of injury: focal traumatic or surgical loss of a particular muscle or muscle groups, Volkmann ischemic contracture, and brachial plexus injury.

Focal Muscle Loss

Reconstruction using FFMT has been described for upper extremity reconstruction after tumor extirpation and traumatic injuries to muscle

Disclosures: The authors have no financial or conflicts of interest to disclose.
Division of Plastic and Reconstructive Surgery, Washington University School of Medicine, 660 South Euclid Avenue, Campus Box 8238, Saint Louis, MO 63110, USA
* Corresponding author.
E-mail address: tungt@wustl.edu

Hand Clin 32 (2016) 243–256
http://dx.doi.org/10.1016/j.hcl.2015.12.010

groups.[3] Donor muscles include the gracilis, extensor digitorum brevis, flexor carpi ulnaris (FCU), and latissimus dorsi muscles to reconstruct functions, such as thenar function, shoulder adduction, and wrist and finger extension.[4–7] The focal nature of tissue loss in patients with traumatic or postoncologic soft tissue excision allows for the availability of a larger variety of donor nerves closer to end-target to power the FFMT. Often, the native nerve to the missing muscle group is preserved and available for direct coaptation.[3]

Volkmann Ischemic Contracture

FFMT for the reconstruction of finger flexion was first described in 1976 using the pectoralis major muscle and then in 1978 using the gracilis muscle after devastating traumatic soft tissue loss or after Volkmann ischemic contracture.[8,9] Independent finger and thumb flexion has been described using gracilis FFMT by splitting the muscle in a bipennate fashion and performing internal neurolysis of the gracilis motor branch of the obturator nerve to provide 2 independently innervated slips that can be tenodesed to the flexor pollicis longus (FPL) and flexor digitorum profundus (FDP) as separate motors.[10] A Volkmann ischemic contracture has unique considerations, including soft tissue constraints from the extent of injury and the pediatric population, and considerations for growth in the future that are beyond the focus of this article but are covered in-depth elsewhere.[11]

Brachial Plexus Palsy

FFMT enables surgeons to restore upper extremity function in patients with brachial plexus palsy who have either exhausted potential nerve transfer options and have persisting deficits, delayed presentation, or complete plexus injuries.

Following the report of Manktelow and McKee[9] of the use of FFMT for finger flexion, Ikuta and colleagues[12] described the reconstruction of elbow flexion in late brachial plexopathy in 1979. Few surgical options existed for the late or complete brachial plexus injury before those studies.[13] Primary excision and grafting in brachial plexus injuries affecting hand function had disappointing results because the surgical reconstruction was too distant from the target muscles to provide meaningful reinnervation before motor endplate deterioration. Terzis and Kostopoulos[13] described the historical approach by Seddon[14] to severe plexopathy, which suggested that the aim of early surgery was to clarify the level of injury and recommended amputation of the extremity in injury patterns without recovery potential.

The development of the FFMT allowed a shift in focus of brachial plexus surgery. Although the principles of shoulder stabilization and restoration of elbow flexion remain unchanged, increased effort is now focused on restoring elbow extension and hand function as well. Nerve transfers are often used for restoration of proximal targets, including shoulder function, elbow flexion, and extension, while FFMT is important to restore hand function. Some centers advocate for FFMT to restore both elbow flexion and finger flexion or extension in a single muscle transfer.[15–19] The multistage approach to brachial plexus reconstruction using combinations of nerve transfers and FFMT has now replaced primary excision and grafting as the preferred technique for severe adult brachial plexus injury.[20]

PATIENT EVALUATION

A complete history and physical examination, including mechanism of injury and concomitant trauma, such as fractures, vascular injuries,[21] and brain injury,[22,23] are important in determining which reconstructive options are available. A brachial plexus diagram to record testing of all major muscle groups organized by nerve roots is helpful to identify the level of injury, severity, and recovery (**Fig. 1**). Muscle strength is documented using the British Medical Research Council (MRC) scale.[24] Evaluation of sensation using 2-point discrimination can provide insight into preganglionic or postganglionic level of injury. Identification of Horner syndrome (eyelid ptosis, miosis, and anhidrosis) signifies likely avulsion of the T1 root. Possible donor nerves of intraplexal and extraplexal origin should also be assessed.

Key diagnostic tests are obtained early, including chest radiographs, extremity radiographs (if humerus or forearm fractures occurred at the time of injury or patient has history of previous bony fixation), electromyography (EMG), and nerve conduction studies. The chest radiograph will identify rib fractures and the functional status of the phrenic nerve.

Electrodiagnostics, including EMG, are ordered outside of the acute period, usually at 3 months and immediately preoperatively for the first stage of brachial plexus intervention. Evidence of denervation (muscle fibrillation) without evidence of reinnervation (motor unit potentials) indicates more severe injury that requires operative intervention for functional return.[25] EMG should also evaluate potential donor nerves for nerve transfers or FFMT.[26] The investigators ask for specific evaluation of the trapezius, pectoralis major, and latissimus dorsi because they provide excellent nerve donors when available.[27]

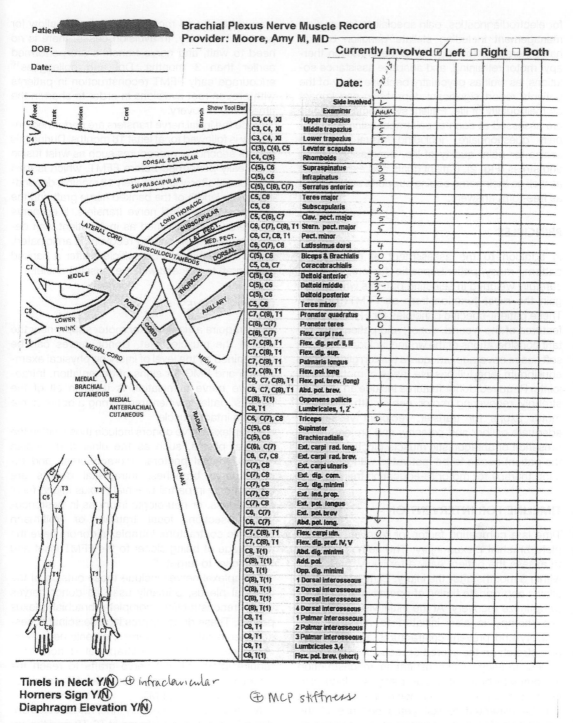

Fig. 1. Brachial plexus diagram for recording functional status of all muscle groups to evaluate injury level, severity, and potential donors for nerve or muscle transfer.

In addition to the EMG, nerve conduction studies are also obtained and assist in localizing the brachial plexus injury. The presence of sensory nerve action potentials (SNAPs) but lack of compound motor action potentials (CMAPs) indicates root avulsion injury. The lack of both SNAPs and CMAPs indicates an injury to the brachial plexus distal to the roots. These findings help guide expectation of recovery.

At the authors' institution, a multidisciplinary team approach is used to treat complex brachial plexus patients. They collaborate with neurologists for electrodiagnostics, pain specialists for medical management including stellate ganglion blocks, hand therapists for ongoing range of motion therapy, motor retraining, and adaptive assistance solutions, as well as psychiatry because many of the patients report significant depression and impact on their quality of life. Patient symptoms and goals are assessed at each appointment using a patient pain questionnaire, including visual analogue scales for pain, quality of life, depression, anger, and stress (**Fig. 2**). Patient goals and expectations as well as their home coping supports are included as free-form answers.

PRINCIPLES

In addition to the assessment of nerve injury pattern, many patient-specific factors must be carefully weighed in selecting patients who will regain the most function from an FFMT (**Box 1**). These patient-specific principles for FFMT include features of the wound, donor, and patient. Important considerations of the wound include adequate soft tissue coverage, adequate tendon glide/tissue equilibrium, and full passive range of motion of all joints. Required donor features include an intact or strongly recovering motor nerve with adequate motor axons for transfer, recipient vessels of adequate caliber and patency, and preferably the presence of antagonistic muscle function. Finally, the patient needs to be motivated with access to hand therapy for motor re-education training.

TIMELINE FOR INTERVENTION

Time is a competing factor for recovery in complete brachial plexus injury. The authors' goal is to assess the patient early after injury, preferably within 3 months after the injury. Early assessment allows appropriate timing of operative procedures to optimize recovery. At the initial visit, preoperative therapy is also initiated to maintain joint mobility and prevent contractures and/or excessive stretch on the injured or recovering muscles.

Despite early initial consultation, reconstruction in complete brachial plexus palsy is a long process, and a clinical relationship with the patient can be expected to last years because of the scheduling of multiple operative stages. In general, intervention is dependent on the severity of the injury and the availability of nerve donors. In complete brachial plexus palsy, nerve transfers to restore elbow flexion and/or shoulder external rotation are pursued. The authors also recommend during this first surgery that a long nerve graft is "banked" for future FFMT (**Fig. 3**). If avulsion is not suspected, these procedures are

pursued by 3 to 4 months after injury to allow for potential recovery. In avulsion cases, there is no need to wait, and nerve transfers are performed earlier than 3 months. Doi and colleagues[16] encourage early FFMT reconstruction in patients with proven root avulsions in order to shorten the timeline to recovery.

Once the initial nerve transfers are performed, recovery is followed for at least 18 months. During this period, secondary procedures such as wrist fusion are ideally performed before FFMT, which is then considered after approximately 18 months, depending on the length of the banked nerve graft and the recovery of the initial nerve transfers. If no nerve transfers were performed as in a patient with delayed presentation and no recovery is anticipated, then 12 months may be sufficient after a banked nerve graft to proceed with the muscle transfer.

DONOR NERVES

FFNT require a viable donor motor supply near the site of the muscle inset. Donor nerves can be determined by the level of injury on physical examination and EMG for signs of denervation. Intraoperative nerve stimulation is used in all of the authors' patients when transferring a donor nerve from an intact muscle.

Intraplexal nerve donors include those within the brachial plexus, such as the ulnar and median nerves, medial pectoral, thoracodorsal, and triceps nerve branches. Intraplexal donors are options only in partial brachial plexus injury, focal muscle loss, or neurologic injury as in postoncologic resection, focal trauma, or Volkmann ischemic contracture. Intraplexal donors have the advantage of being closer to the FFMT inset and thus closer to target.[28]

Extraplexal nerves include those outside of the brachial plexus, primarily used as donor nerves when reconstructing complete brachial plexus palsies. These donor nerves include spinal accessory nerve, intercostal nerves, phrenic nerve, and contralateral C7 root. Extraplexal donors may require interpositional nerve grafts to reach the target and can be donor sources for "banked" nerve grafts for an FFMT.

Nerves to the segmentally innervated rectus abdominis muscle can be found at T6-T8, and the authors' preliminary histomorphometric data show that their axon counts are up to twice as much as intercostal nerves (Tung, unpublished data, 2015). They provide an additional donor motor option if the patient has had multiple ipsilateral rib fractures, putting the function of the higher intercostal nerves in question. If ipsilateral hemidiaphragm function is compromised because of involvement of the

A

Name _____ Date ____ / ____ / ____

Age____ Sex: ☐ Male ☐ Female Dominant Hand: ☐ Right ☐ Left Diagnosis _____

1. **Pain is difficult to describe. Check the words that best describe your symptoms:**

☐ Burning ☐ Throbbing ☐ Aching ☐ Stabbing ☐ Tingling ☐ Twisting ☐ Squeezing
☐ Cramping ☐ Cutting ☐ Shooting ☐ Numbing ☐ Vague ☐ Stinging ☐ Indescribable
☐ Pulling ☐ Smarting ☐ Pressure ☐ Coldness ☐ Dull ☐ Other_____

LEVEL OF SYMPTOMS

Check to indicate the level of your pain, with zero being no pain and 10 the most severe pain you can imagine having.

2. **Mark your average level of pain in the last month:**

No Pain   Most Severe Pain

3. **Mark your worst level of pain in the last week:**

Right   No Pain   Most Severe Pain

Left   No Pain   Most Severe Pain

4. **Where is your pain? (Draw on diagram):**

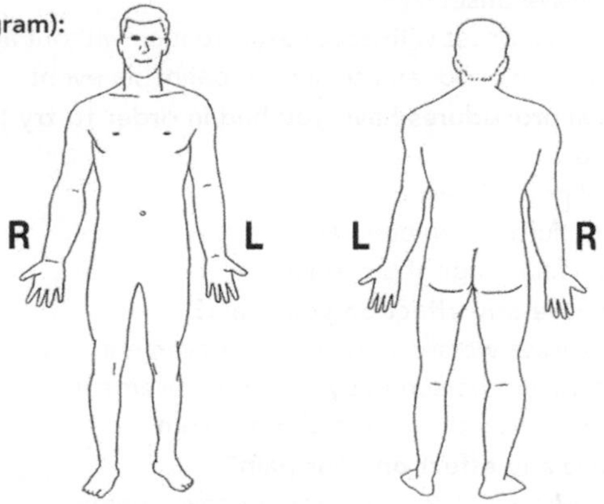

R   L   L   R

5. **Mark on this scale how your pain has affected your quality of life:**

0% (Not at All)   100% (A Large Amount)

6. **Mark on this scale how <u>sad</u> you are:**

0% (Not at All)   100% (A Large Amount)

7. **Mark on this scale how <u>depressed</u> you currently feel:**

0% (Not at All)   100% (A Large Amount)

8. **Mark on this scale how <u>frustrated</u> you currently feel:**

0% (Not at All)   100% (A Large Amount)

9. **Mark on this scale how <u>angry</u> you currently feel:**

0% (Not at All)   100% (A Large Amount)

Fig. 2. (*A–C*) Three-page pain questionnaire, which includes visual analogue scale and assessment of quality of life, depression, and stress. (*Courtesy of* Washington University, St Louis.)

phrenic nerve in the injury, denervating the intercostal muscles will further compromise respiratory function. In such cases, the rectus abdominis nerves can be used for an FFMT without significantly affecting respiration. If the intercostal nerves have already been transferred for elbow flexion in the initial reconstruction, use of the rectus abdominis nerves could allow a second FFMT to

B

10. Mark on this scale how <u>hopeful</u> you are:

|_____|
0% (Not at All)   100% (A Large Amount)

11. Mark your average level of stress in the last month:

|_____|
At Home   0   10

|_____|
At Work   0   10

12. How well are you able to cope with that stress:

|_____|
At Home   Very Well   Not at All

|_____|
At Work   Very Well   Not at All

13. **How did the pain that you are now experiencing occur?**
    - ☐ a. Sudden onset with accident or definable event
    - ☐ b. Slow progressive onset
    - ☐ c. Slow progressive onset with acute exacerbation without an accident or definable event
    - ☐ d. A sudden onset without an accident or definable event

14. **How many surgical procedures have you had in order to try to eliminate the cause of your pain?**
    - ☐ a. None or one
    - ☐ b. Two surgical procedures
    - ☐ c. Three or four surgical procedures
    - ☐ d. Greater than four surgical procedures

15. **Does movement have any effect on your pain?**
    - ☐ a. The pain is always worsened by use or movement
    - ☐ b. The pain is usually worsened by use and movement
    - ☐ c. The pain is not altered by use and movement

16. **Does weather have any effect on your pain?**
    - ☐ a. The pain is usually worse with damp or cold weather.
    - ☐ b. The pain is occasionally worse with damp or cold weather.
    - ☐ c. Damp or cold weather has no effect on the pain.

17. **Do you ever have trouble falling asleep or awaken from sleep?**
    - ☐ a. No - *Proceed to Question 19*
    - ☐ b. Yes - *Proceed to 18A & 18B*

18A. **How often do you have trouble falling asleep?**
    - ☐ a. Trouble falling asleep every night due to pain
    - ☐ b. Trouble falling asleep due to pain most nights of the week
    - ☐ c. Occasionally having difficulty falling asleep due to pain
    - ☐ d. No trouble falling asleep due to pain
    - ☐ e. Trouble falling asleep which is not related to pain

18B. **How often do you awaken from sleep?**
    - ☐ a. Awakened by pain every night
    - ☐ b. Awakened from sleep by pain more than 3 times per week
    - ☐ c. Not usually awakened from sleep by pain
    - ☐ d. Restless sleep or early morning awakening with or without being able to return to sleep, both unrelated to pain

19. **Has your pain affected your intimate personal relationships?**
    - ☐ a. No   ☐ b. Yes

Fig. 2. *(continued)*

C

20. Are you involved in any legal action regarding your physical complaint?
    ☐ a. No   ☐ b. Yes
21. Is this a Workers' Compensation case?
    ☐ a. No   ☐ b. Yes
22. Are you presently receiving or have you ever received psychiatric/psychological treatment?
    ☐ a. No   ☐ b. Presently receiving psychiatric treatment   ☐ c. Previous psychiatric treatment
23. Have you ever thought of suicide?
    ☐ a. No   ☐ b. Yes   ☐ c. Previous suicide attempts
24. Were you a victim of childhood trauma– emotional or physical?
    ☐ a. No   ☐ b. Yes   ☐ c. No comment
25. Are you a victim of emotional abuse?
    ☐ a. No   ☐ b. Yes   ☐ c. No comment
26. Are you a victim of physical abuse?
    ☐ a. No   ☐ b. Yes   ☐ c. No comment
27. Are you a victim of sexual abuse?
    ☐ a. No   ☐ b. Yes   ☐ c. No comment
28. Are you presently a victim of abuse?
    ☐ a. No   ☐ b. Yes   ☐ c. No comment
29. Are you currently: (Check all that apply)
    Employed for wages   ☐ No   ☐ Yes
    On medical leave   ☐ No   ☐ Yes
    A homemaker   ☐ No   ☐ Yes
    Self-employed   ☐ No   ☐ Yes
    Student   ☐ No   ☐ Yes
    Retired   ☐ No   ☐ Yes
    Volunteer   ☐ No   ☐ Yes
    None of the above   ☐ No   ☐ Yes
30. If you are still working, do you?
    ☐ a. Work every day at the same pre-pain job.
    ☐ b. Work every day but the job is not the same as the pre-pain job with reduced responsibility or physical activity.
    ☐ c. Work occasionally.
31. Are you able to do your household chores?
    ☐ a. Do same level of household activities without discomfort.
    ☐ b. Do same level of household chores with discomfort.
    ☐ c. Do a reduced amount of household chores.
    ☐ d. Most household chores are now performed by others.
32. What medications have you used in the past month?
    ☐ a. No medications
    ☐ b. List medications:_____
    _____
    _____
33. If you had three wishes for anything in the world, what would you wish for?
    1._____
    2._____
    3._____

From: Hendler N, Viernstein M, Gucer P, Long D: A preoperative screening test for chronic back pain patients. Psychosomatics 1979;20:801-808.
Mackinnon SE & Dellon AL: Surgery of the Peripheral Nerve, Thieme Medical Publishers, 1988
Melzack R: The McGill pain questionnaire: major properties and scoring methods. Pain 1975;1:277-299.
Modified by 1/5/2010

Fig. 2. (continued)

provide additional function via a banked nerve graft.

The use of a banked nerve graft alters the timeline to FFMT. The initial surgery includes extraplexal donor nerve preparation and coaptation to a long interpositional graft, usually a long sural nerve graft. The distal nerve is coapted to a nonfunctional nerve distally either end to end (eg,

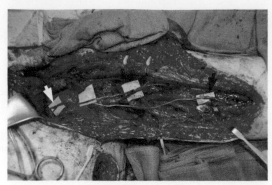

Fig. 4. First-stage brachial plexus reconstruction with motor and sensory transfers, and banked sural nerve graft to medial pectoral nerve branches (*white arrowhead*) and distal coaption to medial antebrachial cutaneous nerve (*black arrowhead*).

medial or lateral antebrachial cutaneous nerves) or end to side to a functioning nerve if available (eg, median nerve) (**Fig. 4**). The distal coaptation assists with revascularization of the distal end of the long graft and theoretically facilitates regeneration.[29] Regeneration is allowed to proceed for at least 12 months postoperatively until an advancing Tinel sign reaches mid arm. During the regeneration period, bony procedures are considered to stabilize the wrist and thumb in preparation for the FFMT.[30,31]

DONOR MUSCLES

Muscle donors for FFMT include gracilis, rectus femoris, latissimus dorsi, gastrocnemius, tensor fascia lata, and serratus anterior.[32] Muscle flaps with a single dominant vascular pedicle, or single dominant and one minor pedicle, are preferred for FFMT to ensure adequate perfusion from a single arterial anastomosis and enable transfer of the entire muscle, including its distal tendon.

In principle, muscle force recovery from a transferred FFMT cannot exceed the maximal tetanic contraction force of the muscle in its pretransfer state.[33] Therefore, the muscle must have sufficient inherent contractile strength and excursion to provide enough force when transferred to the upper extremity for the specific function desired. Sufficient tendinous origin and insertion are necessary in the donor muscle for muscle inset and tenodesis to reconstruct upper extremity motion.

The most popular donor muscle transfer for upper extremity reconstruction is the gracilis. It has a favorable vascular anatomy, reliable and relatively long motor nerve, muscle length, strength, and sufficient tendinous insertion. Donor site morbidity and functional loss are low, and many techniques to improve the ease of harvest and limit donor site morbidity have been described.[10]

RECONSTRUCTIVE GOALS
Upper Plexus (C5-C6)

FFMT has been used to restore elbow flexion historically in patients who had inadequate functional recovery after upper plexus primary excision and grafting.[34] In isolated upper plexus palsy, FFMT is most often used in patients with delayed presentation. Final motor strength of the transferred gracilis muscle as recorded by the MRC grading

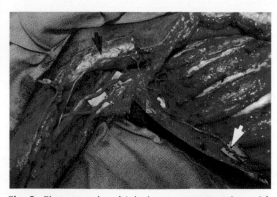

Fig. 3. First-stage brachial plexus reconstruction with motor and sensory transfers, and banked sural nerve graft to rectus abdominis branches as donor nerve supply (*white arrowhead*). The graft is left in a superficial location at the edge of the pectoralis major at the axillary fold to facilitate identification at the second-stage muscle transfer procedure (*black arrowhead*).

classification has exceeded that of a pedicled latissimus dorsi muscle transfer,[35] possibly because of partial injury to the upper plexus contributions to the thoracodorsal nerve.[35] Free muscle transfer is an alternative to Steindler flexorplasty or other muscle transfers (pectoralis major or triceps) to provide independent functional elbow flexion in patients who are candidates for microvascular surgery.

Lower Plexus (C7-T1)

Reconstructive goals in lower brachial plexus palsy include restoration of finger and thumb flexion. If presenting early with available intraplexal donor nerves, hand prehension can be achieved using nerve transfers.[36,37] Otherwise, FFMT has been used for prehension in the patient with lower brachial plexus injury and/or delayed presentation after failed primary excision and grafting. FFMT has also been reported for finger extension in lower brachial plexus palsy.

Complete Plexus (C5-T1)

Primary goals of reconstruction in the complete brachial plexus palsy include elbow flexion and finger prehension. The traditional approach to complete plexus reconstruction has been a proximal-to-distal approach, focusing on establishing elbow flexion at a higher priority than hand function. The FFMT has enabled a modification of the reconstructive priorities in the complete brachial plexus palsy to provide more focus on the recovery of hand function as well as shoulder and elbow function, as practiced by Terzis and colleagues[13,38] in both adult and obstetric brachial plexus palsy. Doi and colleagues[18] developed a double FFMT using 2 gracilis neurotized free flaps to improve hand function.

In complete brachial plexus palsy, proximal nerve transfers are performed to restore function to the elbow and shoulder if feasible. The stabilization of the proximal joints is critical to optimize the outcome of the FFMT used for more distal function. Muscle efficiency is limited by the number of joints crossed. For example, shoulder stabilization improves the efficiency of FFMT for elbow flexion by allowing the transfer to flex the elbow alone without shoulder flexion. Doi and colleagues[39] reported improvement in hand prehensile function in patients with complete brachial plexus avulsions by reconstructing elbow extension using nerve transfers.

Insetting of the muscle will depend on the function or functions targeted for restoration and the level of the donor motor nerve. If performed for elbow flexion, the muscle origin will be anchored to the clavicle; branches of the thoracoacromial vessels will be used; the thoracodorsal nerve, medial pectoral nerves, or a banked nerve graft can provide the motor; and the gracilis tendon is weaved to the biceps tendon. The tension is set such that the muscle, when maximally stretched, will hold the elbow at approximately 30° to 45° of flexion. If being used for elbow and finger flexion, the muscle can be set as above, but a tendon graft will be required to reach the finger flexors in the distal forearm. The lacertus fibrosus can be used as the pulley at the elbow. Alternatively, the muscle can be inset a little more distally with the origin anchored to the proximal humerus; branches of the brachial vessels will be used, and the gracilis tendon is weaved directly to the finger flexors in the distal forearm (**Fig. 5**). With a more distal inset, the motor branch to the gracilis may reach the thoracodorsal nerve and certainly a banked nerve graft, but medial pectoral branches as the motor supply will require a short nerve graft.

Given the lack of donors, reconstruction of elbow extension in the complete palsy is not usually pursued, because elbow extension can be achieved by gravity. However, given Doi's investigation[39] of reconstructed finger flexion without elbow stabilization in the complete brachial plexus palsy, reconstruction of elbow extension should be considered if at all possible. Similarly, arthrodeses are frequently performed to stabilize the wrist and thumb for pinch and provide more efficient pull of FFMT for finger flexion.[29,30]

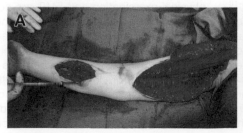
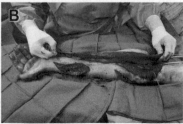

Fig. 5. (*A*) Inset of free gracilis origin to proximal humerus and to finger flexor tendons distally for elbow and finger flexion. (*B*) Low inset to distal humerus proximally and finger flexors distally for primarily finger flexion.

OUTCOMES

Muscle Transfer for Elbow Flexion

In general, use of a single muscle to restore elbow flexion has favorable results, with investigators frequently reporting strength greater than MRC grade 4.[15,35,40–43] Chuang and colleagues[35] reported that the FFMT using gracilis muscle had MRC grade 3 elbow flexion comparable to pedicled latissimus dorsi transfer, and 7 good results of MRC 4 or 5 with intercostal nerve donors for an overall success rate of 41%.[35] They reported difficulty in assessing whether the latissimus dorsi muscle was involved in the brachial plexus injury with subclinical weakness as well as difficulty fixating the latissimus dorsi muscle to the biceps tendon to prevent tendon pull-out with elbow flexion.[35] Dodakundi and colleagues[41] reported that perioperative flap ischemia requiring anastomotic revision correlated with an inferior outcome requiring second FFMT and ancillary procedures. At the authors' center, use of intraplexal donor nerves is associated with more reliable restoration of elbow flexion strength than extraplexal donors (Nicoson MC, Franco MJ, Tung TH: Donor nerve sources in free functioning gracilis muscle transfer for elbow flexion in adult brachial plexus injury. Submitted for publication.)

Single Muscle Transfer for Hand Function

In FFMT for finger flexion, Terzis and Kostopoulos[13] found that distal spinal accessory nerve, upper plexal donors, and intercostal nerve donors restored superior mean muscle strength and range of motion compared with contralateral C7 root donors, in that order. For finger extension, use of the distal spinal accessory nerve for FFMT was associated with the strongest functional recovery.

Double Free Functional Muscle Transfer for Hand Function

Doi and colleagues[16] developed a double FFMT using 2 gracilis flaps to improve hand function. The first flap provided combined elbow flexion and finger extension, and the second flap provided finger and thumb flexion. Doi and colleagues[16–18] emphasized the importance of hand function and advocated early intervention with FFMT, often as early as 3 to 6 weeks, in patients with root avulsion injuries. Hattori and colleagues[21] recommended complete vascular workup in brachial plexus patients with root avulsions when considering early FFMT, outlined in their recent article discussing critical upper extremity vascular injuries in this population. They discussed the limitations of the double FFMT because of the requirement for adequate donor arteries of sufficient caliber to support 2 free flaps inset at different levels.

The use of a single FFMT to perform 2 tasks has been described originally by Doi and colleagues for elbow flexion and finger extension, but has also been described for combined elbow flexion and finger flexion.[44,45] Carlsen and colleagues[44] described the modification of insetting the FFMT using an FCU sling as a pulley to enhance elbow flexion when their stage 1 FFMT was designed to provide both elbow flexion and finger extension. Giuffre and colleagues[19] further modified the double muscle transfer described by Doi to provide simultaneous elbow and finger flexion.

Doi and colleagues[18] described excellent results for elbow flexion in 54%, and good results in 42% of patients receiving the double FFMT for combined elbow flexion and finger extension. Elbow flexion was often assisted by biceps brachii reinnervated by nerve transfer. In their study, only 15% of patients had excellent results for total active finger motion, and 50% of patients had good results with total active motion of only 30° to 55°.[18] Barrie and colleagues[15] reported that the FFMT for combined elbow flexion and finger extension resulted in inferior elbow strength function with only 63% of patients recovering M4 or greater elbow flexion compared with the 79% of patients with M4 elbow flexion after FFMT for elbow flexion alone.

THE AUTHORS' ALGORITHM

At the authors' institution, early presentation of partial brachial plexus injury is preferentially treated with nerve transfer procedures. FFMT is primarily used as a secondary reconstructive procedure to restore function after a complete plexus injury. In the following section, the authors provide their algorithm for reconstruction (**Table 1**).

Delayed Presentation of Upper Brachial Plexus Injury (C5-C6)

In the delayed presentation of an upper brachial plexus injury, the authors' primary reconstructive goal is the restoration of elbow flexion. Detailed physical examination and EMG are performed to assess the potential donors. The authors' preference is the thoracodorsal nerve followed by medial pectoral nerves. The physical examination and EMG determine whether these nerves have signs of injury. The thoracodorsal nerve is often a viable option to power an FFMT given the contribution coming from C6, C7, and C8. The medial pectoral nerve is usually spared in an upper plexus injury due to its contributions from C8 and T1. Distal spinal accessory nerve, FCU fascicles of the ulnar

Table 1
Brachial plexus reconstruction algorithm

Injury Level	Goals	Stage 1	Stage 2	Stage 3
Delayed C5-C6	Elbow flexion	Preferred: Thoracodorsal nerve to obturator nerve of gracilis FFMT Alternate: Medial pectoral nerve to obturator nerve of gracilis FFMT	—	—
Delayed C7-T1	Finger flexion	Preferred: Brachialis branch of musculocutaneous nerve to obturator nerve of gracilis FFMT	—	
	Thumb flexion	—	Brachioradialis to FPL tendon transfer	—
	Finger extension	—	—	Medial or lateral pectoral nerve to second FFMT (gracilis)
Complete brachial plexus injury (C5-T1)	Elbow flexion	Intercostal T3-T6 nerves to musculocutaneous (possible interpositional nerve graft)	—	—
	Shoulder stability	Distal spinal accessory to suprascapular nerve transfer		
	Finger and thumb flexion	Intercostal T7-T8 and rectus abdominis motor nerve branches to banked sural nerve graft for future FFMT	Wrist fusion, thumb carpometacarpal fusion, thumb interphalangeal joint fusion	Gracilis FFMT, powered by the banked nerve graft
	Hand sensation	Sensory T4 and intercostal brachial nerve transfer to the lateral cord contribution of median nerve	—	—

nerve, and intercostal plus rectus abdominis nerves have all been used as donors to power FFMT for elbow flexion at their institution. The authors' outcomes support the use of intraplexal donors if available to avoid interpositional nerve grafts with restoration of MRC4 elbow flexion strength (**Fig. 6**) (Nicoson MC, Franco MJ, Tung TH: Donor nerve sources in free functioning gracilis muscle transfer for elbow flexion in adult brachial plexus injury. Submitted for publication.) The shoulder is stabilized using tendon transfers at a later procedure if necessary by one of the shoulder surgeons.[46]

Delayed Presentation of Lower Brachial Plexus Injury (C7-T1)

In the delayed presentation of a lower brachial plexus injury, the reconstructive goal is to restore finger and thumb flexion. The authors recommend transfer of the gracilis muscle for FFMT with the brachialis branch of the musculocutaneous nerve (C5-C6) as their preferred donor nerve. Often the brachioradialis (BR) muscle is preserved (C5-C6

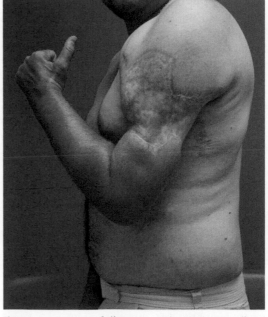

Fig. 6. Long-term follow-up with MRC 4/5 elbow flexion from thoracodorsal nerve donor.

contribution) and a tendon transfer from BR to FPL can be performed at the time of FFMT.

Complete Brachial Plexus Injury (C5-T1)

In a complete brachial plexus injury, careful evaluation for level of injury and potential recovery is important in determining donor nerves. With root avulsions, only extraplexal donors are available. Reconstructive priorities are elbow flexion, shoulder stability, finger and thumb flexion, and restoration of hand sensation.

The first stage of reconstruction includes distal spinal accessory to suprascapular nerve transfer at 3 to 4 months after injury to restore shoulder stability. Intercostal donor motor nerves from T3-T6 are transferred to the musculocutaneous nerve to restore elbow flexion. Upper intercostal nerves will usually reach the transposed proximal musculocutaneous nerve for a direct transfer, whereas an interpositional nerve graft will be required for the lower intercostal nerves. Motor intercostal nerves from T7 and T8 as well as nerve branches to the rectus abdominis muscle from the same level are coapted to a banked sural nerve graft for future FFMT for finger and thumb flexion. Hand sensation is reconstructed using sensory T4 and intercostal brachial nerve transfer to the lateral cord contribution to the median nerve.

Following the first stage of the reconstruction, ancillary procedures are performed, including wrist fusion and thumb carpometacarpal and interphalangeal joint fusions. After at least 1 year following the initial surgery, the second stage of the gracilis FFMT is performed and motored by the banked nerve graft from T7-T8 intercostals and rectus abdominis nerves to power finger and thumb flexion (**Fig. 7**). In the complete palsy, elbow extension and finger extension are usually not reconstructed due to the lack of donor nerves. However, any partial recovery may provide a potential donor motor nerve for a second FFMT to restore elbow or finger extension. After recovery of the FFMT, tenolysis of the gracilis and flexor tendons may further improve finger motion.

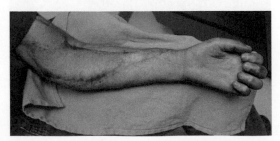

Fig. 7. Long-term follow-up with low inset for finger flexion.

POSTOPERATIVE CARE

As with any free tissue transfer, patients are monitored closely in the postoperative period for signs of flap ischemia, which has been associated with poor recovery of muscle function (**Fig. 8**).[47] A posterior splint is used to maintain the elbow at 90° of flexion to eliminate tension on the muscle and its attachment sites for at least a month. The authors recommend long-term use of a splint or arm sling until muscle recovery is established to avoid overstretching of the transferred muscle and loss of the optimal length tension ratio.[48]

REHABILITATION

Physical therapy is essential for motor rehabilitation after FFMT in the same manner as it is for nerve and tendon transfers to allow the patient to learn how to activate the transferred muscle properly. The source of reinnervation of the transferred muscle is different so the native motor pathways and cortical maps previously established are no longer relevant. New motor patterns and cortical remapping are needed to restore maximum function of the extremity.[49–51]

As in the case of nerve transfers, motor re-education teaches the patient how to correctly and sufficiently activate the transferred muscle. Activation of the reinnervated muscle will not be accomplished by thinking of the intended action intuitively but will require attempted activation of the donor muscle action. For an FFMT reinnervated by intercostal nerves, activation of the transferred gracilis muscle will require contraction or tightening of the ipsilateral chest or abdomen if rectus abdominis nerves were used. If a patient is not able to learn how to activate the reinnervated muscle consistently, he or she will not be able to strengthen it satisfactorily and ultimately use it efficiently.[52]

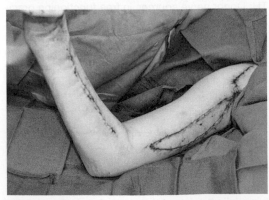

Fig. 8. Postoperative photograph of skin paddle overlying the gracilis muscle for acute monitoring of perfusion.

SUMMARY

FFMT provides a viable option to restore function to the upper extremity after a devastating brachial plexus injury. The identification of donor nerves, tensioning of the muscle at inset, and postoperative splinting and therapy influence the outcome of the FFMT. Adjunctive procedures such as joint arthrodesis and tendon transfers are also important in the reconstructive algorithms for these patients with complex injuries. Having an algorithm and focusing on education of the patient of the timeline and surgical procedures from the beginning will contribute to the commitment of the patient and overall success of the procedures.

REFERENCES

1. Tamai S, Komatsu S, Sakamoto H, et al. Free muscle transplants in dogs, with microsurgical neurovascular anastomoses. Plast Reconstr Surg 1970; 46:219–25.
2. Gordon AM, Huxley AF, Julian FJ. The variation in isometric tension with sarcomere length in vertebrate muscle fibres. J Physiol 1966;184:170–92.
3. Lin SH, Chuang DC, Hattori Y, et al. Traumatic major muscle loss in the upper extremity: reconstruction using functioning free muscle transplantation. J Reconstr Microsurg 2004;20:227–35.
4. Zhu SX, Zhang BX, Yao JX, et al. Free musculocutaneous flap transfer of extensor digitorum brevis muscle by microvascular anastomosis for restoration of function of thenar and adductor pollicis muscles. Ann Plast Surg 1985;15:481–8.
5. Baker PA, Watson SB. Functional gracilis flap in thenar reconstruction. J Plast Reconstr Aesth Surg 2007;60:828–34.
6. Lim AY, Kumar VP, Sebastin SJ, et al. Split flexor carpi ulnaris transfer: a new functioning free muscle transfer with independent dual function. Plast Reconstr Surg 2006;117:1927–32.
7. Doi K, Kuwata N, Kawakami F, et al. Limb-sparing surgery with reinnervated free-muscle transfer following radical excision of soft-tissue sarcoma in the extremity. Plast Reconstr Surg 1999;104:1679–87.
8. Free muscle transplantation by microsurgical neurovascular anastomoses. Chin Med J 1976;57:495.
9. Manktelow RT, McKee NH. Free muscle transplantation to provide active finger flexion. J Hand Surg Am 1978;3:416–26.
10. Zuker RM, Bezuhly M, Manktelow RT. Selective fascicular coaptation of free functioning gracilis transfer for restoration of independent thumb and finger flexion following Volkmann ischemic contracture. J Reconstr Microsurg 2011;27:439–44.
11. Zuker RM, Manktelow RT. Functioning free muscle transfers. Hand Clin 2007;23:57–72.
12. Ikuta Y, Yoshioka K, Tsuge K. Free muscle graft as applied to brachial plexus injury-case report and experimental study. Ann Acad Med Singapore 1979;8:454–8.
13. Terzis JK, Kostopoulos VK. Free muscle transfer in posttraumatic plexopathies: part III. The hand. Plast Reconstr Surg 2009;124:1225–36.
14. Seddon HJ. Surgical disorders of the peripheral nerves. 1st edition. Edinburgh (United Kingdom): Churchill Livingstone; 1972.
15. Barrie KA, Steinmann SP, Shin AY, et al. Gracilis free muscle transfer for restoration of function after complete brachial plexus avulsion. Neurosurg Focus 2004;16:1–9.
16. Doi K, Sakai K, Kuwata N, et al. Double free-muscle transfer to restore prehension following complete brachial plexus avulsion. J Hand Surg Am 1995; 20:408–14.
17. Doi K, Kuwata N, Muramatsu K, et al. Double muscle transfer for upper extremity reconstruction following complete avulsion of the brachial plexus. Hand Clin 1999;15:757–67.
18. Doi K, Muramatsu K, Hattori Y, et al. Restoration of prehension with the double free muscle technique following complete avulsion of the brachial plexus. Indications and long-term results. J Bone Joint Surg Am 2000;82:652–66.
19. Giuffre JL, Kakar S, Bishop AT, et al. Current concepts of the treatment of adult brachial plexus injuries. J Hand Surg 2010;35A:678–88.
20. Yang LJ, Chang KW, Chung KC. A systematic review of nerve transfer and nerve repair for the treatment of adult upper brachial plexus injury. Neurosurgery 2012;71:417–29.
21. Hattori Y, Doi K, Sakamoto S, et al. Complete avulsion of brachial plexus with associated vascular trauma: feasibility of reconstruction using the double free muscle technique. Plast Reconstr Surg 2013;132:1504–12.
22. Stone L, Keenan MA. Peripheral nerve injuries in the adult with traumatic brain injury. Clin Orthop Relat Res 1988;233:136–44.
23. Matsuyama T, Okuchi K, Akahane M, et al. Clinical analysis of 16 patients with brachial plexus injury. Neurol Med Chir (Tokyo) 2000;42:114–21.
24. MacAvoy MC, Green DP. Critical reappraisal of Medical Research Council muscle testing for elbow flexion. J Hand Surg Am 2007;32:149–53.
25. Ray WZ, Mackinnon SE. Management of nerve gaps: autografts, allografts, nerve transfers, and end-to-side neurorrhaphy. Exp Neurol 2010;223:77–85.
26. Schreiber JJ, Feinberg JH, Byun DJ, et al. Preoperative donor nerve electromyography as a predictor of nerve transfer outcomes. J Hand Surg Am 2014;39:42–9.
27. Mackinnon SE. Evaluation of the patient with nerve injury or nerve compression. In: Mackinnon SE, Yee A, editors. Nerve surgery. New York: Thieme; 2015. p. 41–58.

28. Oishi SN, Ezaki M. Free gracilis transfer to restore finger flexion in Volkmann ischemic contracture. Tech Hand Up Extrem Surg 2010;14:104–7.

29. Mackinnon SE, Dellon AL, Lundborg G, et al. A study of neurotrophism in a primate model. J Hand Surg Am 1986;11A:888–94.

30. Terzis JK, Barmpitsioti A. Wrist fusion in posttraumatic brachial plexus palsy. Plast Reconstr Surg 2009;124:2027–39.

31. Giuffre JL, Bishop AT, Spinner RJ, et al. Wrist, first carpometacarpal joint, and thumb interphalangeal joint arthrodesis in patients with brachial plexus injuries. J Hand Surg 2012;37A:2557–63.

32. Seal A, Stevanovic M. Free functional muscle transfer for the upper extremity. Clin Plast Surg 2011;38:561–75.

33. MacQuillan AH, Grobbelaar AO. Functional muscle transfer and the variance of reinnervating axonal load: part II. Peripheral nerves. Plast Reconstr Surg 2008;121:1708–15.

34. Vekris MD, Beris AE, Lykissas MG, et al. Restoration of elbow function in severe brachial plexus paralysis via muscle transfers. Injury 2008;39:S15–22.

35. Chuang DC, Epstein MD, Yeh MC, et al. Functional restoration of elbow flexion in brachial plexus injuries: results in 167 patients (excluding obstetric brachial plexus injury). J Hand Surg Am 1993;18:285–91.

36. Phillips BZ, Franco MJ, Yee A, et al. Direct radial to ulnar nerve transfer to restore intrinsic muscle function in combined proximal median and ulnar nerve injury: case report and surgical technique. J Hand Surg Am 2014;39:1358–62.

37. Ray WZ, Yarbrough CK, Yee A, et al. Clinical outcomes following brachialis to anterior interosseous nerve transfers. J Neurosurg 2012;117:604–9.

38. Terzis JK, Kokkalis ZT. Outcomes of hand reconstruction in obstetric brachial plexus palsy. Plast Reconstr Surg 2008;122:516–26.

39. Doi K, Shigetomi M, Kaneko K, et al. Significance of elbow extension in reconstruction of prehension with reinnervated free-muscle transfer following complete brachial plexus avulsion. Plast Reconstr Surg 1997;100:364–72 [discussion: 373–4].

40. Chin K, Vasdeki D, Hart A. Inverted free functional gracilis muscle transfer for the restoration of elbow flexion. J Plast Reconstr Aesth Surg 2013;66:144–6.

41. Dodakundi C, Doi K, Hattori Y, et al. Viability of the skin paddle does not predict the functional outcome in free muscle transfers with a second ischemic event: a report of three cases. J Reconstr Microsurg 2012;28:267–71.

42. Hosseinian MA, Tofigh AM. Cross pectoral nerve transfer following free gracilis muscle transplantation for chronic brachial plexus palsy: a case series. Int J Surg 2008;6:125–8.

43. Coulet B, Boch C, Boretto J, et al. Free gracilis muscle transfer to restore elbow flexion in brachial plexus injuries. Orthop Traumatol Surg Res 2011;97:785–92.

44. Carlsen BT, Bishop AT, Shin AY. Late reconstruction for brachial plexus injury. Neurosurg Clin N Am 2009;20:51–64.

45. Carlsen BT, Wendt MC, Spinner RJ, et al. Use of a free-functioning muscle transfer from a paralyzed lower extremity to restore upper extremity elbow flexion. J Surg Orthop Adv 2011;20:247–51.

46. ElHassan B. Lower trapezius transfer for shoulder external rotation in patients with paralytic shoulder. J Hand Surg Am 2014;39:556–62.

47. Kuzon WM Jr, McKee NH, Fish JS, et al. The effect of intraoperative ischemia on the recovery of contractile function after free muscle transfer. J Hand Surg Am 1988;13:263–73.

48. Lieber RL. Skeletal muscle architecture: implications for muscle function and surgical tendon transfer. J Hand Ther 1993;6:105–13.

49. Anastakis DJ, Chen R, Davis KD, et al. Cortical plasticity following upper extremity injury and reconstruction. Clin Plast Surg 2005;32:617–34.

50. Malessy MJ, Bakker D, Dekker AJ, et al. Functional magnetic resonance imaging and control over the biceps muscle after intercostal-musculocutaneous nerve transfer. J Neurosurg 2003;98:281–8.

51. Chen R, Anastakis DJ, Haywood CT, et al. Plasticity of the human motor system following muscle reconstruction: a magnetic stimulation and functional magnetic resonance imaging study. Clin Neurophysiol 2003;114:2434–46.

52. Duff SV. Impact of peripheral nerve injury on sensorimotor control. J Hand Ther 2005;18:277–91.

Management of Pain in Complex Nerve Injuries

Gabrielle Davis, MD[a], Catherine M. Curtin, MD[a,b],*

KEYWORDS

• Pain • Nerve injuries • Neuropathic pain • Neuroma • CRPS

KEY POINTS

- Nerve injuries often result in severe pain.
- This pain can prevent recovery and return to preinjury function.
- Those who treat nerve injuries need to have several strategies to address pain to achieve the best results for their patients.

INTRODUCTION

Traumatic nerve injuries can be devastating and life changing events leading not only to functional morbidity but also to psychological stress and social constraints. Advances in nerve regeneration and repair have led to significant improvement in motor and sensory outcomes following traumatic injuries. However, despite these advances, certain patients still develop neuropathic chronic pain syndromes (**Fig. 1**). Even in the event of a successful surgical repair with recovered motor function, pain can result in continued disability and poor quality of life. Pain also significantly limits participation in physical and occupational therapy, leading to inferior outcomes. It is difficult to predict which patients will develop persistent pain, and once incurred, pain can be even more challenging to manage. Although there have been numerous studies evaluating the functional, psychosocial, and quality of life after peripheral nerve injuries, few studies have evaluated chronic pain. This review seeks to define the types of pain following peripheral nerve injuries, investigate the pathophysiology and causative factors, and evaluate potential treatment options.

NEUROPATHIC PAIN

Pain after nerve injury is called neuropathic pain and is defined by the International Association for the Study of Pain as pain directly resulting from a lesion or disease affecting the somatosensory system.[1,2] Neuropathic pain often has distinct qualities that set it apart from the pain from soft tissue injury. It can persist long after the injury has healed. Neuropathic pain can occur spontaneously.[3] Common features to neuropathic pain include allodynia, in which pain is induced by typically an innocuous stimuli such as light touch, and hyperalgesia, which is severe pain induced by a typically painful stimuli. Patients will often describe neuropathic pain as burning, pins and needles, shooting, or electrical-type sensation. However, this pain can also be described as throbbing, so that the description of the quality of the pain cannot differentiate neuropathic pain from other processes. For the provider, a diagnosis of neuropathic pain should be considered in the patient with severe pain or prolonged pain after the soft tissue has healed. When a patient has a known nerve injury, the provider should have a low threshold for diagnosing the pain as neuropathic in origin. Neuropathic pain has a unique treatment algorithm, and early recognition and initiation of therapy are key factors.

CHRONIC REGIONAL PAIN SYNDROME

Complex regional pain syndrome (CRPS) is a severe variant of neuropathic pain, and any article

[a] Department of Surgery, Palo Alto VA, Suite 400, 770 Welch Road, Palo Alto, CA 94304, USA; [b] Division of Plastic Surgery, Stanford University, Suite 400, 770 Welch Road, Palo Alto, CA 94304, USA
* Corresponding author. Suite 400, 770 Welch Road, Palo Alto, CA 94304.
E-mail address: curtincatherine@yahoo.com

Hand Clin 32 (2016) 257–262
http://dx.doi.org/10.1016/j.hcl.2015.12.011
0749-0712/16/$ – see front matter Published by Elsevier Inc.

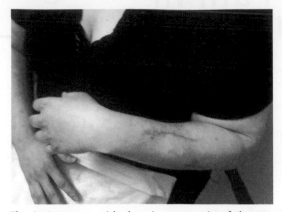

Fig. 1. A woman with chronic nerve pain of the arm after prior nerve injury.

on nerve injuries and pain must include a discussion of CRPS. CRPS is a syndrome with a constellation of symptoms. The one feature common to all patients with CRPS is pain out of proportion that is not explained by any other conditions. To meet the criteria for a diagnosis of CRPS, there must also be other features, including changes in blood flow, disturbed cold or warm perceptions, sudomotor activity, edema, and pigmentation changes[4] (**Fig. 2**). CRPS has been subdivided into 2 types. Type I is not associated with an identifiable nerve

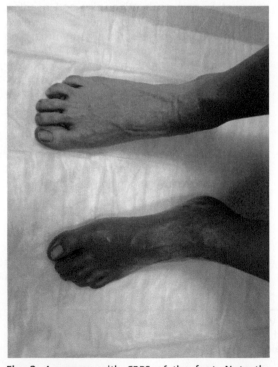

Fig. 2. A woman with CRPS of the foot. Note the changes in the color of the foot.

lesion, and type II is the result of a detectable nerve injury. The symptoms can develop immediately after injury or several months later, and commonly involved nerves include the median, ulnar, sciatic, and tibial nerves. The somatosensory profiles between CPRS I and II are almost identical.[5] Often CPRS II patients are misdiagnosed for CPRS I because of missed nerve injuries. CRPS generates fear among surgeons, but if there is a nerve injury, it will not get better until the nerve is dealt with. To address this, surgeons may be called on to assist in the treatment of this condition.

MECHANISM OF NEUROPATHIC PAIN

The exact pathophysiology or mechanism of neuropathic pain has not been completely elucidated. However, what is known is that it involves complex interactions of both the peripheral and the central nervous system. Similarly to the normal wound-healing pathways, immediately following nerve injury, a cascade of local inflammatory cytokines and neurotrophic factors are released that promote tissue healing and regeneration. Depending on the extent of injury, programmed cell death occurs at the disrupted ends in the form of Wallerian degeneration to create more favorable environment for nerve reinnervation. Reinnervation can occur via axonal sprouting at nerve ends to reconnect the proximal and distal nerve stumps. Although neuroplasticity plays a critical role in functional adaption after peripheral and central nervous system injury, it can also lead to unfavorable circuitry that can predispose to the development of neuropathic pain. The release of trophic factors by an injured cell can lead to chronic stimulation of uninjured neighboring neurons. These changes can lead to increased activity or dysregulation of ion channels in these neurons, lowering action potential thresholds and even leading to the development pacemaker activity.[3] Hyperexcitability can be generated by upregulation of sodium channels and calcium-gated voltage channels and downregulation of potassium channels in involved neurons.[6] These modifications occur not only occur at the site of injury but also at other remote sites, including at the spinal cord level. Another mechanism for chronic pain is that the persistent sensory input to the dorsal horn neurons leads to frequent depolarization and release of neurotransmitters glutamate and norepinephrine, which leads to dorsal horn excitability.[7] Pain is the result of a system with competing influences of excitatory and inhibitory pathways. Not only can nerve injury result in increased excitability but also the inhibitory pathways can be decreased, resulting in augmentation of the pain pathway. For example, in animal studies, GABA expression in the dorsal horn (an inhibitory pathway) is decreased after nerve injury, further supporting this theory.[8]

The constant bombardment of the nervous system with pain signals changes the physiology of the cells of the peripheral nerve, spinal cord, and brain. The resulting persistent state of high reactivity of the central nervous system is called central sensitization. Central sensitization leads to changes on a cellular transcriptional level and lasts for extended periods of time.[9] Chronic regional pain syndrome in part can be explained by central sensitization because the chronic pain, peripheral in origin, is further perpetuated by central mechanisms.[3] This data suggest that early breaking of the excitability pathways by decreasing the painful simulation may limit these adverse changes of the somatosensory system and allow for pain relief. The message continues to be that early recognition and treatment are key factors to treating neuropathic pain.

NEUROMA

Traumatic nerve injuries that result in pain may be caused by the development of painful neuromas. Neuromas are not always painful and can be discovered incidentally on imaging or nerve repair.[10] The incidence of neuromas causing significant symptoms after nerve injuries is reported to be relatively low, ranging from 3% to 5%.[11] However, when they provoke pain, they can lead to the same process of central sensitization described in the prior paragraph. Neuromas result from sprouting axons that become entrapped in scar tissue, not reaching its proximal or distal targets.[12] Pain elicited by neuromas may be secondary to mechanical traction on the axons within the neuroma, compression or chemical irritation of axons of local nerves, or development of ectopic ion channels.

Painful neuromas can be treated surgically with good results.[13] There are several strategies to the treatment of neuroma. The first is resection of the neuroma and repair with nerve grafts. This treatment is ideal because it restores the nerve's continuity and gives the axons a path to their end organs. When reconstruction of the nerve is not possible, the goal is to place the neuroma in a friendlier environment. This placement is done by first resecting the old neuroma, resetting the injury, and then placing the new nerve stump deep to the skin in either local bone or muscle.[14] The neuroma should not have traction so it should not be crossing a joint or held under tension. Surgical

outcomes have been superior to pharmacologic treatments and sclerosing agents in improving pain.[11] Neuroma treatment is yet another painful injured nerve process that may require surgical care.

BRACHIAL PLEXUS INJURIES

Brachial plexus injuries have a high incidence of neuropathic pain. Brachial plexus injuries can result in either preganglionic lesions or postganglionic lesions. The preganglionic injuries are a unique type of injury cared for by peripheral nerve surgeons because the injury occurs more centrally between the spinal cord and the dorsal root ganglion. The proximal brachial plexus injuries, which include avulsions of the nerves, are highly associated with the development of neuropathic pain.[15] A theory on why these injuries are so prone to development of pain includes the lack of sensory afferent inputs leading to the spontaneous activation of neurons in the dorsal horn.[16] Pain from avulsion injuries are difficult to treat, usually only responding to imaging-guided nerve blocks or ablative procedure like DREZtomy. Pain management is part of the treatment of care for patients with brachial plexus injury.

PHARMACOLOGIC TREATMENT
Anticonvulsants

Antiepileptic agents have long been used for the treatment of neuropathic pain.

The gabapentinoid class of medications (Neurontin and Lyrica) is the most commonly used anticonvulsant medications for neuropathic pain. These medicines are effective with tolerable side effects. Randomized trials of gabapentinoids in patients with nerve injuries have found better results treating neuropathic pain when compared with a placebo.[17] The mechanism of action for these drugs is thought to be related to binding and antagonizing specific subunits of voltage-gated calcium channels. These medications have few serious side effects, but adverse reactions, including fatigue, dizziness, and weight gain, are common. The side effects of the gabapentinoids are related to the speed of titration of the medication. Thus, for better compliance with these medications, they should be started at a low and ineffective dose and slowly titrated to efficacy. It is critical that the patient understands that patience is required when initiating these medications.

Several other antidepressants, including carbamazepine, oxycarbazepine, and lamotrigine, have been used to treat neuropathic pain with some efficacy. These medications are thought to achieve their beneficial effects by stabilizing the neurons by blocking Ca-gated voltage ion channels and preventing presynaptic release of glutamine.[18] Unfortunately, this class of medicines has numerous drug interactions and undesirable adverse effects, thus limiting their use for the treatment of pain.[19]

Antidepressants

Tricyclic antidepressants (TCA) are effective at decreasing neuropathic pain, by central mechanisms of inhibition of noradrenaline and serotonin uptake as well as N-methyl-D-aspartate receptor antagonism and sodium channel inhibition.[3,20] These medications are an attractive option because many patients with neuropathic pain suffer concomitant mental health disorders, and there is potential to address both conditions with one medication. The issue with these medications is the broad side-effect profile. These medications can have serious side effects, including cardiac arrhythmias with higher doses. Thus, titrating up these medications to effective doses requires careful monitoring of blood levels and electrocardiograms. The nonpain specialist may be comfortable initiating TCAs at a low dose and sending the patient to a pain management specialist for titration.

Serotonin-norepinephrine reuptake inhibitors such as duloxetine (trade name Cymbalta) have been found to be effective against neuropathic pain, and these medications do not have the anticholinergic or cardiac side effects.[20,21]

There was a comparative trial of pregabalin versus amitryplyine for the treatment of diabetic neuropathy. Both drugs demonstrated similar efficacy; however, amitriptyline had more reported adverse events.[22] On the other hand, studies of combined treatment of TCAs with gabapentin demonstrated significantly improved pain relief compared with single agents alone, with no serious adverse effects.[23] Most studies investigating the use of antidepressants have been performed in patients with diabetic neuropathy, and therefore, it is unclear if they have similar efficacy in nerve injury–induced neuropathic pain.

Opioids

The teaching had been that opioids analgesics had little benefit in the management of neuropathic pain. However, a recent meta-analysis proved compelling results. In evaluating randomized controlled trials of opioid use in neuropathic pain from all causes including posttraumatic nerve injuries, opioids were effective compared with a placebo in reducing spontaneous pain in intermediate term studies (median 28 days).[24] However, opioids have decreasing efficacy over time and present a risk for abuse. These medications should be considered an adjunct but not primary treatment of neuropathic pain.

Topicals

A lidocaine 5% patch is currently US Food and Drug Administration approved for the treatment of neuropathic pain related to postherpetic neuralgia. A prospective, placebo-controlled randomized control trial conducted on patients with postherpetic neuralgia assessed the impact of topical lidocaine using the neuropathic pain scale. This scale is a subjective measurement of pain qualities specific to neuropathic pain. The assumption is that the lower scores seen in this trial could suggest efficacy to other neuropathic pain conditions.[25]

To date, there has been no large randomized control trials demonstrating one pharmacologic modality has better efficacy with respect to trauma-induced neuropathies. The current European Federation of the Neurological Societies guidelines on pharmacologic treatment on general neuropathic pain recommends first-line treatment with TCA, gabapentinoid, or serotonin-norepinephrine reuptake inhibitors, and second-line treatment with a weak opioid like tramadol, and third-line treatment, strong opioids.[19]

SURGERY

Studies have demonstrated that early nerve repair and grafting have been associated with lower incidences of neuropathic pain.[26] Bertelli and Ghizoni[15] demonstrated that brachial plexus root grafting in avulsion injuries significantly reduced pain by 80% within the first 3 weeks, and these results persisted at least by 24 months with a 95% reduction in pain. However, the surgeon must carefully evaluate the decision of early grafting versus allowing for spontaneous reinnervation to minimize any unnecessary surgery.

How surgery fits into the treatment of CRPS still remains unclear. The fear has been that nerve surgery to treat CRPS would exacerbate the pain and therefore had not been advocated. However, if a compressed nerve can be identified, a release can reduce pain.[27] A study evaluating CPRS resulting from lower extremity injuries demonstrated surgical intervention led to decreased pain and function at least a year after surgery.[28] The general thinking seems to be changing: for the patient with CRPS, judicious use of surgery for clear nerve injuries is appropriate.

Dorsal root entry zone lesioning, or DREZ procedure, can be used to treat intractable pain. In this procedure, the peripheral sensory nerve inputs are disrupted at the spinal cord level by coagulation of dorsal root entry zone. This procedure has provided durable results for pain after brachial plexus injuries. One study of 52 patients found that 70% of patients had 75% pain reduction with a 2-year follow-up.[29] This procedure has most commonly been used for the severe pain after brachial plexus injuries because there are serious risks to this surgery, including motor loss of the ispilateral leg. However, the DREZ procedure can be very effective for those challenging patients with severe intractable pain.

NEUROSTIMULATION

Neurostimulation can be an effective treatment for pain that has not responded to more conservative measures. The mechanism of action remains unknown, but the use of stimulation is based on the Gate theory. The Gate theory states that non-painful signals can close the "gate," preventing other painful signals from being processed.[30] There are a variety of different stimulators available with increased interest on more distal peripheral nerve stimulators. The spinal cord stimulator is best known and has been used for decades. There have been numerous studies showing that spinal neurostimulation can reduce pain by 50%.[31] There have also been reports of stimulators helping with the intractable pain after brachial plexus injuries.[32,33] Effective current stimulators still require leads, which can migrate, break, or become infected. Neurostimulation can be an effective tool for the patient with severe intractable pain after nerve injury.

OUTCOMES

The development of neuropathic pain yields to poor outcomes with respect to functional rehabilitation and quality of life.[34] Taylor and colleagues[35] evaluated patients that suffer complete median nerve transection followed by repair. They demonstrated that patients that developed neuropathic pain after nerve repair had worse overall motor function. Novak and colleagues[36] found that pain was the most significant independent predictor of disability in patients suffering from brachial plexus injuries. Pain and nerve injuries are often comingled, and good results require treatment of both the nerve injury and the associated pain.

SUMMARY

There is a paucity of literature that specifically addresses pain after complex nerve injuries,

and thus, the human toll is likely underappreciated. In a survey administered to peripheral nerve surgeons, only half of the participants noted that they formally assessed for pain.[37] One reason is that formal assessment of pain has been difficult as this is a subjective complaint, and until recently, there were no quantitative testing methods for neuropathic pain. This gap has led to the development of The Leeds Assessment of Neuropathic Symptoms and Signs, Neuropathic Pain Questionnaire, and Neuropathic Pain Scale. All are validated, self-reporting measurements to allow for more quantitative assessment of pain. The European Federation of the Neurological Societies recommends using these validated testing methods as screening tools for neuropathic pain and to gauge treatment responses. Beyond better measurement, there is also a need for randomized control trials to better predict treatment outcomes and identify potential responders to treatment. As more patients are screened, the hope is the initiation of randomized control trials to guide more selective treatment modalities.

Pain after nerve injury can prevent recovery and return to preinjury life. There are treatments that are effective. Both patient and provider need to work together to tailor right treatment combination.

REFERENCES

1. Marchettini P, Lacerenza M, Mauri E, et al. Painful peripheral neuropathies. Curr Neuropharmacol 2006;4(3):175–81.
2. Treede RD, Jensen TS, Campbell JN, et al. Neuropathic pain: redefinition and a grading system for clinical and research purposes. Neurology 2008; 70(18):1630–5.
3. Gilron I, Watson CP, Cahill CM, et al. Neuropathic pain: a practical guide for the clinician. CMAJ 2006;175(3):265–75.
4. Harden RN, Bruehl S, Perez RS, et al. Validation of proposed diagnostic criteria (the "Budapest Criteria") for complex regional pain syndrome. Pain 2010;150(2):268–74.
5. Gierthmühlen J, Maier C, Baron R, et al, German Research Network on Neuropathic Pain (DFNS) Study Group. Sensory signs in complex regional pain syndrome and peripheral nerve injury. Pain 2012;153(4):765–74.
6. Haroutounian S, Nikolajsen L, Bendtsen TF, et al. Primary afferent input critical for maintaining spontaneous pain in peripheral neuropathy. Pain 2014; 155(7):1272–9.
7. Laired JMA, Bennett GJ. An electrophysiological study of dorsal horn neurons in the spinal cord of

rats with an experimental peripheral neuropathy. J Neurophysiol 1993;69:2072–85.

8. Moore KA, Kohno T, Karchewski LA, et al. Partial peripheral nerve injury promotes a selective loss of GABAergic inhibition in the superficial dorsal horn of the spinal cord. J Neurosci 2002;22(15):6724–31.

9. Woolf CJ. Dissecting out mechanisms responsible for peripheral neuropathic pain: implications for diagnosis and therapy. Life Sci 2004;74(21):2605–10.

10. Rajput K, Reddy S, Shankar H. Painful neuromas. Clin J Pain 2012;28(7):639–45.

11. Stokvis A, van der Avoort DJ, van Neck JW, et al. Surgical management of neuroma pain: a prospective follow-up study. Pain 2010;151(3):862–9.

12. Navarro X, Vivó M, Valero-Cabré A. Neural plasticity after peripheral nerve injury and regeneration. Prog Neurobiol 2007;82(4):163–201.

13. Novak CB, van Vliet D, Mackinnon SE. Subjective outcome following surgical management of upper extremity neuromas. J Hand Surg Am 1995;20:221–6.

14. Mackinnon SE, Dellon AL, Hudson AR, et al. Alteration of neuroma formation by manipulation of its microenvironment. Plast Reconstr Surg 1985;76(3): 345–53.

15. Bertelli JA, Ghizoni MF. Pain after avulsion injuries and complete palsy of the brachial plexus: the possible role of nonavulsed roots in pain generation. Neurosurgery 2008;62(5):1104–13.

16. Teixeira MJ, da Paz MG, Bina MT, et al. Neuropathic pain after brachial plexus avulsion–central and peripheral mechanisms. BMC Neurol 2015;15:73.

17. Gordh TE, Stubhaug A, Jensen TS, et al. Gabapentin in traumatic nerve injury pain: a randomized, double-blind, placebo-controlled, cross-over, multicenter study. Pain 2008;138(2):255–66.

18. Eisenberg E, Lurie Y, Braker C, et al. Lamotrigine reduces painful diabetic neuropathy: a randomized, controlled study. Neurology 2001;57(3):505–9.

19. Attal N, Cruccu G, Baron R, et al, European Federation of Neurological Societies. EFNS guidelines on the pharmacological treatment of neuropathic pain: 2010 revision. Eur J Neurol 2010; 17(9):1113-e88.

20. Sindrup SH, Bach FW, Madsen C, et al. Venlafaxine versus imipramine in painful polyneuropathy: a randomized, controlled trial. Neurology 2003;60(8): 1284–9.

21. Wernicke JF, Pritchett YL, D'Souza DN, et al. A randomized controlled trial of duloxetine in diabetic peripheral neuropathic pain. Neurology 2006; 67(8):1411–20.

22. Bansal D, Bhansali A, Hota D, et al. Amitriptyline vs. pregabalin in painful diabetic neuropathy: a randomized double blind clinical trial. Diabet Med 2009;26(10):1019–22.

23. Gilron I, Bailey JM, Tu D, et al. Nortriptyline and gabapentin, alone and in combination for neuropathic pain: a double-blind, randomised controlled crossover trial. Lancet 2009;374(9697):1252–61.

24. Eisenberg E, McNicol ED, Carr DB. Efficacy and safety of opioid agonists in the treatment of neuropathic pain of nonmalignant origin: systematic review and meta-analysis of randomized controlled trials. JAMA 2005;293(24):3043–52.

25. Galer BS, Jensen MP, Ma T, et al. The lidocaine patch 5% effectively treats all neuropathic pain qualities: results of a randomized, double-blind, vehicle-controlled, 3-week efficacy study with use of the neuropathic pain scale. Clin J Pain 2002;18(5):297–301.

26. Kato N, Htut M, Taggart M, et al. The effects of operative delay on the relief of neuropathic pain after injury to the brachial plexus: a review of 148 cases. J Bone Joint Surg Br 2006;88(6):756–9.

27. Placzek JD, Boyer MI, Gelberman RH, et al. Nerve decompression for complex regional pain syndrome type II following upper extremity surgery. J Hand Surg Am 2005;30(1):69–74.

28. Dellon L, Andonian E, Rosson GD. Lower extremity complex regional pain syndrome: long-term outcome after surgical treatment of peripheral pain generators. J Foot Ankle Surg 2010;49(1):33–6.

29. Haninec P, Kaiser R, Mencl L, et al. Usefulness of screening tools in the evaluation of long-term effectiveness of DREZ lesioning in the treatment of neuropathic pain after brachial plexus injury. BMC Neurol 2014;14:225.

30. Melzack R, Wall PD. Pain mechanisms: a new theory. Science 1965;150:971–9.

31. Deer TR, Skaribas IM, Haider N, et al. Effectiveness of cervical spinal cord stimulation for the management of chronic pain. Neuromodulation 2014;17:265–71.

32. Abdel-Aziz S, Ghaleb AH. Cervical spinal cord stimulation for the management of pain from brachial plexus avulsion. Pain Med 2014;15:712–4.

33. Chang Chien GC, Candido KD, Saeed K, et al. Cervical spinal cord stimulation treatment of deafferentation pain from brachial plexus avulsion injury complicated by complex regional pain syndrome. A A Case Rep 2014;3:29–34.

34. Wojtkiewicz DM, Saunders J, Domeshek L, et al. Social impact of peripheral nerve injuries. Hand (N Y) 2015;10(2):161–7.

35. Taylor KS, Anastakis DJ, Davis KD. Chronic pain and sensorimotor deficits following peripheral nerve injury. Pain 2010;151(3):582–91.

36. Novak CB, Anastakis DJ, Beaton DE, et al. Relationships among pain disability, pain intensity, illness intrusiveness, and upper extremity disability in patients with traumatic peripheral nerve injury. J Hand Surg Am 2010;35(10):1633–9.

37. Novak CB, Anastakis DJ, Beaton DE, et al. Evaluation of pain measurement practices and opinions of peripheral nerve surgeons. Hand (N Y) 2009; 4(4):344–9.

Donor Activation Focused Rehabilitation Approach
Maximizing Outcomes After Nerve Transfers

CrossMark

Lorna Canavan Kahn, BSPT, CHT[a], Amy M. Moore, MD[b],*

KEYWORDS

- Nerve transfer • Rehabilitation • Hand therapy • Physical therapy • Occupational therapy
- DAFRA • Exercise

KEY POINTS

- Donor activation focused rehabilitation approach (DAFRA) is a rehabilitation model that recognizes the altered neural pathways created with nerve transfers and attempts to maximize functional outcomes by strengthening these pathways.
- There is no predetermined timeline for the progression of the rehabilitation program; the 3 phases of rehabilitation are adapted to the individual and their rate of motor recovery.
- Preservation of muscle length following a denervating injury is achieved with positioning and splinting to aid in countering the forces of antagonist muscles and gravity.

 Video content accompanies this article at http://www.hand.theclinics.com

INTRODUCTION

Over the past 20 years, a paradigm shift toward the use of nerve transfers in peripheral nerve surgery has occurred. This shift has brought about a plethora of research and published articles focused on surgical innovation and outcomes; however, a concomitant interest in rehabilitation following nerve transfers is lacking. In a recent literature review involving 12 papers addressing nerve transfers for upper trunk plexopathies, rehabilitation models and outcomes following nerve transfers were compared.[1] Three groups were identified: papers in which no rehabilitation is mentioned, papers that refer to nonspecific or a generic physical therapy approach, and papers describing a donor activation focused rehabilitation approach (DAFRA). Beers and colleagues[1] found there was a significantly increased percentage of excellent outcomes in the DAFRA group following nerve transfers for elbow flexion.

DAFRA is a rehabilitation model that recognizes the altered neural pathways created by the nerve transfer and focuses on strengthening these pathways in an attempt to maximize functional outcomes. This approach emphasizes the importance of cortical plasticity, familiarity with the anatomic aspects of the surgery, and strong patient education regarding the altered control mechanism for movement. These components are vital to a successful motor re-education program. In this article, the factors influencing outcomes after nerve transfers are reviewed, including preoperative and postoperative interventions. Rehabilitation protocols for specific nerve transfers also are addressed. Although not

---

Disclosure: The authors have no conflict of interests to disclose.
a Milliken Hand Rehabilitation Center, The Rehabilitation Institute of St. Louis, 4921 Parkview Place, Suite 6F, St Louis, MO 63110, USA; b Division of Plastic and Reconstructive Surgery, Washington University School of Medicine, 660 South Euclid Avenue, CB 8238, St Louis, MO 63110, USA
* Corresponding author.
E-mail address: mooream@wustl.edu

Hand Clin 32 (2016) 263–277
http://dx.doi.org/10.1016/j.hcl.2015.12.014
0749-0712/16/$ – see front matter © 2016 Elsevier Inc. All rights reserved.

all-inclusive, the general principles presented can be applied to any nerve transfer performed.

FACTORS INFLUENCING RETURN OF FUNCTION AFTER NERVE TRANSFERS
Cortical Plasticity

It is widely accepted that adaptive changes occur at the sensory-motor cortex in response to motor learning.[2] Numerous investigators have demonstrated change or expansion in the sensorimotor cortex in response to training, and this has been seen with musicians, legally blind participants, and patients with limb amputations (and subsequent replants).[3–5] Anastakis and colleagues[6] suggest that the functional success of nerve transfers may require pre-existing interconnection on a cortical level between the donor and recipient muscles. From this, one may surmise that strengthening this pre-existing interconnectivity may improve functional outcomes.

The work of Nudo and colleagues[7] has demonstrated a clear relationship between cortical adaptation and acquisition of new skills. After-injury training, which involves developing new motor skills, has been shown to effectively correlate with neuroanatomic changes on a cortical level.[8] Based on their research using functional MRI with nerve transfers, Anastakis and colleagues[6] suggest several strategies to maximize functional outcomes. These strategies include the following:

1. Activate the nerve transfer with preoperative exercise instruction.
2. Educate the patient regarding the need for continued compliance with the home exercise program (HEP).
3. Activate the recipient muscle early using gravity-lessened planes.
4. Work with a hand therapist in the early stages of recovery, focusing on functional movements and repetition.
5. Plan for strengthening and endurance exercises for up to and possibly beyond 2 years following signs of reinnervation.

Exercise

In addition to cortical changes that occur following nerve transfer, the concepts that drive muscle recovery following peripheral nerve injury and repair must be kept in mind. Much of what is known regarding the effect of exercise on recovering peripheral nerve repair is from animal models. van Meeteren and colleagues[9] have shown that physical activity encourages functional motor and sensory recovery and increased motor nerve conduction velocity following sciatic nerve injury.[9]

Udina and colleagues[10] demonstrated that maintaining activity in muscle with active or passive exercise may increase trophic factor release on regenerating motor neurons.

The level of intensity of exercise is also an important consideration when working with the peripheral nerve and brachial plexus–injured patient population. Although Sabatier and colleagues[11] demonstrated low-intensity training increased the length of regenerating axons after peripheral nerve repair, Herbison and colleagues[12] noted that intense training and exercise may have negative effects on axonal regeneration. As the recipient muscle gains strength following a nerve transfer, an effort should be made to limit the patient from overwhelming the muscle with high-intensity exercise and thereby potentially limiting his functional outcome.

Positioning

Following a denervating injury, muscle length may change because of the unopposed force of the antagonist muscle, improper positioning, or the weight of the limb due to gravity. Once the muscle begins to regain function following a nerve transfer, a muscle that is overly stretched or shortened may have difficulty generating force. The length-tension relationship has been clearly described by Gordon and colleagues[13] (**Fig. 1**). The ability of a muscle to generate tension is directly related to the overlap of the actin and myosin filaments. A muscle will contract with the largest amount of tension when it is close to its ideal length. Therefore, when shortened or stretched beyond this ideal length, the maximum active tension generated will decrease.

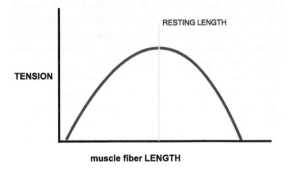

Length-Tension Curve

Fig. 1. The length tension curve. This curve illustrates the concept of muscle having an ideal length at which it can develop the greatest contraction force.[13] This concept applies to denervated muscle in which the length should be protected from the unopposed forces of antagonist muscles and gravity while awaiting reinnervation.

After nerve transfer, it is important to educate the patient regarding positioning. The use of slings and/or splints to preserve ideal resting sarcomere length is important. Patients may presume that once their muscle shows early signs of recovery that they can then eliminate the support. In reality, keeping them in the shortened position in the sling (or other support) may help regain control and strength faster because of the preserved length of the involved muscles. In addition, the support will limit drag on the plexus, reduce arm pain, and decrease hand edema, which is often correlated to dependent positioning.

PREOPERATIVE THERAPY

In the ideal setting, a preoperative physical/occupational therapy evaluation is performed. The surgical plan is shared with the therapist to maximize this preoperative visit. Baseline measures of range of motion (ROM) and strength of potential muscle donors are obtained. This documentation will enable the therapist to accurately monitor postoperative functional recovery of both donor and recipient muscles as well as neighboring muscles (which may also benefit from increased use of the limb following nerve transfers). The patient is also taught exercises that activate the donor muscle(s) before surgery. Although it is not yet clear whether greater strength of the donor muscle has an effect on nerve transfer outcomes, the ability to activate the donor muscle is inherently important.

Furthermore, any issues of joint limitation, muscle length, and edema are addressed at this preoperative visit with patient education, positioning, splinting, and exercise. Early conservative management of edema may improve pain and comfort of the involved extremity. Elevation, maintenance of joint ROM, and compression garments are effective in pain and edema management.[14]

POSTOPERATIVE THERAPY

The DAFRA model encompasses 3 phases of rehabilitation: early, middle, and late. The timeline of phase entry is not predetermined. These phases should be adapted to the individual as they recover from each specific nerve transfer.

Early Phase

Patient education
Anatomy The importance of adequate patient education following nerve transfers cannot be overstated. The authors have witnessed patients who attended their first therapy visit 1 year after transfer with the assumption of surgical failure only to find

that function existed once they were given adequate instruction in the new control mechanism for that movement. This finding underscores the importance of motor re-education and the possibilities of recovery if the patients learn how to activate their nerve transfer.

In order to adequately educate the patient, the operative report should be provided for the therapist—because often the preoperative plan and intraoperative procedures differ. If possible, include the therapist in the first patient postoperative visit as details of the case are discussed with the patient, allowing the physician-therapist-patient unit to be on the same page.

On the initial postoperative therapy visit, significant time should be spent instructing the patient about the involved anatomy of the nerve transfers and how the muscle innervation has been altered. The primary goal is for the patients to demonstrate a heightened understanding of their surgery by identifying the "donor" and "recipient" muscles. When describing the involved nerves and muscles, they are referred to as "donors" and "recipients." Labeling the nerve transfers by the muscle involved may improve patient understanding because these are more familiar words than the involved nerves. For example, in the case of the double fascicular transfer (DFT) for elbow flexion, there are 2 "donors": wrist flexors (ulnar fascicles) and finger flexors (median fascicles). A brief description of the involved muscles' function (ie, finger bending) is given to improve patient understanding. By the end of the first visit, the patient should be able to describe what donor muscle(s) must be fired in order to send a "message" to the recipient muscle.

When describing the altered neural pathway of a nerve transfer, the use of metaphors can be very helpful. The authors use a simple "lamp and electrical cord" metaphor to describe the basic relationship between the muscle and nerve. The patients begin to understand why their arm does not flex on command, that is, when the cord is cut or unplugged the lamp will not turn on. Furthermore, use of familiar language, such as "rewiring a lamp" or "diverting lanes of a highway on a detour," can aid in their understanding of the surgery and thereby improve their ability to actively participate in their recovery (Video 1).

Timeline for motor recovery One of the greatest challenges for a patient after undergoing nerve transfers is waiting for a functional outcome. Patients often get frustrated, depressed, and/or give up when no motor response is seen for months postoperatively. By adequately explaining expectations on a time line, the patient is more likely to be more compliant and dedicated to their HEP. Using a linear model of the manual muscle testing (MMT) scores, one can demonstrate 5/5 strength on an uninvolved limb and 0/5 with the involved muscle (**Fig. 2**). Using this model as a starting point, the first step in "success" is getting to a 1/5 because it means that nerve regeneration has reached the muscle and reinnervation has begun. This first step is an important milestone for patients who often dismiss a muscle twitch as unimportant.

The time frame to advance from 0/5 strength to 1/5 is described in relation to the distance from the nerve coaptation to the recipient muscle; this is a good segue to introduce the concept of axonal growth of "a millimeter a day," "an inch a month," and "a foot and a half a year." With information from the operative note and/or the surgeon, one can estimate when the first twitch or advancement to 1/5 on the timeline might happen. From there, it is helpful to describe the remaining MMT scores in relation to the expected movement and their corresponding time frame. Although often first broached by the surgeon, it important to set and/or reinforce realistic expectations.

Home exercise program Once the concept of donor and recipient muscles is understood, the specific home exercise instruction is initiated. The primary focus during the first phase of the postoperative period is to activate the donor muscles frequently in an effort to encourage neural activation and growth. Following a brief postoperative rest period of 10 to 14 days, the patient is instructed to contract the donor muscle. This contraction should be a simple movement that the patient can do easily without equipment, such as making a fist. They are advised to repeat the movement 10 to 20 times hourly. Passive ROM exercises for the involved joints should also be performed 2 to 3 times a day; this will not only limit joint contractures but also stimulate the motor cortex and regenerating neurons.[10]

Flood the donor High repetition with low resistance exercises for the donor muscles will limit fatigue while "flooding" the new neural pathway with "demand." This exercise is based on an extrapolation of the work of van Meeteren and colleagues,[9] who demonstrated that exercise training involving high repetition improves functional recovery and motor nerve conduction velocity after a peripheral nerve crush lesion in the rat. The concept of "more is more" is described to the patient at this time to encourage maximizing "messages sent" to the donor muscle. Follow-up visits will advance the HEP to exercises that combine resisted donor muscle contractions with passive or assisted recipient muscle contractions. Repetitive co-contractions also aid in strengthening the new altered motor pathway for the recipient muscle.

Once the patient demonstrates an understanding of the importance of donor activation and is accurate and compliant with their HEP, follow-up visits are scheduled monthly, often corresponding to the physician postoperative visits. Given the limitations set by insurance and the expected lengthy recovery time, it is best to use therapy visits judiciously. In the early phase of recovery, the HEP is important, but no progression is made until a response is noted in the recipient muscle.

Middle Phase

Monitoring for return of function
During monthly visits, MMT is performed on both the donor and the recipient muscles. The donor muscle strength is monitored and documented for (in most cases) return to normal strength. When the entire donor nerve is taken (vs only fascicles), obviously no return is expected in the donor muscle. To test for return of function in the recipient muscle, strong resistance is applied to the donor muscle while palpating the recipient muscle or tendon (**Fig. 3**). Depending on the muscle, it may be easier to palpate movement of the tendon than a muscle contraction in the early phase of recovery. Demonstrating and having the patient feel the contraction is a helpful, motivating tool; this is often the first time they "believe" that the nerve transfer is going to work.

Advancing the home exercise program
Once a twitch is perceived in the recipient muscle, the focus of the program advances to gravity lessened exercises. Active-assisted exercise is performed while simultaneously demanding a strong contraction of the donor. Every effort is made to

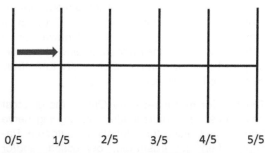

Fig. 2. The linear model of the MMT grading scale is a helpful visual aid when describing motor recovery in terms of the progression and time frame after nerve transfer. *Red arrow* depict direction of motion.

0/5   1/5   2/5   3/5   4/5   5/5

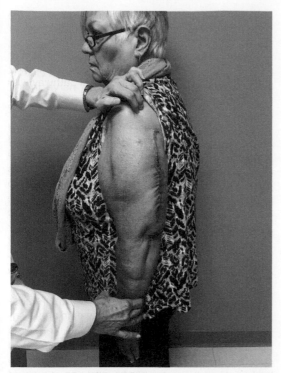

Fig. 3. To assess for recipient muscle return, strong resistance is applied to the donor muscle(s) while palpating the recipient muscle. Here the triceps is resisted while palpating the recipient deltoid muscle belly.

make the movement easier for the weak recipient muscle. To limit drag, one may use a slick surface or an arm skate (**Fig. 4**, Video 2). Positioning the limb in a gravity-assisted position may also help

the patient demonstrate early control of the movement.

Continuation of donor activation exercises is also encouraged in effort to "flood" the recipient muscles for several months. Developing strength and muscle bulk in the recipient muscle is the goal. Separation of the 2 movements (donor contraction to restore recipient function) is generally easier and added to the HEP once there is significant strength in the recipient. The time period for this may be more than 12 months or when a 3+/5 or greater muscle grade is acquired. In some patients, donor activation persists indefinitely, but most patients are able to lessen the need to perform the combined motion with time.

When functional recovery moves beyond a twitch toward 2−/5 strength, the use of aquatic therapy can provide tremendous assistance and encouragement for the nerve transfer patient. By using the benefits of a buoyant environment, the patients experience some early active control in the formerly paralyzed muscle. Floatation devices such as a kick board, inflatable "water wings," and/or dumbbells may be used to aid in these exercises (**Fig. 5**).

Once the patient has progressed to 2+ to 3−/5 muscle strength (incomplete joint range of movement against gravity), instruction is given in "place-and-hold" exercises against gravity. To do this, the patient places the joint in an end range position with the uninvolved arm while strongly contracting the donor muscle. The support of the uninvolved hand is gradually lessened while they attempt to hold the position with the recipient muscle. Patients are encouraged to do this routinely throughout the day (**Fig. 6**).

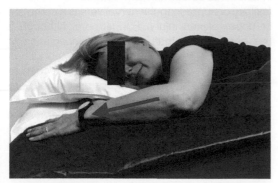

Fig. 4. A sheet of nylon provides a decreased friction surface for the weak recipient muscle to successfully move the limb in the middle phase of motor re-education. Following a triceps to axillary nerve transfer, this setup may be used to train the reinnervating deltoid. *Red arrow* depict direction of motion.

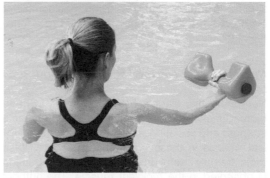

Fig. 5. When available, use of a pool for exercise will provide a buoyant environment in which the patient can successfully move the injured limb. In this example, elbow flexion is achieved under water by holding the dumbbells while activating the donor muscles.

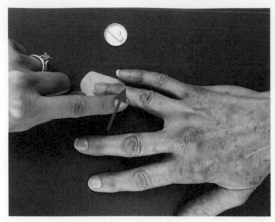

Fig. 6. The "place-and-hold" exercise applied to the ulnar intrinsic muscles following an AIN to deep ulnar nerve transfer. The finger is placed into end range abduction and the patient is asked to pronate the hand into the table while attempting to hold this position. *Red arrow* depict direction of motion.

Late Phase

Resisted exercise

Use of resistive equipment such as hand-held weights and elastic bands is initiated once a 3/5 muscle strength (full active elbow flexion against gravity) is achieved. Attempts before this may lead to early fatigue, pain, and frustration. Once again, reviewing the muscle strength progression timeline is helpful (see **Fig. 2**). With knowledge of the timeline, the patient may be more compliant and have a more realistic expectation for recovery.

If the recipient muscle recovers greater than 3/5 muscle strength, the HEP is progressed gradually. Keep in mind that due to the anatomic limitations of the nerve transfer (fewer motor nerve fibers than the original source), the end point of strength gains will vary and may take as much as 2 to 3 years. In addition, fatigue is a common complaint even once the strength has recovered to a functional level.

Neuromuscular electrical stimulation and biofeedback

Neuromuscular electrical stimulation (NMES) and biofeedback may be helpful in advancing muscle strength and assisting with activation of the recipient muscle in the nerve transfer patient. These tools are only useful once a significant contraction is observed in the recipient muscle. The authors emphasize that these therapies can augment the strength program but do not replace the existing HEP. Use of this modality may be especially helpful for patients with cognitive or emotional issues, such as those found with brain injuries, fear of

pain, and limb dissociation. Increased muscle fatigue with NMES use is common. If used early in the recovery phase, keep in mind that it is best to avoid excessive fatigue in neurologically weak muscle. There is not a consensus for use of electrical stimulation following peripheral nerve injury. Some studies suggest it may impair functional recovery and accentuate skeletal muscle atrophy.[15]

When available, biofeedback can also be helpful as motor recovery becomes evident by aiding in activation of the recipient muscles. Once the muscle is innervated, the patient will often struggle to attain control of volitional contractions. Combining biofeedback with donor activation may enhance the patient's ability to improve the function of their recipient muscle.

THERAPY REGIMENS FOR SPECIFIC NERVE TRANSFERS

In the remaining discussion, the DAFRA therapy approach to common nerve transfers is described: shoulder, elbow, and hand. Nuances, considerations, tips, and tricks are presented for the specific therapy programs. The intervention is broken down by early, middle, and late phases of recovery.

Nerve Transfers to Regain Shoulder Function

The loss of shoulder function following peripheral nerve injury is life altering. Although the average healthy individual requires less than full active ROM to perform many common activities of daily living (ADL), adaptations for work and extracurricular activities may be needed for the patient with the paralyzed shoulder.[16] Nerve transfers to regain shoulder function have been successful.[17] However, it is important to keep in mind the variability in functional outcomes from isolated nerve injuries (axillary or suprascapular nerve) versus a complete or upper plexus injury. Furthermore, although it has been shown that increased reinnervation of the shoulder musculature improves abduction and external rotation,[18] it is important to recognize that the more "donors" that are used, the more "normal" strength structures are removed from the overall shoulder complex. For the therapist, it is important to recognize that the patients will present differently after nerve transfers to restore an isolated injury than one performed in a complete upper trunk injury.

Spinal accessory to suprascapular nerve transfer

Considerations Ideally, the lower branch of the spinal accessory nerve is donated to the suprascapular nerve, and branches and/or fascicles to the upper, middle, and lower trapezius are left to preserve function of the remaining muscle. In the past, the entire lower branch was harvested; however, the authors found the complete harvest left an unstable scapular base on which to build the newly transferred glenohumeral strength. In either situation, building strength in serratus anterior muscle (if available) is important to aid in stability and upward scapular rotation strength postoperatively.

Early phase Donor activation can be achieved early on with instruction in shoulder shrugs and backward shoulder rolls or "pulls," that is, squeezing the blades together. These exercises should be performed hourly with at least 10 repetitions. To pattern the newly combined motor functions, the patient uses the uninvolved hand to passively externally rotate the arm while performing active scapular retraction (**Fig. 7**). In addition, the patient is encouraged to position the arm in partial external rotation and abduction for parts of the day to maintain the ideal length of the supraspinatus/infraspinatus muscles.

Middle phase In the supine position, exercises that combine active-assisted shoulder abduction

and external rotation with active scapular retractions are added to their routine once early motor return is noted. Motor return can also be achieved in sitting with a dowel or cane to assist external rotation/abduction with active scapular elevation and retractions (**Fig. 8**). When pool access is available, patients are encouraged to use the buoyancy of the water to advance early control of supraspinatus function with arm raises under water. Inflatable rings or flotation devices may aid this control. Donor activation continues to accompany all recipient muscle activation attempts. Prone and side-lying positioning are used for manually assisted middle and lower trapezius strengthening exercises as well as assisted external rotation and abduction exercises (**Fig. 9**).

Late phase Once supraspinatus/infraspinatus strength approaches 3/5 strength, wall slides are introduced. These exercises will aid in both trapezius and infraspinatus/supraspinatus strengthening. Patients with an isolated suprascapular nerve injury may advance more quickly to light resistive exercises. The dual function of the intact deltoid and teres minor muscles with the supraspinatus and infraspinatus may blur the accuracy of strength measures. Typically, the amount of resistance as measured by the single repetition maximum strength test (in the against gravity positions) will better capture the differences between involved and uninvolved sides. Those patients who demonstrate difficulty raising the arm over 90° may have incurred greater loss to their lower trapezius. Without this muscle action, it is very difficult to complete the scapulothoracic phase of shoulder abduction.

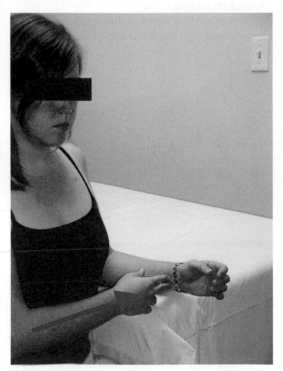

Fig. 7. Passive external rotation combined with active scapular retractions provides early patterning of the donor muscle (trapezius) and the recipient muscle (infraspinatus). *Red arrow* depict direction of motion.

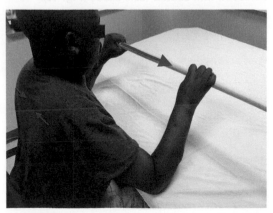

Fig. 8. Following a spinal accessory to suprascapular nerve transfer, combined active donor and passive or assisted recipient muscle exercise is achieved by squeezing the scapulae together while pushing the involved arm into external rotation with the uninvolved arm using a dowel. *Red arrow* depict direction of motion.

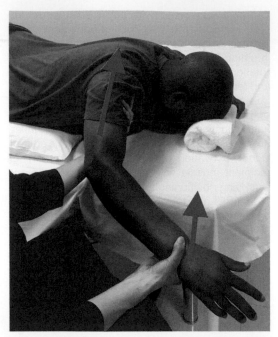

Fig. 9. Following the spinal accessory to suprascapular nerve transfer, the strength of the middle and lower trapezius muscles is often downgraded. Manual assistance is applied to the scapula for place-and-hold exercises to aid in strengthening and retraining. *Red arrow* depict direction of motion.

Triceps branch to axillary nerve transfer

Early phase A simple way to achieve donor activation of the triceps branch is to instruct the patient to slide his hand on the thigh toward the knee. Isometric triceps activation is another option and can easily be performed sitting or standing. Combined active donor and passive recipient action is achieved with seated table slides (**Fig. 10**).

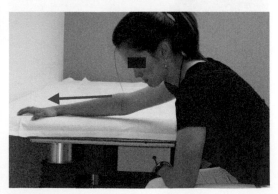

Fig. 10. In the early phase following a triceps to axillary nerve transfer, combined donor and recipient patterning is achieved with seated shoulder flexion slides. This patient actively extends her elbow while passive shoulder flexion and abduction are achieved with trunk flexion. *Red arrow* depict direction of motion.

Middle phase Because of the anatomic course of the axillary nerve running from posterior to anterior, re-innervation of the posterior head of the deltoid muscle typically occurs first. To test for this, the patient will contract the triceps muscles while attempting shoulder extension and abduction. One can palpate the deltoid along the posterior aspect of the acromion. Having the patient perform exercises in the prone position will encourage co-contraction with triceps and limit pectoralis major substitution. Shoulder extension exercises will primarily work triceps at first (as this also crosses the shoulder joint and aids in extension), but as more power returns to the deltoid, it will contribute to this motion. In the prone position, the patient is also instructed in shoulder abduction exercises (**Fig. 11**).

With the understanding that increased recipient output is correlated with increased effort of the donor muscle contraction, the therapist is challenged to position the patient in the appropriate way to achieve this. For example, in supine triceps, effort increases by extending the straight arm into the bed/floor while abducting the shoulder. In addition, performing the movement bilaterally with resistance to uninvolved deltoid can aid in training and increase muscle activation on the affected side.[19] The patient lies supine close to a wall on the uninvolved side and presses against it during bilateral abduction.

In the side-lying position, the weak deltoid can be exercised with the shoulder in 90° of abduction

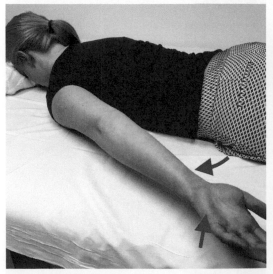

Fig. 11. A patient with a triceps to axillary nerve transfer is instructed to extend the elbow, activating the triceps, while attempting to abduct the shoulder. With the patient positioned in the prone position, there is greater demand on the triceps (donor), and the pectoralis muscle is at a disadvantage for substitution. *Red arrow* depict direction of motion.

with the elbow straight. Therapist support is given to the proximal arm as an attempt is made to move it in a circular motion ("arm circles"). This position puts reasonable demand on the triceps while gaining some assisted control of the deltoid.

Task-oriented activities are helpful in patterning this new combined shoulder movement. For example, slide the arm up an inclined surface on a slick cloth or use the crank or ladder tool on the BTE rehabilitation tool (Corporate Headquarters & Rehabilitation Equipment, Hanover, MD, USA) (**Fig. 12**). These activities can be set to provide greater demand on the donor (triceps) while achieving shoulder elevation. The functional orientation and repetitive nature of BTE activities follow the tenets of cortical plasticity to aid in motor re-education. Patients also tend to be motivated by the visual computer feedback given by the BTE.

Late phase Once the patient demonstrates increased deltoid strength with gains in arm elevation against gravity, the exercises are gradually advanced to light strengthening. Often patients with an isolated axillary nerve injury can raise the arm to some degree against gravity before their nerve transfer; this typically occurs in young men who have a well-developed supraspinatus muscle. The challenge for this group of patients is to carefully tease out actual deltoid recovery and to adjust exercise advancement accordingly. Use of the single repetition maximum test is one way to measure progress beyond the 3/5 strength.[20]

Nerve Transfers to Restore Elbow Flexion

Elbow flexion is vitally important to all aspects of ADLs. Performing basic functional tasks, including

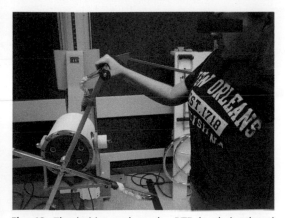

Fig. 12. The ladder tool on the BTE (tool simulator) provides graded resistance to the donor triceps (elbow extension) while assisting recipient deltoid in arm elevation. *Red arrow* depict direction of motion. (*Courtesy of* BTE, Hanover, MD.)

opening a door, eating, and using a telephone, requires anywhere from 30° to 130° of elbow flexion and approximately 50° of supination.[21] Without elbow flexion, a functional hand is made useless.

Double fascicular nerve transfer

Considerations The DFT refers to transferring fascicles of the flexor digitorum superficialis (FDS) to the brachialis branch and the flexor carpi ulnaris (FCU) fascicles to the biceps branch of the musculocutaneous nerve (MC). Working with patients following a DFT for elbow flexion restoration is a rewarding experience for a therapist. DFT is one of the most successful nerve transfers, with papers citing outcomes with an average of 4/5 elbow flexion strength.[22] Given the fact that most humans have been fisting and bringing their hands to their mouths since the womb, one would infer that there is a clear cortical interconnectedness, as Malessy and colleagues[2] described, between these functions. Thus, motor re-education is relatively easy and successful after this transfer. Recovery of muscle twitch has been seen as early as 2.5 months postoperatively given the short distance from the donor to the recipient nerve.

Furthermore, although the transfer has been successfully performed with the FCU fascicle to brachialis branch and FDS fascicle to biceps branch, the authors recommend the originally described orientation of the transfer (ulnar to biceps and median to brachialis). The median nerve controls pronation (pronator teres [PT] and pronator quadratus), and thus, using the median nerve to also control supination with biceps function is theoretically antagonistic and could lead to increased difficulty with motor re-education and potentially decreased efficacy of the transfer.

Early phase Considering that the nerve transfer is performed in the proximal arm and without tension on the repair, activation of the distal donor muscles can start as early as day 1 or 2 postoperatively without compromising the repair. Active fisting and wrist ROM within the postoperative sling will discourage postoperative hand edema while creating early demand on the donor motor efferents. At the 2 to 4 week postoperative initial visit, a hand gripper or Theraputty may be issued to increase this demand and start to restrengthen the potentially weak FDS muscle. Instruction in wrist flexion curls with a 1-pound weight may also be initiated. The concept of high-frequency exercise with low resistance is encouraged.

At 3 to 4 weeks postoperative, exercises that combine active donor contraction with passive recipient motion are introduced. Specifically, this includes the following 2 options:

a. Supine bilateral elbow flexion with forearms supinated using a dowel; a foam buildup may be added to the involved side of the dowel to encourage simultaneous active donor fisting.
b. Active fist and wrist flexion while passively flexing the elbow with the uninvolved arm.

Middle phase Once a muscle twitch is present, gravity-lessened exercises are added to the exercise program. With the arm on a surface at shoulder height, active-assisted elbow flexion is performed while gripping and flexing the wrist simultaneously. A slick cloth or skate to lessen the frictional force of the surface and assist the weak elbow flexors is also encouraged (see **Fig. 4**, Video 2). Donor activation and motor patterning exercises, as with the dowel, are continued as well (Video 3).

When elbow flexion strength approaches a 2+/5, advancement to place-and-hold exercises against gravity is initiated with the uninvolved arm flexing the involved arm to 90+ degrees. Strong donor muscle contractions are made as they attempt to keep the arm flexed while support is gradually removed. This exercise can be performed anywhere, and patients are encouraged to do this frequently throughout the day.

Use of elbow flexion support (such as a sling) and activation of the donor muscles with the elbow flexed continue to be important and emphasized in this phase of therapy. Although the patient may be able to fully flex against gravity without simultaneous gripping, elbow flexion force will continue to increase when there is co-contraction of the donor muscles.

Late phase Use of resistive equipment such as hand-held weights and elastic bands is initiated once 3/5 strength is achieved. Attempts before this may lead to early fatigue, pain, and frustration. As elbow flexion strength increases, dependency on donor muscle contraction will lessen. Patients generally see a separation of function by 1 year as their functional use of the arm improves.

Intercostal nerves to musculocutaneous nerve
Early phase There are 3 functions to consider with the intercostal (IC) muscle donor: inhalation, exhalation, and trunk flexion. Chalidapong and colleagues[23] looked at these 3 functions in patients with IC to MC nerve transfers and found that trunk flexion correlated with the highest response in the recipient muscle electromyography. By the end of the first month, patients are instructed to activate the donor by performing trunk curls in supine and sitting with forced exhalation. Combined donor-

recipient exercises are performed with the patient in the seated position with the forearm on a table next to them. In this position, active trunk flexion will passively flex the elbow.

The regenerative distance from the nerve coaptation to muscle motor endplates is longer in this transfer than the DFT. Often the surgeon is able to perform the transfer proximal to the MC branch to the coracobrachialis muscle. Therefore, when testing for a muscle twitch, one should palpate the proximal medial humerus for this muscle as the patient flexes the trunk with exhalation. Typically, the coracobrachialis muscle is not considered important to shoulder function; however, when no other shoulder muscles are intact, it can provide limited shoulder flexion. Active assistance to this muscle is provided when the patient performs shoulder flexion slides with the arm on a table as he trunk flexes/exhales.

Middle phase Once a twitch is noted in the elbow flexors, the program should be expanded to include supine or sitting trunk curls with dowel-assisted bilateral elbow flexion. This exercise is performed in a supine or sitting position. Alternatively, in the side-lying position, elbow and shoulder flexion is enhanced when practiced on a downward sloped bolster (gravity assisted) with simultaneous trunk flexion (**Fig. 13**). During the middle phase of recovery, use of a pool can be helpful and motivating by allowing independent arm movement in this buoyant environment.

Late phase This phase is identical to the DFT late phase. Once adequate elbow flexion strength against gravity is achieved, separation of recipient muscle action from donor co-contraction occurs with minimal effort.

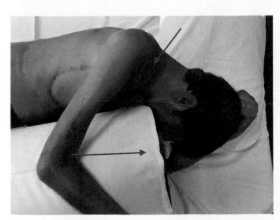

Fig. 13. Intercostal to MC transfer: the patient is positioned in side lying position with the arm supported on a slick bolster. Combined trunk flexion with forced exhalation is performed with active shoulder and elbow flexion. *Red arrow* depict direction of motion.

Nerve Transfers to Restore Hand Function

Median nerve

A proximal median nerve injury limits pronation, which in the modern digital world compromises the ability to communicate via keyboard and computers. When the biceps and supinator are left unchecked, strong supination can become dominant, thereby limiting hand and wrist function. Loss of finger and wrist flexion as well as thumb opposition will further compromise the function of the hand as it demonstrates dominant intrinsic positive posturing.

Extensor carpi radialis brevis to pronator teres nerve transfer

Early phase Active wrist ROM should be started after a 2-week resting period. In this transfer, the nerve coaptation is performed in close proximity to the muscles involved. Care should be taken to avoid complications such as a seroma or hematoma during the early postoperative phase by limiting hand and wrist activity. The patient is instructed to rest the arm, elevated on a pillow or in a sling, with the forearm pronated to maintain muscle length. Following the rest period, patients may begin active wrist extension exercises hourly. For donor and recipient patterning, light resisted wrist extension with passive forearm pronation exercises are performed daily.

Middle phase As active pronation returns, functional exercises such as the BTE steering wheel tool are helpful in simulating a task that involves both donor and recipient muscle action. A lightweight bat or dowel may be used to combine wrist extension and pronation with minimal resistance for the donor and gravity assistance for the recipient pronator. Cues are given for strong donor contraction throughout the pronation portion to provide increased response in the recipient muscle.

Late phase Testing pronation strength with the elbow flexed (isolating PT) versus extended (isolating pronator quadratus) may clarify the amount of force contribution provided by each pronator muscle. Resistance to the functional exercises should be added gradually, making sure the elbow is kept in 90° of flexion to limit substitution and ensure PT contribution.

Flexor digitorum superficialis branch to anterior interosseous nerve

Considerations There are consistent strategies to deal with the unopposed finger and thumb extension in anterior interosseous nerve (AIN) palsy. Regardless of the donor used, the patient will benefit from finger-based splints to block hyperextension of the distal interphalangeal (IP) joints of the index and thumb. This splint not only preserves muscle length, but also can improve fine motor opposition by limiting fingertip collapse during pinch activities (**Fig. 14**).

Early phase The beauty of this transfer is that there is a clear synergistic relationship between the flexor digitorum profundus, flexor pollicus longus (FPL), and the FDS muscles. Donor activation is initiated at 2 to 4 weeks postoperatively and achieved with simple gripping exercises. Light resisted donor exercises may begin once all postoperative edema is resolved. Patients are encouraged to wear finger splints blocking the distal joints as able during the day and to perform passive flexion exercises to the fingers and thumb. Thumb IP joint and index finger distal interphalangeal (DIP) joint restriction are common with AIN palsy. Exercises should encompass both composite flexion as well as blocked DIP flexion to ensure stretch to the oblique retinacular ligament.

Middle phase A twitch may be noted in the recipient muscle as early as 3 months postoperatively. Training advances to include place-and-hold exercises to the thumb and index tips while fisting tightly (Video 4). Resistive donor exercises with a gripper or putty are also strongly encouraged.

Late phase Although signs of reinnervation, that is, a twitch, develop early, recovery of greater than 3/5 strength or resistance through the thumb and index tip may take another 12 to 15 months. Persistence with gripping exercises and protection

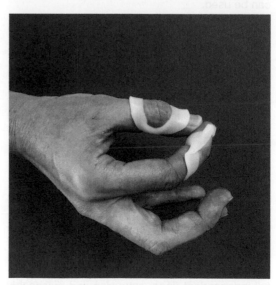

Fig. 14. Finger-based splints are used to limit IP joint hyperextension in patients with AIN palsy. The splints improve function by limiting IP collapse with pinch activities and preserve joint and muscle length.

of FPL length may enhance this time line. Functional activities that demand IP joint flexion, such as spherical grasp, peg boards, and wide-handled gripping (dowel pulls through putty), should be included in the HEP. Success is seen when patients report ability to once again unbutton a shirt or pull up a zipper (Video 5).

Brachialis branch of the musculocutaneous to anterior interosseous nerve

Considerations In this transfer, the nerve coaptations are in the upper arm. The distance from coaptation to the recipient muscle is long. Patient education regarding this timeline is useful to maintain compliance of the HEP.

Early phase Elbow movement is restricted in the first 2 weeks to protect the nerve repair and limit edema. Active elbow flexion with the forearm in pronation will promote donor activation and can be advanced to resisted elbow curls by the end of the first month. When hand function is absent, a splint may be fabricated to support the wrist and position the thumb and index finger in distal joint flexion. Resistance tubing is used for these exercises.

Middle phase Splinting is encouraged to position the hand in pinch for support in order to initiate function with active elbow flexion. Advanced patterning with donor and recipient muscle action can be achieved with the BTE lever tool; this may require a mitt or taping to support the hand placement for resisted elbow flexion. To simulate this at home, a resistance band with a foam tube handle can be used.

Late phase Once the patient has gained isolated movement, putty exercises may be added for resisted pinch and finger flexion exercises. In addition, by grasping a short dowel to pull through the resistance putty, functional demand is placed on the AIN muscles and elbow flexors simultaneously. Buttoning and pulling zippers should be achievable at this point.

Radial nerve

Median to radial nerve transfers

Considerations Median to radial nerve transfers are described as the transfer of the flexor carpi radialis branch to restore finger and thumb extension (posterior interosseous nerve, PIN) and transfer of the FDS branch to restore wrist extension (ECRB). Nerve transfer patients have the potential to regain full independent finger extension and reasonably strong wrist extension.[24] The time line is typically 4 to 5 months to achieve muscle twitch and 10 to 12 months to regain functional movement.

Early phase Postoperative dressings are replaced with a forearm-based "P1 block" splint with thumb extension to support the wrist, thumb, and the proximal fingers in extension. This splint is worn for 2 weeks for tissue rest (**Fig. 15**). Following this period, intermittent use of static or dynamic extension splinting is strongly encouraged until active control of the reinnervating muscles is achieved. The splints maintain recipient muscle length and improve hand function during this time.

Donor activation exercises begin after the first 2 weeks. The exercises include finger IP flexion and isometric wrist flexion. Resisted finger flexion exercises are added when postoperative edema is resolved. Although the authors encourage splint use, the exercises may be performed in or out of the splint. Active use of the hand is encouraged.

It should be noted that some surgeons may opt to perform a PT to ECRB tendon transfer at the same time as this nerve transfer. In these cases, the protocol is deferred to the tendon transfer guidelines in order to protect the tendon repairs.

Middle phase Exercises are advanced once the presence of muscle activation is noted. Patients may begin resisted donor exercises with putty. The following exercises will provide resistance to the donor muscles while passively assisting the recipient muscles. These exercises include (Videos 6 and 7) the following:

1. Log rolls are performed on the table and then turned sideways into a vertical cylinder. Place the palm on top of putty and flex the wrist to flatten putty allowing the putty to passively extend the thumb and fingers.
2. Finger digs are performed with the forearm on a table creating assistance to wrist extension with resisted finger flexion.

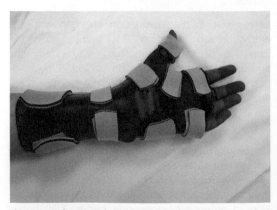

Fig. 15. A forearm-based "P1 block" splint is used to maintain wrist and finger extension muscle length in patients with radial nerve palsy.

When treating an isolated PIN palsy (intact wrist extension), a hand-based P1 block splint may be useful with training extensor digitorum communis to pull into end range metacarpal phalangeal joint (MP) extension with active wrist flexion. Patients may provide resistance to the wrist flexors with their uninvolved hand for this. These patients are followed monthly for monitoring return of function and advancing HEP.

Late phase When control of the extension function is attained, strengthening may be advanced with light resistance. One-pound eccentric wrist extension with full assist during the concentric phase is an example that stresses the donor finger flexors while working to achieve end range wrist extension. Theraputty or resistance bands are used to provide resistance for thumb and finger extension.

Ulnar nerve
Anterior interosseous nerve to pronator quadratus transfer to ulnar motor nerve
Considerations Ulnar nerve palsies result in claw deformity. It is important to address (and prevent) the proximal interphalangeal joints (PIP) contractures perioperatively with splinting and exercise.

Early phase A neutral wrist splint is used for the first 2 weeks postoperatively to limit edema and overuse.

Patients are generally instructed to limit hand use during the first month to light activity. Active forearm pronation exercises are initiated, and baseline measures are taken to monitor changes in motor control, hand girth, and claw deformity. Use of an anti-claw splint is advised to help maintain length of the intrinsic muscles and limit PIP contractures (**Fig. 16**).

Middle phase Because of the distance from coaptation in the distal forearm to the intrinsic muscles, expectation for a twitch is often 6 months. The patient is asked to spread the fingers while resisting forearm pronation. One may see a small twitch of tendon bulge at the radial and ulnar aspects of the proximal fingers. The authors follow responses along the path of ulnar nerve, that is, intrinsics to the small finger recover before the ring finger, and so forth.

Patients are instructed in individual interossei exercises for both passive and active assisted finger abduction/adduction. Place and hold exercises in the intrinsic plus position are used to aid in regaining lumbrical muscle function. In order to increase recipient muscle effort, the patient is instructed to press the radial aspect of the hand into a wad of putty for resisted pronation (**Fig. 17**). Furthermore, finger extension splints are helpful in isolating intrinsic function and aid in correcting substitution patterns. An IP flexion block splint for the thumb will allow isolated pinch strengthening while limiting contribution of the FPL (**Fig. 18**).

Late phase As strength improves and control of the intrinsic muscles improves, resistance exercises are introduced. Resistance putty is used for a series of exercises, which include the following:

1. Log roll with fingers adducted
2. Abduct/adduct: place the "log" between the fingers and gently abduct/adduct and pull with 2 fingers at a time

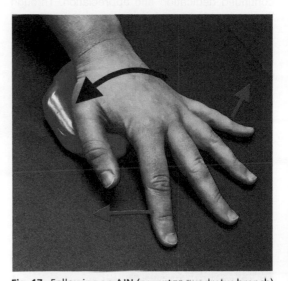

Fig. 17. Following an AIN (pronator quadratus branch) to ulnar motor nerve transfer, intrinsic muscle exercises are enhanced by resisted donor activation with pronation into putty. *Black arrow* depicts forearm pronation and red arrows depict finger finger abduction. *Red arrows* depict direction of motion.

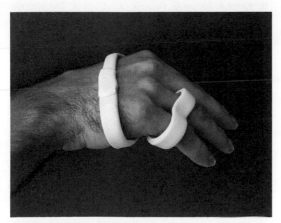

Fig. 16. The anti-claw splint limits hyperextension of the MP joints of the ring and small fingers while encouraging active IP extension.

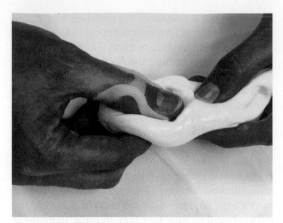

Fig. 18. A thumb-based IP joint extension splint blocks the contribution of the FPL during pinch activity. With the substitution pattern removed, there is greater isolation of the adductor pollicus muscle during pinch strengthening exercises.

3. Intrinsic plus "card draw": place fingers on the putty and pull hand up into MP flexion with IP extension (**Fig. 19**)
4. Various diameter dowels gripped and pulled through putty

SUMMARY

As nerve transfers become the mainstay in treatment of brachial plexus and isolated nerve injuries, the preoperative and postoperative therapy performed to restore motor function requires continued dedication and appreciation. Through the understanding of the general principles of muscle activation and patient education, the therapist has a unique impact on the return of function in patients with nerve injuries. As surgeons continue to develop novel nerve transfers, the

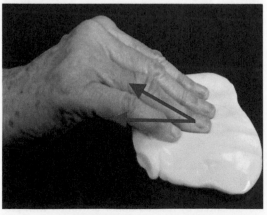

Fig. 19. Resistance putty is used to resist intrinsic plus positioning during lumbrical strengthening exercises. *Red arrows* depict direction of motion.

perioperative training, education, and implementation of the DAFRA model are critical to ensure successful outcomes.

SUPPLEMENTARY DATA

Videos related to this article can be found at http://dx.doi.org/10.1016/j.hcl.2015.12.014.

REFERENCES

1. Beers A, Ivens R, Kahn L, et al. Functional outcomes following nerve transfer surgery for a C5-C7 brachial plexus palsy are improved with DAFRA rehabilitation technique. American Association for Hand Surgery Annual Meeting. Paradise Island, Bahamas, January 21–24, 2015 (poster).
2. Malessy MJ, Bakker D, Dekker AJ, et al. Functional magnetic resonance imaging and control over the biceps muscle after intercostal-musculocutaneous nerve transfer. J Neurosurg 2003;98(2):261–8.
3. Jenkins WM, Merzenich MM, Ochs MT, et al. Functional reorganization of primary somatosensory cortex in adult owl monkeys after behaviorally controlled tactile stimulation. J Neurophysiol 1990; 63(1):82–104.
4. Elbert T, Pantev C, Wienbruch C, et al. Increased cortical representation of the fingers of the left hand in string players. Science 1995;270(5234): 305–7.
5. Pascual-Leone A, Torres F. Plasticity of the sensorimotor cortex representation of the reading finger in Braille readers. Brain 1993;116(1):39–52.
6. Anastakis DJ, Malessy MJ, Chen R, et al. Cortical plasticity following nerve transfer in the upper extremity. Hand Clin 2008;24(4):425–44.
7. Nudo RJ, Plautz EJ, Frost SB. Role of adaptive plasticity in recovery of function after damage to motor cortex. Muscle Nerve 2001;24(8):1000–19.
8. Karni A, Meyer G, Rey-Hipolito C, et al. The acquisition of skilled motor performance: fast and slow experience-driven changes in primary motor cortex. Proc Natl Acad Sci U S A 1998;95(3):861–8.
9. van Meeteren NL, Brakkee JH, Hamers FP, et al. Exercise training improves functional recovery and motor nerve conduction velocity after sciatic nerve crush lesion in the rat. Arch Phys Med Rehabil 1997;78(1):70–7.
10. Udina E, Puigdemasa A, Navarro X. Passive and active exercise improve regeneration and muscle reinnervation after peripheral nerve injury in the rat. Muscle Nerve 2011;43(4):500–9.
11. Sabatier MJ, Redmon N, Schwartz G, et al. Treadmill training promotes axon regeneration in injured peripheral nerves. Exp Neurol 2008;211(2):489–93.
12. Herbison GJ, Jaweed MM, Ditunno JF. Effect of swimming on reinnervation of rat skeletal muscle.

J Neurol Neurosurg Psychiatry 1974;37(11): 1247–51.

13. Gordon AM, Huxley AF, Julian FJ. The variation in isometric tension with sarcomere length in vertebrate muscle fibres. J Physiol 1966;184(1):170–92.

14. Villeco JP. Edema: a silent but important factor. J Hand Ther 2012;25(2):153–62.

15. Gigo-Benato D, Russo TL, Geuna S, et al. Electrical stimulation impairs early functional recovery and accentuates skeletal muscle atrophy after sciatic nerve crush injury in rats. Muscle Nerve 2010;41(5):685–93.

16. Khadilkar L, MacDermid JC, Sinden KE, et al. An analysis of functional shoulder movements during task performance using Dartfish movement analysis software. Int J Shoulder Surg 2014;8(1):1.

17. Yang LJ, Chang KW, Chung KC. A systematic review of nerve transfer and nerve repair for the treatment of adult upper brachial plexus injury. Neurosurgery 2012;71(2):417–29 [discussion: 429].

18. Estrella EP. Functional outcome of nerve transfers for upper-type brachial plexus injuries. J Plast Reconstr Aesthet Surg 2011;64(8):1007–13.

19. Mills VM, Quintana L. Electromyography results of exercise overflow in hemiplegic patients. Phys Ther 1985;65(7):1041–5.

20. Seo DI, Kim E, Fahs CA. Reliability of the one-repetition maximum test based on muscle group and gender. J Sports Sci Med 2012;11(2):221–5. eCollection 2012.

21. Morrey BF, Askew LJ, Chao EY. A biomechanical study of normal functional elbow motion. J Bone Joint Surg Am 1981;63(6):872–7.

22. Mackinnon SE, Novak CB, Myckatyn TM, et al. Results of reinnervation of the biceps and brachialis muscles with a double fascicular transfer for elbow flexion. J Hand Surg 2005;30(5):978–85.

23. Chalidapong P, Sananpanich K, Klaphajone J. Electromyographic comparison of various exercises to improve elbow flexion following intercostal nerve transfer. J Bone Joint Surg Br 2006;88(5): 620–2.

24. Mackinnon SE, Roque B, Tung TH. Median to radial nerve transfer for treatment of radial nerve palsy. J Neurosurg 2007;107(3):666–7.

Index

Note: Page numbers of article titles are in **boldface** type.

Hand Clin 32 (2016) 279–281
http://dx.doi.org/10.1016/S0749-0712(16)30009-9
0749-0712/16/$ – see front matter © 2016 Elsevier Inc. All rights reserved.

Moving?

Make sure your subscription moves with you!

To notify us of your new address, find your **Clinics Account Number** (located on your mailing label above your name), and contact customer service at:

Email: journalscustomerservice-usa@elsevier.com

800-654-2452 (subscribers in the U.S. & Canada)
314-447-8871 (subscribers outside of the U.S. & Canada)

Fax number: 314-447-8029

Elsevier Health Sciences Division
Subscription Customer Service
3251 Riverport Lane
Maryland Heights, MO 63043

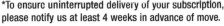

*To ensure uninterrupted delivery of your subscription, please notify us at least 4 weeks in advance of move.